GYNAECOLOGICAL RADIOLOGY

G. H. WHITEHOUSE

MB, BS, MRCP, FRCR, DMRD, AKC
Professor of Diagnostic Radiology
University of Liverpool

BLACKWELL SCIENTIFIC PUBLICATIONS

OXFORD   LONDON   EDINBURGH

BOSTON   MELBOURNE

© 1981 by
Blackwell Scientific Publications
Editorial offices:
Osney Mead, Oxford, OX2 0EL
8 John Street, London, WC1N 2ES
9 Forrest Road, Edinburgh, EH1 2QH
52 Beacon Street, Boston
    Massachusetts 02108, USA
214 Berkeley Street, Carlton
    Victoria 3053, Australia

First published 1981

Printed in Great Britain by
Butler & Tanner Ltd, Frome and London

DISTRIBUTORS

USA
  Blackwell Mosby Book Distributors
  11830 Westline Industrial Drive
  St Louis, Missouri 63141

Canada
  Blackwell Mosby Book Distributors
  120 Melford Drive, Scarborough
  Ontario, M1B 2X4

Australia
  Blackwell Scientific Book Distributors
  214 Berkeley Street, Carlton
  Victoria 3053

British Library
Cataloguing in Publication Data

Whitehouse, G. H.
  Gynaecological radiology.
  1. Diagnosis, Radioscopic   2. Generative
  organs, Female – Diseases – Diagnosis
  3. Radiography in gynecology
  I. Title
  618.1′0757   RG107.5.R3

  ISBN 0–632–00726–5

Contents

Preface

Gynaecological radiology has developed over the last sixty years with the introduction of techniques specific for the diagnosis of the female genital tract. Some of these techniques have remained useful while others have, at least in part, been supplanted by other diagnostic methods. Other widely used radiological procedures such as urography, barium studies and angiography reveal manifestations of diseases of gynaecological origin, especially when they affect other systems of the body. While gynaecological radiology is covered to some extent in several standard text books of gynaecology and radiology, some atlases depicting hysterosalpingographic appearances, and occasional specific articles in radiological journals, there have been few attempts to encapsulate the whole subject in one text book.

The aim of this book is to remedy this deficit. As well as covering the more specific investigations which pertain to the genital tract, I have attempted to show how other standard radiodiagnostic procedures may be applied to the gynaecological patient. It is hoped that this monograph will be useful to both radiologists and gynaecologists, including those in training.

Spectacular advances have occurred over recent years in other methods of organ imaging. Ultrasonography and computed tomography (CT scanning) have particularly extended the role of the radiologist in the investigation of gynaecological disorders, and have provided him with tools which give information impossible to obtain by conventional radiology. I am indebted to Dr Carl Wright for his chapters on ultrasonography and CT scanning, which give an up-to-date appraisal of the role of these modalities in the context of gynaecology.

I also wish to express my gratitude to those who have been closely involved with the production of this book, in particular Miss Mary Hynes who typed the manuscript in its several forms, Messrs David Adkins and Roy Crosby for producing the illustrations, and Miss Jean Dutton and Miss Carol Sausman who as successive Senior Radiographers at the Women's Hospital in Liverpool were very helpful in the gathering of case material. Finally, I wish to thank my family for their cheerful forbearance during the long gestation of this book.

Graham Whitehouse

CHAPTER 1

Radiological Techniques I: Plain Radiographs

The first documented application of radiography in gynaecological practice was a case described by Lewers in 1903, in which a hairpin was located within the uterine cavity. Ludlow in 1909 was able to demonstrate calcification within uterine fibroids by means of X-rays.

TECHNIQUE

For a general view of the abdomen, the film should be of sufficient size to include both the diaphragm above and the pubic symphysis in full expiration. Routinely, the patient should be recumbent and in the supine position. An additional radiograph in the erect position is taken when there is a suspicion of intestinal obstruction, pneumoperitoneum, or ascites.

The pelvic cavity may be shown to better effect by angling the X-ray tube 20°–25° towards the feet, with the central ray entering the patient at 5 cm above the pubic symphysis. Usually an 18 × 24 cm film is of sufficient size. Sometimes a lateral radiograph may be required to aid the localization of foreign bodies, including contraceptive devices, and calcifications within the pelvic cavity.

It is important that the bladder is emptied immediately before radiography, because a full bladder may be confused with a pathological pelvic soft tissue mass (Fig. 1.1).

NORMAL APPEARANCES

A full description of the radiographic appearances of the whole abdomen is beyond the scope of this monograph, but awareness of the soft tissue shadows seen within the pelvic cavity is of prime importance. An anteroposterior radiograph of the pelvic cavity will normally show the ovoid shapes of the bladder and uterus separated by a radiolucent cleavage plane due to surrounding adipose tissue (Fig. 1.2). Characteristically, the uterus, unless it is retroverted, has a lenticular shape on an anteroposterior radiograph, and indents the centre of the bladder dome. The crescentic outlines of the levator ani muscles are sometimes seen directed backwards from the symphysis pubis while the obturator internus muscles, which are likewise delineated by overlying fat, lie lateral and posterior to the levator ani. The sacrospinous ligaments may occasionally be seen between their origin on either side of the coccygeal and lower sacral segments and their insertions onto the ischial spines (Fig. 1.2). The sacrotuberous ligaments are rarely visible, but may form an obstacle to parturition when they occasionally calcify (Levene & Kaufman, 1958). The rectum and sigmoid colon are delineated by the faeces and gas contained within them. However, a circular soft tissue density 2–3 cm in diameter on the left side of the pelvic cavity may be mistaken for a pelvic tumour, but is due to a contracted and empty portion of the sigmoid colon seen in tangential projection (Beranbaum, 1951). On lateral films of the pelvis, cleavage planes due to fatty tissue define the rectum, bladder and space of Retzius.

ABNORMAL APPEARANCES

A large round or ovoid soft tissue pelvic mass is likely to be due to an abnormality of the female genital tract, such as an enlarged uterus or an ovarian cyst or tumour (see Fig. 8.1), only when the bladder is seen as a distinct soft

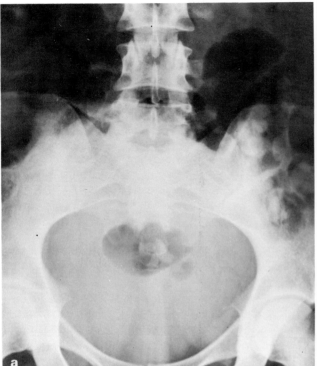

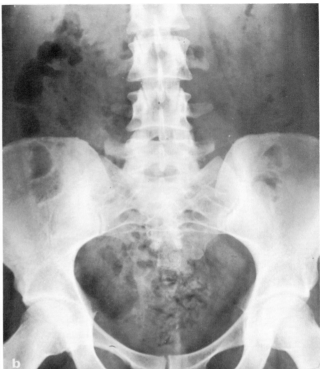

FIG. 1.1   (a) A rounded soft tissue mass extends out of the pelvic cavity into the abdomen.

(b) The 'mass' is no longer apparent after micturition, and was due to a distended bladder.

tissue tumour. Bryk (1966) found a detectable uterine shadow on plain radiography in over half the cases in a series of ovarian masses. A lobulated pelvic mass is far more likely to be due to uterine fibroids than an ovarian lesion (see Fig. 7.1). Difficulty in distinguishing between a uterine and ovarian mass may be due to the obscuring of the pelvic organs by fluid-filled loops of bowel or by ascites. Pelvic infection may obscure the fat planes between the pelvic organs, so that they have a homogenous density on the plain radiograph. Extra-luminal gas collections may occasionally be associated with acute pelvic infections (see Fig. 11.7). Bowel gas shadows may be displaced by a large mass rising out of the pelvic cavity.

Calcified pelvic phleboliths (Fig. 1.2), which are present in a quarter to one third of all European adults and may increase in number with age, are especially diffuse in the female because of their frequent presence in the broad ligament as well as in the rectal and vesical venous plexi. It has been observed by Steinback (1960) that phleboliths

may be displaced by pelvic masses. Midline masses may displace phleboliths laterally, while more laterally situated masses may deviate them in a medial direction. Depending on the position of the pelvic mass, phleboliths may also be displaced upwards or downwards. Serial radiographs may show progressive positional changes of phleboliths in the presence of an actively expanding mass lesion.

Uterine artery calcification (Fig. 1.3) is especially common in diabetic women, and this association is more frequent under the age of 60 years (Fisher & Hamm, 1975).

Calcification in a pelvic mass is an important radiological sign and its diagnostic significance is considered in detail in Chapters 8 and 9.

Uterine fibroids frequently calcify (see Figs. 7.1 and 7.2), and calcification may be visible in a variety of ovarian lesions including cystadenoma and cystadenocarcinoma, dermoid cysts, gonadoblastoma and fibroma

(Chapter 8). Ovarian calcification, and even true bone formation, may occasionally occur in corpora albicantia either in the form of clusters of small foci 0.5 cm in diameter (Buckrow *et al.*, 1966) or as coarser 'popcorn' calcification (Puckette *et al.*, 1969). Complete calcification of the ovary of unknown aetiology is extremely rare, but cases were presented at the Chicago Gynaecological Society in 1921 and have been described by Kamniker (1928) and Coors (1942). Lester & McAlister (1970) reported calcification occurring in a spontaneously amputated ovary which was shown radiologically to be freely mobile. Tuberculosis sometimes causes calcifica-

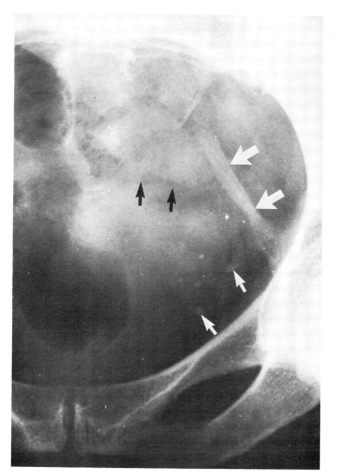

FIG. 1.2 Sacrospinous ligament calcification (large white arrows). The ovoid uterine shadow is separated from the moderately distended bladder by a radiolucent fat line (small black arrows). Phleboliths are present (small white arrows).

tion within the Fallopian tubes (see Fig. 6.11) and pelvi-abdominal lymph nodes (Fig. 1.4). Tubal calcification is otherwise extremely rare and of uncertain cause, although most of these cases appear to be related to elongation and compression of the involved tubes by ovarian or uterine tumours or to kinking and constriction by dense adhesions (Kulka, 1942). The differential diagnosis of pelvic calcification also includes urinary calculi, faecoliths, appendicoliths and vascular calcifications.

The presence of radio-opaque foreign bodies in the genital tract, most commonly in the vagina of children, and the position of contraceptive devices may be ascertained by anteroposterior and lateral films of the pelvic cavity. Ultrasonography is a useful and accurate means of determining whether or not a contraceptive device is in the uterine cavity. Tampons have a radiolucent rectangular appearance (Fig. 1.5). Bubbles of gas within the wall of the vagina are identified as beaded translucencies in vaginal emphysema.

Ascites frequently occurs in association with ovarian malignancy (Fig. 1.6), usually as a result of peritoneal spread of the tumour, but may also be present in benign ovarian conditions (Chapter 8). A generalized homogenous haziness, often more marked in the lower abdomen and pelvic cavity on erect radiographs, with upward displacement and separation of gas-filled bowel loops, obliteration of extraperitoneal fat lines, elevation of the diaphragm and bulging of the flanks, is seen with ascites. Generalized peritonitis may cause a paralytic ileus, with separation of rather ill-defined and moderately distended loops of bowel, obscuration of the properitoneal fat lines and often radiological evidence of free fluid within the peritoneal cavity. A localized abdominal or pelvic abscess may cause an ill-defined soft tissue mass, displacing adjacent bowel which often shows some ileus. A ruptured tubo-ovarian abscess will often cause marked paralytic ileus.

Rupture of a corpus luteum, in the second half of the menstrual cycle of a young woman, may result in a haemoperitoneum. Abdominal radiographs will show free fluid within the pelvic cavity and lateral gutters between the vertical segments of the colon and the lateral abdominal wall, sometimes with associated paralytic ileus. Culdoscopy will confirm the diagnosis (McCort, 1975). Haemoperitoneum with the same radiological findings may also be caused by a ruptured ectopic pregnancy. Rarely, torsion and infarction of an ovarian

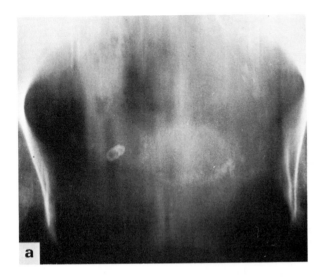

cyst causes intraperitoneal haemorrhage (Taniguchi *et al.*, 1952).

Pneumoperitoneum is a frequent sequel of abdominal surgery and usually disappears within one week of the operation, although it may rarely persist for as long as 24 days (Fig. 1.7). Carbon dioxide is absorbed within a few hours of its introduction into the peritoneal cavity for purposes such as diagnostic pneumography, laparoscopy or tubal insufflation. Air, which disappears more slowly than carbon dioxide, may enter the peritoneal cavity following a vaginal douche with a bulb syringe or effervescent fluid (Walker, 1942; Stilson & Neufeld, 1949). The abnormal patency of the genital tract in the postpartum state may result in a pneumoperitoneum

FIG. 1.3   (a) Calcification is seen within the pelvic cavity on this tomogram.

(b) Excised uterus and adnexa show gross uterine artery calcification. The patient was diabetic. Courtesy of *British Journal of Radiology* (1976), **49**, 797–798.

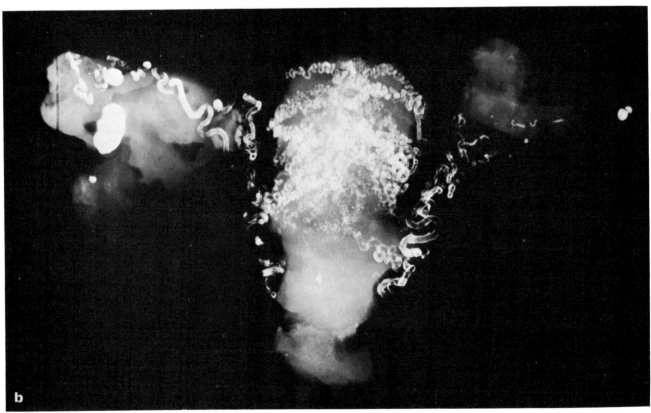

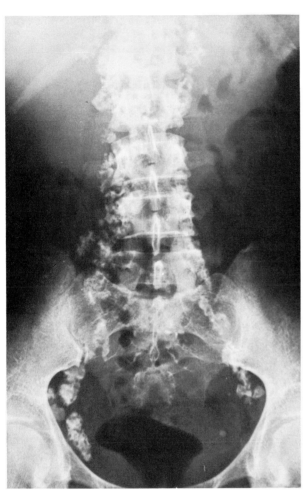

Fig. 1.4 Heavy iliac and para-aortic lymph node calcification, secondary to pelvic or abdominal tuberculosis.

THE CHEST RADIOGRAPH

Kindermann (1967) found some abnormality on routine chest radiographs in 356 out of 1000 women prior to gynaecological operations, although some of these were of little or no immediate clinical significance. In a gynaecological context, chest radiography has some specific indications:

1. To detect the presence of possible pulmonary metastases in cases of pelvic malignant disease.
2. A pleural effusion may be present in a variety of ovarian conditions associated with ascites (Meig's syndrome) (see Fig. 8.24). The reason why pleural effusions are found in combination with ascites in hepatic cirrhosis and Meig's syndrome has been explained by Lieberman & Peters (1970). Severe and prolonged distention of the peritoneal sac by fluid stretches the diaphragm, as well as the closely attached parietal peritoneum and pleura, to such an extent that the fibres of the diaphragm are pulled apart. The widened interstices cause the diaphragm to become permeable to fluid.
3. Tuberculosis is a cause of infertility (Chapter 7).
4. Congenital cardiac abnormalities may be associated with severe anomalies of the genitourinary tract.

Catamenial pneumothorax, or recurrent spontaneous pneumothorax associated with the menstrual period, is a rare condition. It is due to the presence of pleural endometriosis, and occurs in the interval between three days prior to and three days after the onset of menses (Ripstein et al., 1959; Shearin et al., 1974). The right side is most frequently involved, although bilateral pneumothoraces have been described (Laws et al., 1977).

THE PITUITARY FOSSA

Raised levels of prolactin have sometimes been found in association with chromophobe adenomas and occasionally craniopharyngiomas (Saxena, 1977). Secondary amenorrhoea and infertility then occur because of inhibition of progesterone production by granulosa cells, and sometimes galactorrhoea is also present. Ginsberg et al. (1977) found that a quarter of women with primary amenorrhoea and hyperprolactinaemia had radiological evidence of sellar enlargement, while Haesslein & Lamb (1976) found that a quarter of all patients with secondary amenorrhoea for longer than five years had abnormal

when exercises are performed in the knee-elbow position (Conn & La Fon, 1956). A case has been reported in which air was found to have entered the peritoneal cavity via a tubo-vaginal fistula one year after vaginal hysterectomy (Tabrisky et al., 1972). Pneumoperitoneum due to entry of air per vaginam may occur in female water skiers who do not wear wet suits. Cases of spontaneous pneumoperitoneum have been ascribed to the entry of air from a patulous genital tract in women who have no associated pathological condition (Felson & Wiot, 1973).

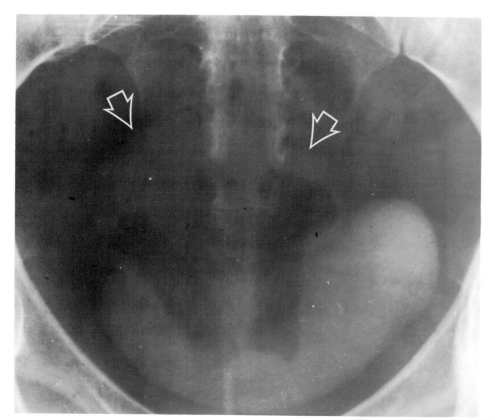

FIG. 1.5 Two tampons within the vagina appear as radiolucent shadows. The bladder is opacified by contrast medium during intravenous urography. The uterus appears as an ovoid soft tissue opacity (arrows) immediately above the bladder.

radiological findings in the sella. Jones & Kemmann (1976) described erosion and enlargement of the pituitary fossa in 3% of anovulatory patients and in 26% when galactorrhoea was associated with absence of ovulation (Fig. 1.8). The use of hypocycloidal tomography in diagnosing prolactin-secreting microadenomas was described by Vezina & Sutton (1974). They found that if these tumours were at least 5 mm and less than 10 mm in diameter, the sella was still of normal size but localized bulging of the anteroinferior wall of one side of the sella was seen with lateralization being an essential criterion. The size of the sella was increased when the adenoma was more than 10 mm in size, the maximum normal length and height being respectively 16 mm and 13 mm.

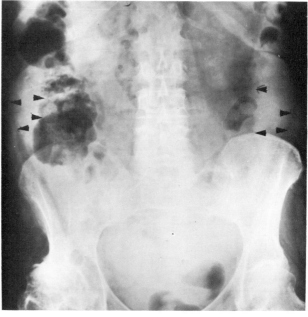

FIG. 1.6 Ascites secondary to ovarian carcinoma. Note the homogenous haziness of the abdomen caused by the ascitic fluid, with distention of the flanks and separation of the properitoneal fat lines from the lateral borders of the colon (arrows).

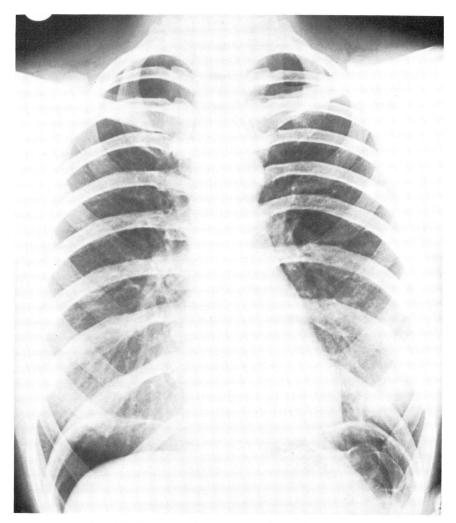

FIG. 1.7 Pneumoperitoneum secondary to laparoscopy.

SKELETON

Bone metastases may occasionally occur secondary to malignancy of the female genital tract, especially from cervical carcinoma.

Deviations of bone age from the normal may be due to gynaecological abnormalities, and can be estimated by the methods of Tanner *et al.* (1975) or of Greulich & Pyle (1959) (Fig. 1.9).

Generalized retardation of skeletal maturation occurs with hypogonadism, for instance Turner's syndrome (Chapter 5), and in hypopituitarism. On the other hand, generalized acceleration of skeletal maturation may be seen in the adrenogenital system, in androgen or oestrogen secreting gonadal tumours, and occasionally with ectopic gonadotropic production from a variety of tumours including teratomas. Accelerated skeletal maturation is also associated with Albright's syndrome, where there is fibrous dysplasia of bone (often unilateral), 'cafe-au-lait' spots, and precocious puberty.

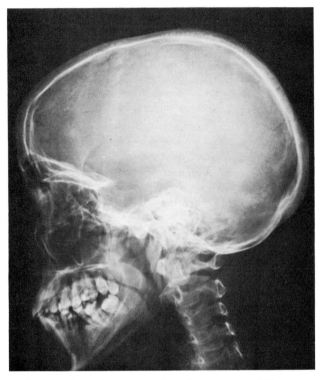

FIG. 1.8 Secondary amenorrhoea in woman aged 34 years. Expanded pituitary fossa with destruction of dorsum sellae.

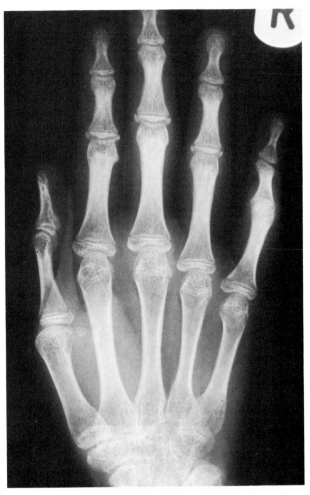

FIG. 1.9 Bone age estimated as 13½ years in girl aged 22 years with Turner's syndrome.

REFERENCES

BERANBAUM S. L. (1951) Fictitious pelvic mass. *Radiology*, **57**, 554–555.

BRYK D. (1966) Roentgen evaluation of large uterine and ovarian masses. *Obst. Gynec.*, **28**, 630–636.

BUCKROW C. J., CARY T. M. & CLARKE W. E. (1966) Ovarian corpora albicantia calcifications. *Radiology*, **87**, 746–747.

CHICAGO GYNECOLOGICAL SOCIETY MEETING PROCEEDINGS (1922) Completely calcified ovary. *Surg. Gynec. Obst.*, **34**, 686.

CONN H. O. & LA FON W. F. (1956) Recurrent spontaneous pneumoperitoneum. *Amer. J. Obst. Gynec.*, **71**, 1342–1347.

COORS G. A. (1942) Calcification of ovaries. *Amer. J. Surg.*, **56**, 492–494.

FELSON B. & WIOT J. F. (1973) Another look at pneumoperitoneum. *Seminars Roentgenol.*, **8**, 437–443.

FISHER M. S. & HAMM R. (1975) Uterine artery calcification. Its association with diabetes. *Radiology*, **117**, 537–538.

GINSBERG J., SCADDING G. & HAVARD C. W. H. (1977) Primary amenorrhoea: the ambiguous non-entity. *Brit. Med. J.*, **2**, 32–35.

GREULICH W. W. & PYLE S. I. (1959). *Radiographic Atlas of Skeletal Development of the Hand and Wrist*. Stanford University Press, Palo Alto, California.

HAESSLEIN H. C. & LAMB E. J. (1976) Pituitary tumors in patients with secondary amenorrhoea. *Amer. J. Obstet. Gynecol.*, **125**, 759–767.

JONES J. R. & KEMMANN E. (1976) Sella turcica abnormalities in an anovulatory population. *Obst. Gynec.*, **48**, 76–78.

KAMNIKER A. (1928) Calcification of the ovary with ossifications. *Zbl. Gynäk.*, **20**, 21–23.

KINDERMANN G. (1967) The value of chest X-rays and pyelography before gynaecological operations. *Geburtsh. u. Frauenheilk.*, **27**, 22–32.

KULKA E. W. (1942). True bone formation in the Fallopian tube. *Amer. J. Obst. Gynec.*, **44**, 383–398.

LAWS H. L., FOX L. S. & YOUNGER J. B. (1977) Bilateral catamenial pneumothorax. *Arch. Surg.*, **112**, 627–628.

LIEBERMAN F. L. & PETERS R. L. (1970) Cirrhotic hydrothorax: further evidence that an acquired diaphragmatic defect is at fault. *Arch. Intern. Med.*, **125**, 114–119.

LESTER P. D. & MCALISTER W. H. (1970) A mobile calcified spontaneously amputated ovary. *J. Canad. Ass. Radiol.*, **21**, 143–145.

LEVENE G. & KAUFMAN S. A. (1958) The diagnostic significance of roentgenologic soft tissue shadows in the pelvis. *Amer. J. Roentgenol.*, **79**, 697–704.

LEWERS A. H. N. (1903) A case of hairpin in the uterus discovered by x-rays. *Brit. Med. J.*, **2**, 814.

LUDLOW I. (1909) Calcification of fibromyomata of uterus. *Cleveland Med. J.*, **8**, 398.

MCCORT J. J. (1975) Ruptured corpus luteum with haemoperitoneum. *Radiology*, **116**, 65–67.

PUCKETTE S. E., WILLIAMSON H. O. & SEYMOUR E. Q. (1969) Calcification in an ovarian corpus albicans. *Radiology*, **92**, 1105.

RIPSTEIN C. B., ROBMAN M. & WALLACH J. B. (1959) Endometriosis involving the pleura. *J. Thorac. Surg.*, **37**, 464–471.

SAXENA B. B. (1977) Human prolactin. In *Endocrinology of Pregnancy*, 2nd edn., ed. F. Fuchs and A. Klopper, Harper & Row, pp. 222–245.

SHEARIN R. P., HEPPER N. G. & PAYNE W. S. (1974) Recurrent spontaneous pneumothorax concurrent with menses. *Mayo Clin. Proc.*, **49**, 98–101.

STEINBACK H. L. (1960) Indentification of pelvic masses by phlebolith displacement. *Amer. J. Roentgenol.*, **83**, 1063–1066.

STILSON R. D. & NEUFELD O. J. (1949) Spontaneous pneumoperitoneum. *California Med.*, **70**, 269–273.

TABRISKY J., MALLIN L. P. & SMITH J. A. (1972) Pneumoperitoneum after coitus. A complication due to uterine tube prolapse after vaginal hysterectomy. *Obst. Gynec.*, **40**, 218–220.

TANNER J. M., WHITEHOUSE R. H., MARSHALL W. A., HEALY M. J. R. & GOLDSTEIN H. (1975) *Assessment of Skeletal Maturity and Prediction of Adult Height. (TW2 Method)*. Academic Press, London.

TANIGUCHI T., KLIEGER J. A. & KUHN M. J. (1952) Surgical emergencies resulting from corpus luteum cysts and hematomas. *Arch. Surg.*, **64**, 516–524.

VEZINA J. L. & SUTTON T. J. (1974) Prolactin-secreting pituitary microadenomas. *Amer. J. Roentgenol.*, **120**, 46–54.

WALKER M. A. (1942) Pneumoperitoneum following a douche. *J. Kansas Med. Soc.*, **43**, 55.

CHAPTER 2

Radiological Techniques II: Hysterosalpingography, Pelvic Pneumography, Vaginography

HYSTEROSALPINGOGRAPHY

The optimum time to perform hysterosalpingography is towards the end of the first week after the menstrual period. At this time the isthmus is at its most distensible and the tubes are most easily filled. The menstrual history must be carefully reviewed so as to avoid investigating a pregnant uterus.

Preparation

Premedication is not required in the majority of cases. The investigation is more likely to be painful, and there is an increased risk of provoking tubal spasm when the patient is very anxious. Reassurance and an explanation of the procedure provide the best form of preparation. When the patient is especially nervous, 5–10 mg of intravenous diazepam is often helpful in allaying anxiety. Morphia, nembutal and pethidine should not be given, as they stimulate the contraction of smooth muscle within the Fallopian tubes (Davids & Weiner, 1950). General anaesthesia, or the emotional distress caused by the thought of it, will often precipitate tubal spasm which will not be relieved under the influence of the anaesthesia (Stallworthy, 1948).

Emptying the bladder immediately prior to hysterosalpingography is of prime importance. A full bladder will elevate the Fallopian tubes and may cause apparent tubal blockage with the spurious radiological appearance of a hydrosalpinx (Bligh & Williams, 1956).

Technique

The patient is placed in the lithotomy position on the screening table and a bimanual pelvic examination is carried out. A vaginal speculum is inserted and the external os is then swabbed with Hibitane or some other suitable non-irritant antiseptic solution. A uterine sound is passed to determine the direction and size of the uterine cavity. Volsellum forceps are placed onto the anterior lip of the cervix. One of a variety of available cannulae is inserted into the external os, followed by the removal of the vaginal speculum.

THE INJECTION CANNULA

The Leech-Wilkinson cannula (Fig. 2.1) has a conical, ridged metallic end which is inserted into the cervical canal with a screwing motion. This action may often be painful, and the junction between cannula and cervix is prone to leakage of the contrast medium. The Green-Armytage type is a popular device, in which a rubber acorn may be altered in its position along the length of the straight metal cannula, and usually provides a fairly watertight junction with the cervix. The plunger attachment of the Green-Armytage cannula is in the form of a screw, one turn of which will cause the injection of 1 ml of contrast medium, thus enabling the operator to know exactly how much of the medium has been injected in a steady flow. There are other varieties of straight or curved metal cannulae with rubber acorns (Figs. 2.2. and 2.3). There are instances where cannulation of the cervix is not possible, such as the presence of tumours deforming the cervix, extensive cervical lacerations and abnormally small cervical canals.

In recent years, the suction type of cannula has come into common usage (Fig. 2.4). Originally described by Kjellman in 1953, this apparatus is generally known in

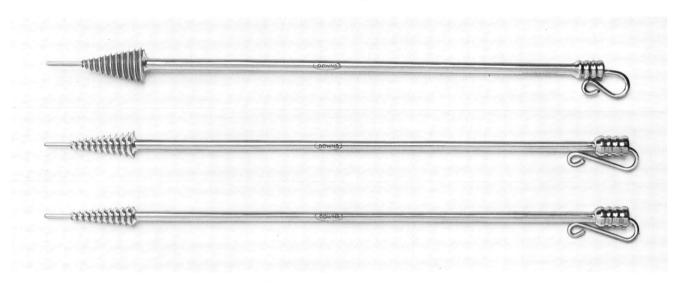

FIG. 2.1   Leech–Wilkinson cannula. Courtesy of Downs Surgical Ltd.

its modified form as the Malström-Westerman vacuum uterine cannula. The technique employed has been well described by both Malström (1961) and by Wright (1961). The special Malström speculum is large enough to accommodate the Malström-Westerman cannula and can be easily removed following insertion of the cannula. Plastic cups, which are in three different sizes, fit over the external part of the cervix. A silicone rubber acorn in the centre of the cup is inserted into the cervical canal. The lumen of the cup is connected by a tube to a unit which will produce a vacuum and consists of a pump, a pressure meter and a vacuum bottle. By establishing a negative pressure of 0.2–0.3 kg/cm², the cervix is drawn into the cup when the tip of the acorn is applied to the external os. An adjustment screw allows the distance of insertion of the acorn into the cervical canal to be controlled, usually 1–2 cm along the cannula being sufficient. With the cannula locked into position in the cervix, the negative pressure is increased to 0.6 kg/cm². The injection cannula will have been connected via a stopcock to a syringe containing contrast medium prior to its application. The whole injection system must contain contrast medium which is free of air bubbles (Fig. 2.5). The stopcock is then opened to allow the

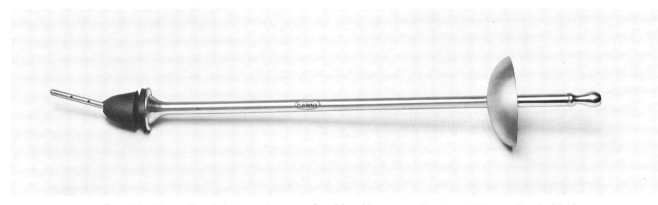

FIG. 2.2   Hayes–Provis intrauterine cannula with rubber cone. Courtesy of Downs Surgical Ltd.

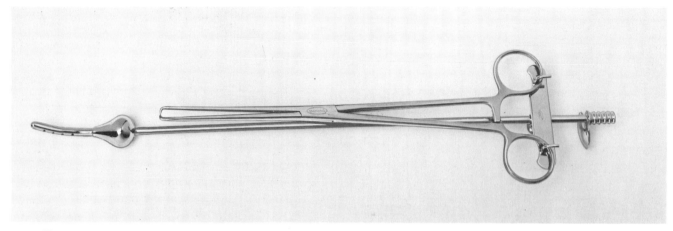

FIG. 2.3   Spackman intrauterine cannula, with adjustable plate for volsellum forceps. Courtesy of Downs Surgical Ltd.

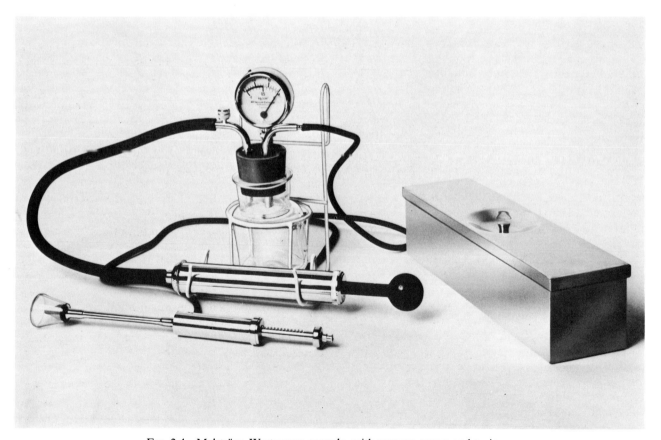

FIG. 2.4   Malström–Westerman cannula, with vacuum pump and syringe.

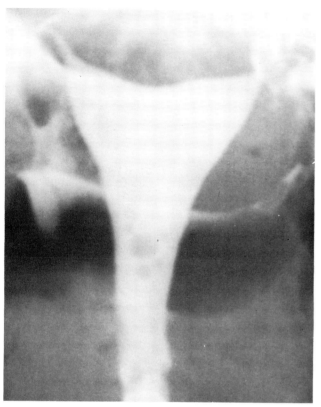

FIG. 2.5   Air bubbles within contrast opacified uterine cavity.

injection of contrast medium. The advantages of the vacuum method is that the painful and traumatic application of volsellum forceps to the cervix is avoided, a water-tight junction is established between the cannula and the cervix, traction may be easily applied to the cannula, the patient may be rotated without fear of dislodging the cannula, the cervical canal is well shown, and traumatic bleeding is a rare occurrence. However, the vacuum cannula is not suitable in cases of severe cervical laceration or effacement. The plastic cups may be sterilized but tend to crack after only a few examinations. Fullenlove (1973) has used cervical cups made of aluminium, and found that they were both durable and radiolucent. Another method of uterine cannulation involves the insertion of a size 16 or 18 Foley catheter into the cervix. Distention of the balloon within the cervical canal is claimed by protagonists of the method

to provide a good watertight junction and satisfactory demonstration of the uterine cavity.

With the use of image intensification, a preliminary radiograph of the pelvic cavity is only required if oily contrast medium from a previous examination or some other opacity is visible on screening. The contrast medium is then injected under screening control. There is no place for the 'blind' injection of contrast medium, which will lead to many diagnostic difficulties during film interpretation and the risk of uterine trauma. The advantage of image intensification over fluoroscopy is better relaxation of the patient who is no longer in complete darkness, with a reduction of the intravaginal dose of irradiation by as much as 86% when compared to fluoroscopy (Dietz, 1956). A lead shield must be provided to protect the operator's hands from irradiation.

Routinely, an undercouch radiograph is taken during uterine filling before the contrast opacification becomes too dense, so that fairly small uterine filling defects and deformities may be seen (Fig. 2.6a). Another radiograph is exposed when the uterus and tubes are delineated and peritoneal spill is just occurring from the fimbrial ends of the tubes (Fig. 2.6b). Using factors of 80 kV and 75 MAS, radiation dosage to the ovaries is 0.45 R, (Barnett & Bewley, 1954) which is equivalent to 30 seconds of image intensification screening time (Altemus et al., 1967). Occasionally, an abnormality may be better shown by oblique or tube lateral views, but these necessitate a higher dosage of radiation. A lateral view is mandatory to show the defect caused by previous Caesarean section. There is generally no need for lateral radiographs in the assessment of uterine retroversion or anteversion. The uterine fundus appears to move in the same direction as a transverse movement of the screen when the uterus is anteverted, and in the opposite direction with retroversion. Malposition of the uterus may make injection difficult and will tend to prevent tubal filling, but good uterotubal filling and correction of the deformity is usually obtained by pulling on both the cannula and the forceps during the injection of contrast medium. Tubal filling may also be obtained by the 'butterfly manœuvre', where the application of alternate relaxation and tension on the instruments may overcome tubal spasm. The injection of contrast medium must always be slow and steady, with constant radiographic visualization through as small an aperture as possible.

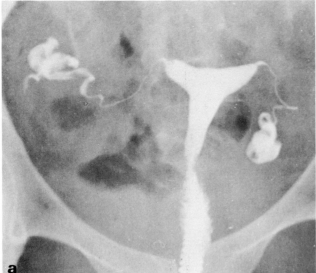

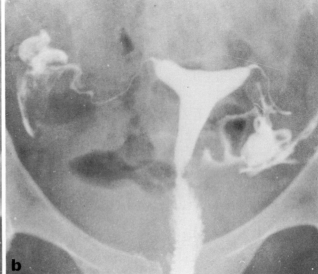

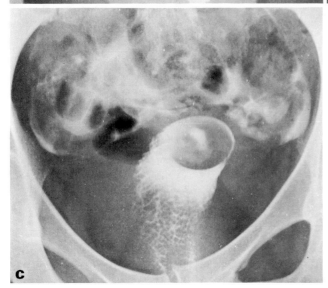

FIG. 2.6   Normal hysterosalpingogram.
(a) Uterus well filled, and Fallopian tubes delineated to ampullae.
(b) A little later, there is full delineation of both tubes with early peritoneal spillage of contrast medium.
(c) Fifteen minutes after withdrawal of cannula. Contrast medium is freely spread over pelvic peritoneal surface. Some contrast medium has flowed back into the vagina.

Atropine is often used as a means of relaxing cornual spasm, but Stallworthy (1948) has found this to be unreliable (Fig. 2.7). Sublingual trinitrin or an inhalation of amyl nitrite may relieve cornual spasm, but they are not universally successful, although Stallworthy claims that their use reduced the incidence of apparent tubal blockage during hysterosalpingography from 21.6% to less than 13% of cases. Gentle manipulation and reassur-ance of the patient as well as prior warming of the contrast medium are important in preventing the onset of cornual spasm. Seibert (1953) has found that the intramuscular injection of dihydroergotamine 1 mg or hydergine 0.3 mg will relax cornual spasm within a few minutes. The vasodilator and antispasmodic agent isoxsuprine hydrochloride has been claimed by Page (1968) to have a significant effect on uterine musculature when 20 mg is given by mouth one hour before hystero-salpingography. Glucagon has recently been found to be an effective tubal spasmolytic agent (Gerlock & Hooser, 1976). The uterine body itself may undergo pronounced spasm with cannulation and injection (Fig. 2.8). Thick tenaceous mucus may be a problem in cervical delineation and may cause spurious filling defects. Irrigation of the vagina with the proteolytic agents papain or bromelain has been found by Hunter et al. (1957) to clear the cervix of mucus.

The injection of water soluble contrast medium is

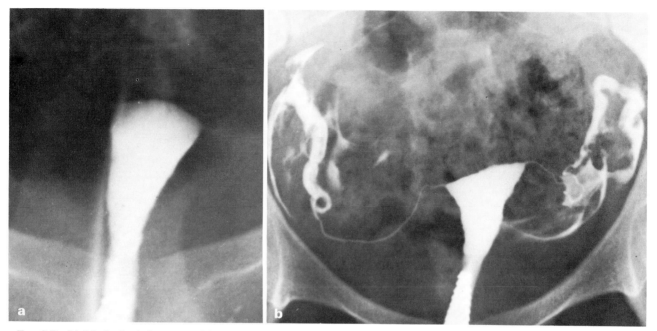

FIG. 2.7 (a) Marked tubal spasm, with rounded and blunted cornual contour. (b) Repeat investigation, following diazapam premedication. Excellent tubal delineation and peritoneal spill.

concluded when either bilateral peritoneal spill or tubal blockage has been shown. Usually 8–12 ml are required, occasionally more. A further radiograph is routinely taken 15–20 minutes later to show the pattern of peritoneal spill (see Fig. 2.6c). This delayed film is usually taken with the patient supine. If any doubt remains concerning the freedom of spillage of contrast medium from the fimbrial ends of the tubes, an additional radiograph in the prone position is often helpful. When peritoneal spill is free, all trace of the contrast agent will have disappeared by one hour after injection, but may be visible for longer in the presence of distal tubal obstruction.

Variations on the basic technique

1. Double contrast hysterography has been described by Deak *et al.* (1958) and by Erbslöh (1959). A small amount of intrauterine water-soluble contrast medium is followed by air insufflation in an attempt to show small mucosal defects. Unfortunately, there is often an uneven adherence of contrast medium to the endometrium.

2. Colpohysterography (Calandra *et al.*, 1959) has been used when conventional hysterosalpingography is impossible, for example in the presence of severely lacerated cervices and vaginocervical malformations. The vagina is first occluded by the inflated balloon of a Foley catheter. Contrast medium is then injected into the vagina and is forced into the uterus and Fallopian tubes with the patient in the Trendelenberg position. The results are inconstant, but users of the method have claimed it to be painless.

3. Pelvigraphy. Jefferis & Samuel (1946) have described the injection of 20–30 ml of water-soluble contrast medium diluted with 10–15 ml of $\frac{1}{2}\%$ novocaine through the cervical cannula and into the peritoneal cavity. The contrast medium collects in the pouch of Douglas and the lateral pelvic recesses, where it may give an assessment of pelvic tumours and inflammatory disease. The method has now been superseded by direct viewing techniques.

The choice of contrast medium

Rindfleish in 1910 was the first to attempt the radiographic delineation of the uterine cavity when he injected bismuth emulsion through the cervical canal. Collargol was used

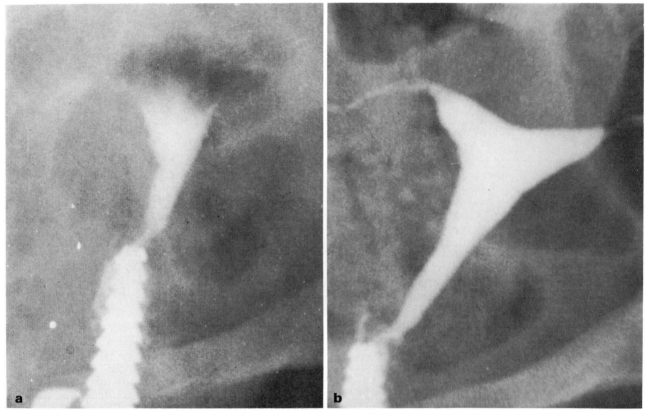

FIG. 2.8 (a) Pronounced spasm of uterine body.   (b) Good relaxation after intravenous diazapam.

as a hysterosalpingographic contrast medium by both Cary (1914) and Rubin (1914). Rubin criticized collargol because it was not absorbed and caused peritoneal irritation. Thorium (Polak, 1920), sodium bromide (Kennedy, 1923) and emulsions of barium sulphate and bismuth (Williams & Reynolds, 1925) were also used in the early days of hysterosalpingography.

Sicard and Forestier in 1922 considered the potential use of Lipiodol in diagnostic radiology. However, it was Hauser who first reported the use of Lipiodol as a hysterographic contrast medium in 1925, employing the investigation solely for the diagnosis of pregnancy. Forsdike (1925) was the first in Great Britain to use Lipiodol for the investigation of sterility.

Lipiodol is a stable compound of iodine in poppy seed oil, which is a glycerin ester, and has a 40% iodine content by weight. Gradually the original Lipiodol com-

pound was supplanted in Europe, and latterly in America, by a modified and less viscous form known as Lipiodol Ultra-Fluid (Ethiodol or Lipiodol F) which has a similar composition to Lipiodol but differs in being an ethyl alcohol ester. Passage along the Fallopian tubes and eventual peritoneal spill is slow, the patient being required to return 24 hours after hysterography for a further radiograph to determine tubal patency and the pattern of peritoneal spillage.

Rubin & Bendick in 1926 were the first to consider that Lipiodol was a peritoneal irritant and suspected, with no convincing evidence at that time, that it could possibly cause adhesions within the peritoneal cavity. The iodine component of Lipiodol is absorbed within several months. However, the radiolucent oily vehicle persists until it is slowly broken down to absorbable fatty acids, having remained localized in lipoid granulomas within the submucosa of the Fallopian tubes and on the peritoneal surface for several years (Elliott *et al.*, 1965). There is a distinct risk of provoking acute salpingitis, peritonitis or pelvic abscess, and therefore a chance of causing infertility, when Lipiodol is used as a contrast medium in hysterosalpingography (Rubin, 1928). Cases where there is stasis in the Fallopian tubes due to previous pelvic inflammation are particularly at risk when Lipiodol is used, and a partially closed tube may develop a complete blockage secondary to stasis of flow of the oily medium and the onset of local chronic inflammation (Royals *et al.*, 1950; Freeth, 1952). Oil granulomas have been found in endometrial curettings taken at three weeks after Lipiodol hysterosalpingography (Aaron & Levine, 1954).

Intravasation of contrast medium, an occasional

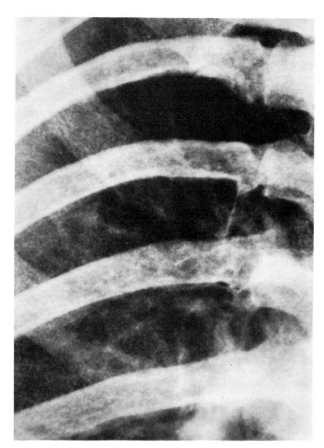

FIG. 2.10   Multiple, dense, punctate opacities in lower lung field following intravasation at hysterosalpingography of Lipiodol.

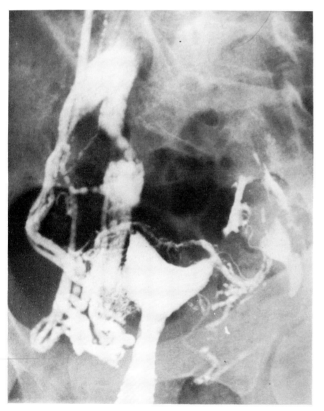

FIG. 2.9   Marked intravasation of Lipiodol during hysterosalpingography. Extensive opacification of pelvic veins with Lipiodol. Note the globular nature of the contrast medium.

occurrence in hysterosalpinography (Fig. 2.9), is hazardous when oily media are used because of the risk of pulmonary oil embolism. The patient may be entirely symptomless when this occurs, but there is often pain and a feeling of constriction within the chest, nausea and perhaps vomiting, rigors, a persistent cough and haemoptysis. Cerebral irritation may develop if some of the oil emboli pass through the lungs. Symptoms usually subside within a week, but death has been reported after the intravasation of Lipiodol (Faris & McMurray, 1947). In most cases, a chest radiograph taken immediately after the intravasation shows dense, punctate opacities widely disseminated through the lung fields (Fig. 2.10). Occasionally, the pulmonary arteries are delineated by the contrast agent (Grossman, 1946). There may also be small pleural effusions and solitary or multi-focal areas of consolidation consistent with pulmonary infarction (Ingersoll & Robbins, 1947).

A high incidence of conception has been claimed in the weeks following hysterosalpingography with an oily contrast medium, suggesting both a therapeutic potential and a diagnostic use. The breaking down of small tubal adhesions, a direct stimulant effect on cilia within the Fallopian tubes, and a mild antiseptic effect were postulated by the protagonists of Lipiodol. On the other hand, it is well recognized that pregnancy may occur after any diagnostic procedure for infertility. Oily hysterosalpingographic agents have now been abandoned by most gynaecologists and radiologists.

There was a gradual introduction of water-soluble contrast media following the increased recognition of the serious side effects of Lipiodol. The first of these media was an aqueous solution of lithium iodide (Jaroschka, 1926). Swick (1929) used Uroselectan, but the low viscosity of this water-soluble contrast agent allowed such rapid passage through the uterus and Fallopian tubes that their delineation was inadequate. Neustaedter *et al.* (1933) found that the viscosity could be satisfactorily increased by adding 50% glucose to Uroselectan B, but there was an unacceptable incidence of pelvic irritation. Skiodan, with acacia added for increased viscosity, was claimed by Titus (1938) to combine good radiographic contrast, rapid absorption, adequate viscosity and a low incidence of pelvic irritation. Rubin (1941) introduced Viscorayopaque, the combination of a complex organic iodine salt in polyvinyl alcohol, and found that while the medium was fairly viscous because of the heavy alcohol vehicle, the iodine concentration was low and pain on peritoneal spill was frequently severe.

Post-war developments in the field of water-soluble hysterosalpingographic media continued to follow two lines in an attempt to increase their viscosity. One group of substances has utilized a large molecular size or high concentration of the medium, while additives have been used as 'stiffeners' to increase viscosity in the other group of contrast media. Satisfactory contrast density, an absence of inflammatory reaction, rapidity of absorption in the genital tract and peritoneal cavity, and lack of pain on peritoneal spill are other requirements in the search for the 'ideal' contrast medium.

All water-soluble contrast media are rapidly absorbed,

no trace being seen after one hour except in cases of tubal occlusion where they may be persistent for up to four hours, with subsequent excretion through the kidneys. Contrast density is less than that of Lipiodol, but most water-soluble media are usually regarded as satisfactory in this respect. However, this relative lack of viscosity and density may be an advantage because there will be an increased chance of delineating tubal and uterine filling defects and narrow crypts or sinuses. Reflux into the vagina should not be a problem provided there is good contact between the cannula and the cervix.

A modification of Viscorayopaque was Viskiosol 6, a mixture of 50% diodone and 6% polyvinyl alcohol, which was regarded for many years as being a satisfactory medium (Freeth, 1952). However, Viskiosol 6 was withdrawn from use when the polyvinyl alcohol was suspected of having a carcinogenic action. Diodone without the additive had too low a viscosity (Reiss & Grossman, 1958).

Methylglucamine iodipamide 50% was marketed as the cholangiographic contrast medium Biligrafin, and has been used in hysterosalpingography. Endografin (Fig. 2.11), the 70% solution of the same substance, has had much use as a hysterosalpingographic agent because of its greater contrast density and viscosity, but it is considered to be associated with a high incidence of pelvic pain due to peritoneal irritation (Sandler, 1956; Reiss & Grossman, 1958; McNabb, 1959). Sinografin, a mixture of 40% diatrizoate and 20% iodipamide as methylglucamine salts, is associated with a low incidence of pain, although its very low viscosity makes it an unsuitable contrast medium. Another contrast medium which depends on molecular size and concentration for its viscosity is Urografin 370 (10% sodium diatrizoate and 66% methylglucamine diatrizoate) which is still a popular agent (Reiss & Grossman, 1958; McNabb 1959). Hypaque 90 (30% sodium diatrizoate and 60% methylglucamine diatrizoate) and a 60% solution of sodium iothalamate (Conray 60) have also been considered by some to be satisfactory (Freedman *et al.*, 1959; Catalano, 1966) but experience with these agents is more limited than with Urografin 370.

As regards currently used water-soluble contrast media with viscous additives, Salpix* (53% sodium acetrizoate and polyvinyl pyrrolidone) and Diaginol viscous (40%

*Salpix is no longer obtainable in the United Kingdom, but is still available in the USA and some other countries.

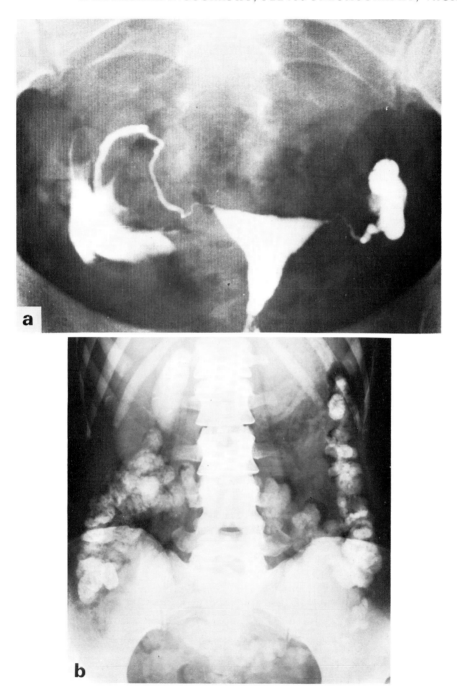

FIG. 2.11   (a) Hysterosalpingogram with Endografin.
(b) 24 hours later the contrast medium has been absorbed from peritoneum and in gall bladder and colon.

sodium acetrizoate and dextran) have been in use for many years. Salpix has the advantage of a higher contrast density. Earlier reports were unequivocal in their praise of Salpix (Rubin et al., 1953; Thomas & Dunn, 1956) but like all water-soluble media it does cause some peritoneal irritation, although it has been claimed by Griffiths (1969) that the pelvic pain is less than that provoked by Urografin 370 while the two media have equal diagnostic value. Crystal formation occurs, but is readily overcome by heating Salpix to body temperature prior to its use. Some difficulty has been found in the injection of Salpix due to its high viscosity (McNabb 1959; Sheach, 1959). Salpix fell temporarily into disrepute when Kantor et al. (1956) attributed pelvic foreign body granulomas to its use. However, this work was held in doubt because no other example of pelvic granulomas has been found (Henry & Hunter, 1960) and Salpix has failed to provoke peritoneal granulomas in animal experiments. Suspicion of a possible carcinogenic action of polyvinyl pyrrolidone in animals (Hueper, 1957) has not been substantiated by wide clinical use of this substance. Histological examination of curettings after Salpix hysterography have failed to reveal any endometrial response that could be attributed to the contrast agent (Seegar Jones & Woodruff, 1960). On the other hand, carboxymethylcellulose which has been used as a viscogenic agent in combination with iodopyracet (Umbradil) and with sodium ortho-iodohippurate (Medopaque H) has been found to stimulate foreign body granulomas in the myometrium, Fallopian tubes and on the ovaries (Bergman et al., 1953).

None of the current available contrast media are entirely satisfactory. Safety is a prerequisite, and the risks to the patient were much lessened by the abandonment of oily media. Overall, a wide and well documented clinical experience shows that Salpix and Urografin 370 are both acceptable contrast media in hysterosalpingography. The optimum benefits from the contrast medium, however, do depend on a satisfactory technique. Diagnostic inaccuracies may be attributable to insufficient or excessive contrast medium, or to a poor junction between cannula and cervix.

Indications for hysterosalpingography

INFERTILITY

The two causes of infertility which are most likely to be seen on hysterosalpingography are maldevelopment of the uterus and occlusion of the Fallopian tubes, which together constitute 60% of all abnormalities demonstrated when this investigation is performed for infertility (Robins & Shapira, 1931; Abbas, 1954). Congenital abnormalities account for 20% of positive findings in primary infertility cases, the most frequent being hypoplasia of the uterus, although various degrees of the bicornuate anomaly are also common (Pontifex et al., 1972). In secondary infertility, as would be expected, evidence of tubal disease is more common than congenital abnormalities. The uterus and Fallopian tubes must be demonstrated before any attempted surgical correction to these organs.

RECURRENT ABORTION

The main cause of repeated abortions is cervical incompetence, the investigation of which is discussed in Chapter 9. Cervical incompetence apart, Behrman & Poppy (1957) found a higher incidence of uterine polyps, fibroids and mild anomalous conditions in patients with habitual abortion than in infertile women.

ABNORMAL UTERINE BLEEDING

Hysterosalpingography complements curettage in the investigation of menstrual disorders, and likely pathological causes of abnormal uterine bleeding may be found in approximately 75% of cases (Wexler et al., 1949). In a survey of cases with metrorrhagia, Kohane & Schwartz (1961) found that 40% had abnormalities (fibroids, endometrial polyps and adenomyosis) diagnosed on hysterography but missed on diagnostic curettage. Oligomenorrhoea may be associated with uterine hypoplasia or intrauterine adhesions.

DYSMENORRHOEA

Isthmic spasm and hypoplasia of the uterus have now been discarded as causes of dysmenorrhoea on the basis of hysterographic studies (Clitheroe, 1964). A significant number of patients with dysmenorrhoea are found to have fibroids or chronic salpingitis (Dutton & Stapleton, 1963).

POST-CAESAREAN SECTION (Chapter 9)

The integrity of the uterine scar following Caesarean section may be accurately shown by hysterography. Assessment on the feasibility of subsequent pregnancies being delivered by the vaginal route, or whether or not further uterine section will be required, may be confidently given on the basis of hysterographic findings employing the lateral view.

AFTER LAPAROSCOPIC STERILIZATION

Following electrocoagulation or clipping of the Fallopian tubes, hysterosalpingography will show whether there is tubal patency or occlusion. The investigation should be performed at least twelve weeks after the operation (Jordan *et al.*, 1971).

BEFORE ARTIFICIAL INSEMINATION

Hysterosalpingography is a prerequisite when artificial insemination is being considered, to rule out structural abnormalities of the genital tract.

LOCALIZATION OF INTRAUTERINE CONTRACEPTIVE DEVICES (Chapter 12)

The partial or complete extrusion of these devices through the uterine wall may be determined by hysterography or ultrasonography.

MALIGNANT UTERINE CONDITIONS

Jarcho (1929) was the first to suggest that hysterosalpingography was contraindicated in malignant uterine disease, because of the potential hazard of disseminating the tumour. However, no cases in which this has happened have been described to date. The location and extent of the tumour may be assessed more accurately by hysterography than by uterine sounding and curettage, and this information may influence the case management if radium is to be inserted into the uterus.

Contraindications

HYSTEROSALPINGOGRAPHY DURING PREGNANCY

Although Heuser in 1925 originally reported the use of Lipiodol in the diagnosis of pregnancy without any apparent ill effects, it was soon realized that hysterosalpingography carried a risk of abortion (Witwer *et al.*, 1930). Awareness of the teratogenic hazards of radiation to the early fetus and a possible increased chance of developing childhood leukaemia is a relatively recent development (Stewart *et al.*, 1958).

When hysterosalpingography is inadvertently performed during the first two months of pregnancy, the

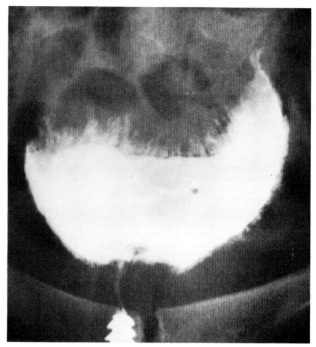

FIG. 2.12 Pregnant uterus on hysterogram. Ovum produces a filling defect in a globular uterus which is lined by thickened endometrium.

uterine cavity is found to be enlarged, atonic and globular, with the ovum as a filling defect (Fig. 2.12). The edges of the uterine shadow are often ill-defined due to the permeation of the contrast medium into the thickened endometrium. At three or four months, the contrast medium delineates only part of the growing ovum and the contrast shadow takes on a meniscus shape (Fig. 2.13). When the ovum is older, no contrast medium can enter the uterus.

ECTOPIC PREGNANCY

There are no reported cases of precipitate haemorrhage following hysterosalpingography in cases of ectopic pregnancy. Nevertheless, the manipulation and the contrast injection are potentially hazardous and may theoretically cause dislodgement of the extrauterine pregnancy. The contrast medium may either envelope the blood mole within the lumen of the Fallopian tube to a varying extent, or may diffusely spread through the

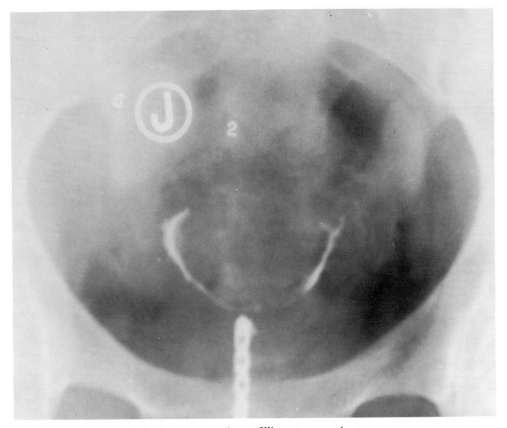

FIG. 2.13 Large ovum almost filling uterus on hysterogram.

intervillous spaces or through larger channels in the blood mole (Ekengren & Ryden, 1954).

PELVIC INFECTION

A history of salpingitis in the previous six months precludes hysterosalpingography until a course of antibiotics has been given and a clinical assessment of successful treatment has been made. Acute vaginitis and cervicitis carry a risk of ascending infection and are also contra-indications.

IMMEDIATE PRE- AND POST-MENSTRUAL PHASES

The thickened or denuded endometrium respectively, which is present before and after the menstrual period, increases the chance of intravasation. This is of no significance in the case of water-soluble contrast media, except that it may obscure the contours of the uterus and adnexa. During the premenstrual phase there is a risk of performing hysterosalpingography in early pregnancy. Spasm of the isthmus and cornua is least likely to occur at mid-cycle.

SENSITIVITY TO CONTRAST MEDIUM

Water-soluble contrast media are absorbed from the peritoneum into the vascular system, so there is a risk of a hypersensitivity response in the susceptible. Where there is a previous history of sensitivity to contrast media or to other substances, it is necessary to consider the advisability for performing the procedure or the need for antihistamine or steroid cover.

Complications of hysterosalpingography

PAIN

The most common complaint described by patients undergoing hysterosalpingography is pain, which may occur at various stages of the examination.

Passage of the speculum, uterine sound and injection cannula may all cause transient lower abdominal discomfort. Almost every patient experiences a brief episode of pain when the anterior lip of the cervix is grasped by the volsellum.

Patients with a low pain threshold and those in an apprehensive state may feel a low central abdominal discomfort or pain when the uterus is distended with contrast medium. A similar sensation may be felt to one side of the midline in the pelvic region with similar distention of Fallopian tubes. A rapid rate of injection will also provoke these symptoms, which usually subside within 10 minutes. Pain, which may be severe, is also frequent when tubal spasm or organic tubal obstruction is present and is maximal just lateral to the midline.

Water-soluble media may be associated with painful peritoneal spillage. This pain usually lasts for about one hour, is relieved by mild analgesics, and is an especially frequent symptom when the contrast medium is methylglucamine iodipamide (Biligrafin) although it also occurs with any of the other water-soluble agents. This pain on peritoneal spillage has been attributed to an inflammatory response in the peritoneum, being probably related to the hypertonicity and amount of the contrast medium. Scila et al. (1962) found on animal experiments that several standard hysterosalpingographic contrast media caused hyperaemia, and that the equivalent effect could be simulated by 0.1% formaldehyde solution on the peritoneum.

Pain may uncommonly commence within an hour or two of the procedure, but usually disappears within twenty-four hours although it may occasionally persist for several days. This type of pain is often attributed to peritoneal irritation, but Smitham (1959) considers that it usually occurs in patients who have dysmenorrhoea. This type of pain is especially common with the use of methylglucamine iodipamide. Clinically, the pain of delayed onset must be differentiated from pain caused by either an exacerbation of pelvic infection or by uterine perforation.

PELVIC INFECTION

It has been estimated that 0.25–2% of patients have pelvic infection following hysterosalpingography (Nielsen, 1946; Arnet & Elkin, 1967). This is usually the result of an acute exacerbation of a pre-existing chronic pelvic infection, but may occur de novo. This complication was especially likely to occur when oily contrast media were used, but pelvic infection may also follow the use of water-soluble agents. Hysterosalpingography should therefore not be performed until it has been ensured that recent or current episodes of pelvic infection have been eradicated by antibiotics. Acute salpingitis, pelvic cellulitis and pelvic peritonitis, and exacerbation of tuberculous peritonitis may all occur after hysterosalpingography (Measday, 1960).

HAEMORRHAGE

Slight spotting is a common consequence of hysterosalpingography, the origin being the site of volsellum application on the cervix. Bleeding from the uterine cavity after hysterosalpingography suggests the presence of an organic lesion, such as a polyp or carcinoma. Vigorous uterine sounding or the use of a cannula whose tip extends for more than 1 cm beyond the acorn may cause endometrial irritation and hence bleeding (Siegler, 1967).

PERFORATION OF UTERUS

The sounding prior to hysterosalpingography is the most frequent cause of uterine perforation. Rough application of the cannula may cause severe laceration of the cervix. (Fig. 2.14.)

ALLERGIC PHENOMENA

As described in the previous section, all contrast media are potential causes of hypersensitivity reactions in susceptible subjects, the adverse effects including urticaria, asthma and laryngeal oedema.

MISCELLANEOUS SYMPTOMS

These symptoms include nausea, vomiting and headache. They may be directly due to the contrast medium, but when delayed in onset may be part of the systemic manifestations of a provoked acute pelvic infection.

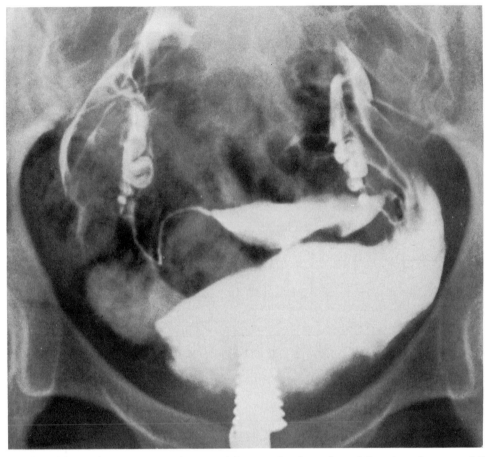

FIG. 2.14   Perforation of the uterine cervix during hysterosalpingography. Apart from delineation of uterus and Fallopian tubes, there is a large extrauterine, extraperitoneal collection of contrast medium.

VASOVAGAL ATTACKS

Sometimes with syncope, but with rapid recovery, vaso-vagal attacks occur in 0.18% of cases (Woltz *et al.*, 1958). The patient may very rarely have mild convulsions.

VENOUS INTRAVASATION

The occurrence of intravasation of contrast media into the venous system of the uterus delineates a fine, inter-lacing network adjacent to the borders of the opacified uterine cavity, within the myometrium. More extensive intravasation results in the delineation of a number of larger superficial uterine veins and those veins which run along the broad ligament (Fig. 2.15). Occasionally,

opacification may extend to the iliac veins and pampini-form plexi. The incidence of venous intravasation has been estimated as 0.6–3.7%. It is of little significance when associated with water soluble contrast media, but pulmonary and cerebral embolization occurred following intravasation of oily media. There are several predispos-ing factors to venous intravasation:

1. Direct trauma to the endometrium from the inject-ing cannula, especially when the cannula projects for a long distance beyond the acorn. Occasionally a short cannula may injure the cervix, particularly if the cervix is deformed by a fibroid or other lesion, and cause intra-vasation. In the severely anteverted, retroverted or

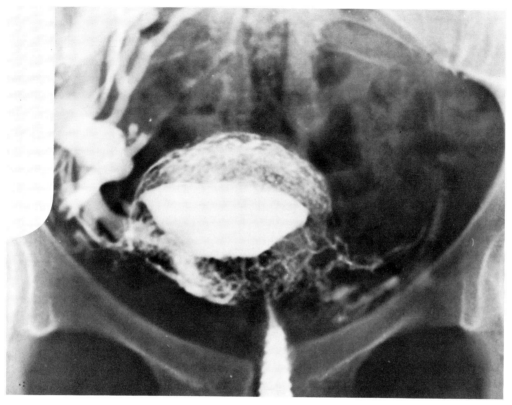

FIG. 2. 15   Gross intravasation of water-soluble contrast medium during hysterosalpingography, with delineation of veins of uterine wall and pelvic cavity.

laterally flexed uterus, the uterine wall may be in direct contact with the cannula tip.

2. Hysterosalpingography performed within a few days of menstruation, when the endometrium is thick and vascular, or in a denuded state.

3. If hysterosalpingography is carried out soon after curettage, before endometrial regeneration has taken place.

4. Certain abnormalities of the uterus, namely endometrial tuberculosis, uterine carcinoma, uterine hypoplasia and fibroids may predispose to intravasation.

5. Tubal occlusion is associated with a high incidence of intravasation. This presumably follows a high pressure of contrast medium within the uterine cavity.

6. Excessive pressure injection, more than 200 mmHg, may play only a secondary role in the causation of uterine intravasation, except when there is occlusion of

the Fallopian tubes. Druckman & Rozin (1951) have found intravasation to be a common occurrence with a low pressure injection, even in the absence of pre-existing uterine disease or tubal occlusion. Moreover, intravasation always occurred in these cases at the same site on repeated hysterosalpingography. A superficial vascular abnormality may account for this repeated intravasation.

LYMPHATIC INTRAVASATION

Uterolymphatic intravasation was first described by Erbslöh in 1949. Other cases have been reported subsequently, usually with oily contrast media, and occurred either as an isolated phenomenon or in association with venous intravasation. The opacified lymphatic system of the uterine wall has a much finer reticular pattern than the venous channels, and the contrast medium flows much more sluggishly in lymphatics than in veins. Lymphatic channels may be seen leaving the uterus, and oily media may be taken up by the draining lymph nodes. The predispositions to lymphatic intravasation are common to venous intravasation, especially tuberculous disease (Kika, 1954), bilateral tubal occlusion (Hipona & Ditchek, 1966), uterine hypoplasia, fibroids and carcinoma. Lymphatic intravasation may also be seen without any apparent predisposing cause (Fisher, 1966).

DEATH

Fatal outcomes of hysterosalpingography are fortunately very rare, especially with the superseding of oily contrast media by water-soluble agents. In the past, deaths have been attributed to pulmonary embolism, and pelvic infection with peritonitis in almost equal proportions (Siegler, 1967). Very occasionally, a severe allergic reaction may result in death. In one case, the rupture of a pelvic abscess associated with choriocarcinoma had a fatal outcome (Chuang *et al.*, 1971).

RUPTURE OF A PYOSALPINX

The spontaneous rupture of a silent pyosalpinx, several hours after hysterosalpingography, has been reported by Brantley *et al.* (1960).

INTESTINAL OBSTRUCTION AFTER
HYSTEROSALPINGOGRAPHY

Becker *et al.* have reported a case of peritonitis following hysterosalpingography with Medopaque-H (sodium orthoiodohippurate and sodium carboxymethylcellulose), where the ensuring pelvic adhesions resulted in acute ileal obstruction seven weeks later.

EFFECT ON THYROID FUNCTION TESTS

Oily contrast media caused a marked depression of iodine up-take for up to four months after hysterosalpingography, with elevated protein bound iodine for several months. Water-soluble contrast media cause marked elevations of the protein bound iodine level within 5–60 minutes after injection, with reversion to normal levels within 24–48 hours (Slater *et al.*, 1959). These effects must be borne in mind if thyroid assay tests are contemplated.

ENDOMETRIOSIS

Teilum & Madsen (1950) found seven cases in which hysterosalpingography was followed by laparotomy and where endometriosis was found on the surface of the ovary or Fallopian tube in close association with lipoid granulomas. This finding raises the possibility of translocation of endometrium resulting from the use of oily contrast media, or even the development of endometriosis as a result of peritoneal irritation.

Radiological anatomy

CERVIX

The cervical canal is best demonstrated in hysterography by the use of the vacuum injector (see Fig. 2.3). The size of the cervical canal is very variable, but is usually 3–4 cm in length, although it tends to become shorter after childbirth. On average, the cervical canal is one third of the entire length of the uterus (Fig. 2.16). It is often spindle shaped, but may be cylindrical or flask shaped, with the

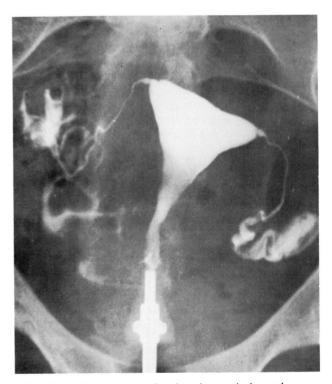

FIG. 2.16 Hysterogram showing the cervical canal as a distinct narrow tubular segment.

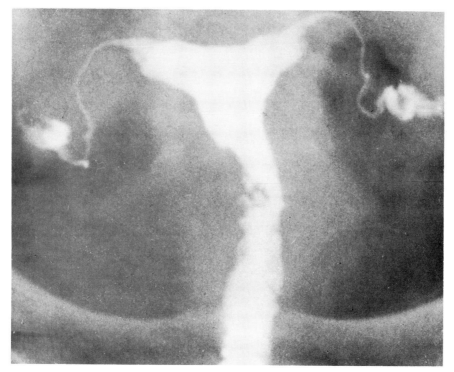

FIG. 2.17 Prominent plica palmata and filling of cervical glands.

width tending to increase in the proliferative phase of the menstrual cycle. Hysterography may reveal longitudinal ridges on the anterior and posterior walls. The cervical mucosa is thrown into a series of small parallel folds, the plicae palmatae, which arise from the longitudinal ridges and tend to give the contrast delineated cervical canal a serrated contour. The plicae palmatae may hypertrophy in the proliferative phase, but often disappear after childbirth. Tubular and racemose glands may fill with contrast medium from the cervical canal (Fig. 2.17).

UTERINE ISTHMUS

Between the inferior ('histological') and superior ('anatomical') internal os lies the isthmus. It is seen as a distinct segment which is narrower than the uterine body and cervical canal in only half of all normal hysterograms (Asplund, 1952). When definable, the isthmus has the shape of a smooth inverted truncated cone of variable length and width. In hysterograms in which the isthmus is indefinite, the cervical canal may blend imperceptibly

with the uterine body. However, in many cases the site of the inferior internal os, the point beyond which typical cervical mucosa is not present, is marked by a short constriction of the lumen (Fig. 2.18). The width and distensibility of the internal os is larger in the proliferative phase than in the secretory phase of the menstrual cycle. Width of more than 8 mm causes suspicion of isthmal incompetence, which is definitely present when the width is 12–14 mm.

UTERINE BODY

The radiographic outline of the contrast-filled cavity of the uterine body is triangular in shape, its walls are normally regular and are straight or concave (see Figs 2.16 and 2.17), although the fundal surface is occasionally convex. The average length of the uterine body is 3.5 cm which is also a mean value for the intercornual diameter, but may be larger (Fig. 2.19). The cornual sphincters are pear or spindle shaped, and may be separated from the uterine body cavity by a short dark line which is due to

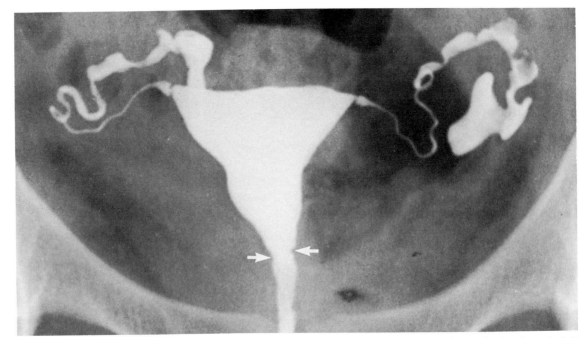

FIG. 2.18 Indentation (arrows) due to internal os. Triangular cornua, separated from uterine cavity by short dark line.

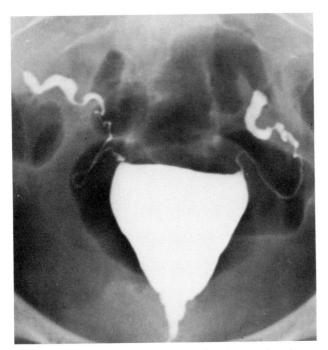

FIG. 2.19 Large globular uterine cavity. A normal variant.

the obliquity of the region or to a localized muscle contraction (Fig. 2.18).

FALLOPIAN TUBES

The interstitial portion of the Fallopian tube is 1.5–3.5 mm long and usually runs an oblique and tortuous course through the myometrium (Fig. 2.20). The apex of the cornua is continuous with the tubal lumen. Anatomically, the cornual sphincter is not a distinct structure and cornual closure is due to contraction of the surrounding myometrium, especially the inner circular muscle component, which causes direct occlusion or kinking of the interstitial portion of the Fallopian tube. The tubal muscle itself probably plays little part in closure.

Some variants of normal hysterographic appearances

SPICULATED OUTLINE TO UTERINE CAVITY (Fig. 2.21)

Slezak & Tillinger (1973a) have drawn attention to a fine saw-toothed pattern which may occasionally be seen on the outline of a contrast-filled uterine cavity. This has to be differentiated from the larger jagged projections

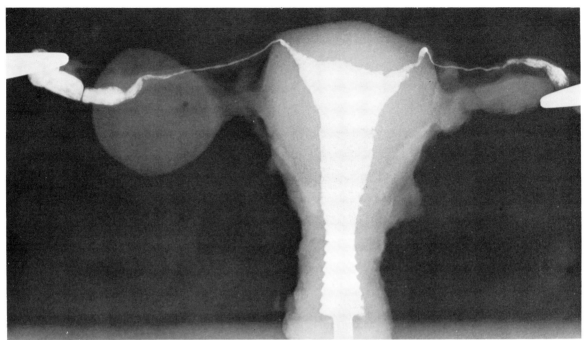

FIG. 2.20 Injection of resected uterus, Fallopian tubes and ovaries. The oblique and tortuous course of the interstitial portion of the Fallopian tubes is seen.

which may be seen in adenomyosis and endometrial carcinoma. The saw-tooth appearance occurs mainly in women approaching the menopause, and is attributed to contrast medium entering mucosal gland openings in an atrophic endometrium. When it is seen in younger women, an abnormal cause for endometrial hypoplasia should be suspected, although it may be found with oral contraception.

ENDOMETRIAL THICKENING IN THE FUNDUS

Sweeney (1958) has found that some cases interpreted as arcuate uteri on hysterography were of normal shape when sectioned after hysterectomy. The wide convex filling defect in the fundal region was due to localized marked endometrial thickening across the fundus.

BROAD UTERINE LONGITUDINAL FOLDS

These are usually 5–10 mm wide, have distinct outlines, and run parallel to the longitudinal contours of the

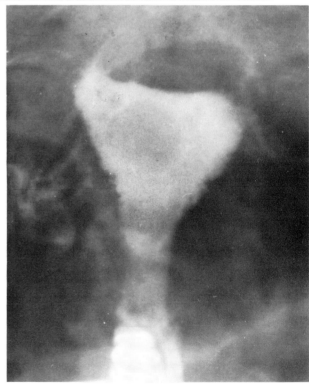

FIG. 2.21 Spiculated outline to uterine cavity. There are also air bubbles within the uterine cavity.

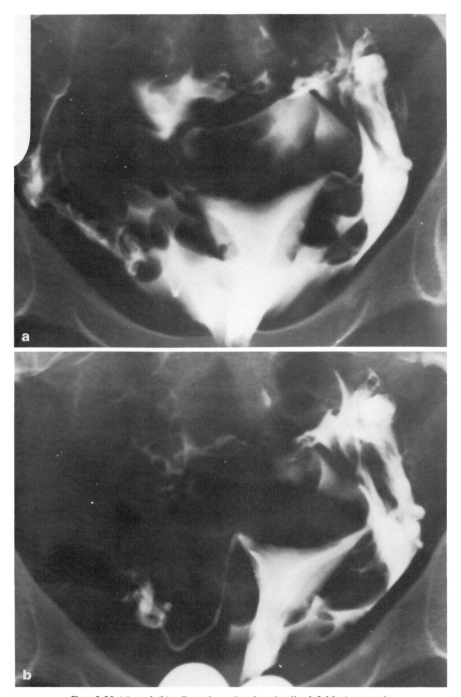

FIG. 2.22 (a) and (b)   Broad uterine longitudinal folds (see text).

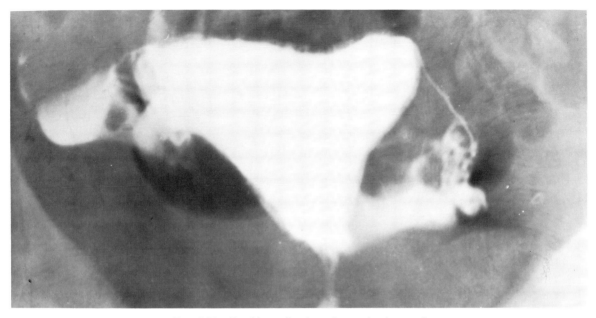

Fig. 2.23   Double outlined uterine cavity (see text).

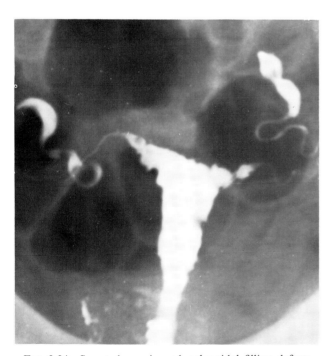

Fig. 2.24   Serrated margin and polypoidal filling defects occurring as a normal variant.

uterine cavity (Fig. 2.22). Pathological investigation has shown these to be undulations of the inner surface of the myometrium, probably remnants of the Müllerian ducts (Slezak & Tillinger, 1973b).

DOUBLE OUTLINED UTERINE CAVITY

Slezak & Tillinger (1968) found that 41% of all hysterograms performed in the second half of the secretory phase of the menstrual cycle showed a double outline to the uterine cavity (Fig. 2.23). They considered this phenomenon to be due to penetration of endometrial glands to a depth of 1–2 mm by contrast medium. A similar change is also seen in early pregnancy.

POLYPOID FILLING DEFECTS IN UTERINE CAVITY

Histologically normal endometrium may be associated with polypoidal filling defects on hysterography (Fig. 2.24) usually during the secretory phase but occasionally in the proliferative phase in the absence of abnormal uterine bleeding. This appearance has no clinical significance (Slezak & Tillinger, 1975).

CYSTIC SPACES WITHIN UTERINE WALL

Cavities within the wall of the upper half of the uterus are often due to adenomyosis. Slezak & Tillinger (1976) consider that cystically dilated cervical glands, and probably the less common but similar finding in the isthmus, may be regarded as a normal variant (see Fig. 2.17).

Diagnostic errors in hysterosalpingography

1. Air bubbles may be mistaken for polypoid lesions within the uterine cavity, but are freely mobile and often do not persist (see Fig. 2.5).

2. Underfilling of the uterus may fail to demonstrate an abnormality, and will possibly result in failure to delineate the Fallopian tubes.

3. Intrauterine filling defects may also be missed when too much contrast medium is injected, when the injection rate is too rapid, or when insufficient radiographs have been taken.

4. Cornual spasm may be mistaken for an organic obstruction to tubal filling (see Fig. 2.7). Patience will often be rewarded by tubal filling if a few minutes are allowed to elapse after uterine distention with contrast medium and with the cannula still in position.

5. Pathological features may be overlooked if the uterus is not fully displayed because of anteversion or retroversion. Traction and oblique radiographs will help to give a fuller demonstration.

6. Diffusion of contrast medium within a large hydrosalpinx may initially be mistaken for free peritoneal spill. A delayed radiograph will differentiate tubal dilatation from the normal state.

7. Mucus in the cervical canal may be misinterpreted as a pathological lesion, such as carcinoma. Subsequent dilatation and curettage or repeated hysterography will differentiate between them. Apparent transient filling defects in the cervical canal may be due to a flow phenomenon.

8. Traces of unabsorbed oily contrast medium from a previous hysterosalpingogram may be mistaken for medium which has been introduced in the current investigation. Differing densities, and a preliminary radiograph or careful screening before the introduction of contrast medium, should minimize the problem.

PELVIC PNEUMOGRAPHY

Pelvic pneumography consists of the induction of a pneumoperitoneum followed by radiography to specifically demonstrate the gas-delineated female pelvic organs. The term 'gynaecography' is sometimes regarded as being synonymous with pelvic pneumography, but should strictly be used to describe the combined simultaneous use of hysterosalpingography with pneumography.

Wuber (1913) was the first to combine artificial pneumoperitoneum with a radiographic examination, while Goetz (1918) used this method for assessing the female genital system. Subsequent refinement of the technique and definition of the role of pelvic pneumography in the investigation of infertility and amenorrhoea has been largely due to the work of Stein (1937). Nowadays pelvic pneumography is not performed as often as previously, mainly due to the widespread use of diagnostic laparoscopy. However, there is still a limited place for the procedure in gynaecological diagnosis.

Technique

The patient has nothing by mouth for twelve hours, a cathartic agent and a cleansing enema being given prior to the examination. The bladder is emptied immediately before establishment of the pneumoperitoneum. Usually no premedication is required, but intramuscular pethidine may be given to the anxious patient.

A preliminary radiograph is taken with the patient lying with her head down in the prone position, the X-ray table being tilted 45° to the floor. A radiograph is then exposed with the beam perpendicular to the floor and centred on the coccyx, and with as long a focus-film distance as possible (usually 100 cm) to limit magnification. If necessary, radiographic factors and positioning are then corrected on the basis of this control radiograph which will also show any faecal masses or bladder distention.

The table is restored to the horizontal plane and the patient turns into the supine position. The abdomen is exposed, palpated and daubed with antiseptic. The puncture site is selected immediately lateral to the left border of the rectus sheath where it intersects a line between the umbilicus and the anterior superior iliac spine. This selected point must be free from any scars or underlying abdominal mass. Infiltration by local anaesthetic of the skin and subcutaneous tissues down to the peritoneum at the chosen point precedes a small skin incision by a scalpel blade. A short-bevelled 10 cm long No. 18 or 20 spinal needle is introduced through this point, and its tip is considered to be within the peritoneal cavity when the needle meets a sudden lack of resistance and the trochar can readily be replaced following its removal. Tension in the abdominal musculature may be increased by elevating the patient's head from the table top, and this manœuvre helps with the insertion of the needle. The trochar is removed and the needle is connected by rubber tubing to an apparatus suitable for the introduction of gas. Air and oxygen have been abandoned as agents in induced pneumoperitoneum because of the risk of embolism when there is puncture of a blood vessel. Carbon dioxide does not have this disadvantage and, although it is rapidly absorbed from the peritoneal cavity within 15–20 minutes, there is usually enough time to perform a satisfactory examination. Nitrous oxide is another safe, but rapidly absorbed, gaseous agent which has many advocates. An apparatus which allows a metered amount of gas to be introduced, such as the Maxwell pneumothorax machine, is used to establish the pneumoperitoneum. When carbon dioxide is used, 1200 ml of gas from a Sparklet cylinder is allowed to enter the peritoneal cavity over 10 minutes. In the case of infants 600 ml are used, and 800 ml in children. If gas is inadvertently introduced into the abdominal wall, palpable crepitus and a lack of a free rise in gas pressure will be evident. Rarely, gas may enter the bowel, but this does not result in any side effects apart from intestinal colic. Shoulder tip pain indicates correct needle placement, and may be alleviated by tilting the patient's head downwards on the table top. Generalized abdominal resonance and distention also indicate a successful pneumoperitoneum. The needle is removed, a plaster placed on the puncture site, and the patient is then turned prone. The patient is then positioned as before and radiographs are taken as described for the control film, and with the tube angled 10° in caudad and cephalad directions. Sometimes a lateral beam may be utilized in a further view.

The gas may be introduced into the peritoneal cavity by uterotubal insufflation, using a vacuum cannula or a Foley catheter within the cervical canal. This method is, of course, unsuccessful in cases of tubal occlusion, where cervical intubation is impossible, and in the young. Ansari (1970) has described a technique for introducing the gas by needle puncture *per vaginam* into the pouch of Douglas.

Complications

1. Pain due to diaphragmatic irritation from the pneumoperitoneum usually disappears as soon as the patient is put in the head down position.

2. Occasionally nausea and vomiting occur, but these symptoms are transient.

3. Inadvertent injection of gas into the abdominal wall results in some discomfort, but the gas is rapidly resorbed without any damage.

4. Occasionally the gas may be injected into the bowel, but without any ill effects.

Normal appearances (Fig. 2.25)

The uterus should lie towards the centre of the correctly positioned radiograph, with the broad ligaments containing the Fallopian tubes running between the uterus and the lateral pelvic walls, and the ovaries are situated laterally on the posterior aspects of the broad ligaments. The round ligaments run anterolaterally from the uterine body towards the internal inguinal ring. The bladder is seen anterior to the uterus and the rectum is posteriorly situated beyond the pouch of Douglas. There should be no loops of small bowel obscuring the pelvic organs, unless peritoneal adhesions are present.

The ovaries should be smooth and ovoid in outline. The ovarian index provides a rough rule of thumb in the estimation of their size, and is estimated by multiplying the length of each ovary by the maximum breadth. The normal range of the ovarian index is 4–14 cm (Kreel *et al.*, 1969). A rough estimation of uterine area (Weigen & Stevens, 1967) by multiplying the smallest height by the width in centimetres gives a wide normal variation of between 15 and 55 (average 33.7).

Uses of pelvic pneumography

Pelvic pneumography has largely been superseded by laparoscopy. The pneumoperitoneum which is established during laparoscopy does allow the radiographic technique described above to be employed immediately afterwards. If laparoscopic facilities are not readily

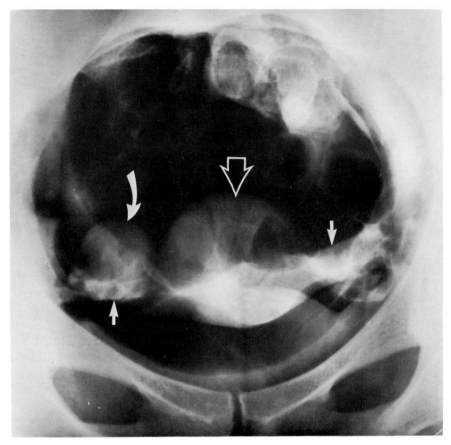

FIG. 2.25 Pelvic pneumogram showing the uterus towards the centre of the pelvic cavity (open arrow). The board ligaments (small arrows) run laterally to the pelvic wall and are overlapped by the ovaries. Small cyst of right ovary (curved arrow). The bladder lies in front of the uterus and the rectum is at the back of the pouch of Douglas.

available, there are then several indications for primary pelvic pneumography:

1. The technique may be used to delineate the external appearances of the internal genitalia if hysterosalpingography cannot be performed; for instance in cases of vaginal or cervical atresia and stenosis, tubal obstruction, and in children.

2. When pathology of the adnexa is suspected or cannot be excluded on pelvic examination, for instance in the obese.

3. In intersex states, the presence or absence of a uterus may be ascertained on pelvigraphy. The presence or absence of ovaries or abdominal testes may be diagnosed, although differentiation of ovaries from atypically situated testes and ovotestes is not possible. (Lunderquist, 1968). Many intersex cases require a diagnostic laparotomy to determine their exact gonadal state, coupled with the removal of abdominal testicular structures which are prone to malignant change.

4. Pelvic pneumography is nowadays rarely required in the evaluation of precocious puberty, as urinary gonadotrophic and oestrogen estimations followed by laparotomy is usually the procedure of choice. The premature release of gonadotrophin will cause uterine enlargement as well as symmetrical enlargement of the ovaries, but sometimes an ovarian tumour may be shown.

Likewise in gonadal dysgenesis, there are now other criteria such as chromosomal studies for confirming or excluding the diagnosis.

5. In cases of uterine carcinoma, pelvic pneumography may be used in the planning of radiotherapy, the protagonists (Sala *et al.*, 1967; Brascho, 1970) claiming that radium application suitable for uterine size can be given and that complications may be minimized by awareness of the relative position of other pelvic viscera. Also, the parametrial spread from carcinoma of the cervix may be demonstrated by this technique.

6. Ovarian status in cases of amenorrhoea may be shown. In primary amenorrhoea, the ovaries may be small or streaked, or totally absent. The polycystic ovaries of the Stein-Leventhal syndrome may be demonstrated (Lea Thomas *et al.*, 1968), but this condition is discussed in Chapter 8.

7. When infertility is the problem, pneumography may show the underlying cause. Congenital abnormalities, such as hypoplasia and aplasia of the uterus or ovaries, are seen, and differentiation of a bicornuate uterus from a septate type may be made. Other visible causes of infertility include ovarian atrophy, polycystic ovaries, endometriosis, and pelvic inflammatory disease. Stevens (1967) claims that a reasonable explanation for infertility is found in a third of patients subjected to pelvic pneumography, while contributory or confirmatory information will be given in a further third of cases, leaving the cause of infertility unexplained in the remaining third.

Contraindications

1. The presence of pelvic infection or peritonitis.

2. Gas in the peritoneal cavity reduces the patient's vital capacity, especially in the head down position, so pelvic pneumography is contraindicated in patients with severe cardiac or respiratory disease. Furthermore, the mechanism for the excretion of carbon dioxide is impaired in patients with cor pulmonale or emphysema.

3. Large masses which completely fill the pelvic cavity or extend into the abdomen result in an unsatisfactory investigation due to lack of gaseous dissemination.

4. Ascites results in poor visualization of the pelvic organs.

VAGINOGRAPHY

Technique

A Foley catheter is inserted into the vagina, and a 30 ml balloon is distended by air (Fig. 2.26). It is imperative that the inflated balloon fits snugly into the lower vagina. The catheter is then gently tugged to ensure that the inflated balloon fits securely above the introitus. When a fluid-tight junction is established between the balloon and the vagina, water-soluble contrast medium is injected into the vagina. Usually, 20–30 ml are required and spot radiographs are then obtained in the anteroposterior, lateral and requisite oblique positions. During the injection of contrast medium, steady traction is applied to the catheter.

Indications

Vaginography may demonstrate:

1. Fistulae between the vagina and ureter, bladder or rectum (Wolfson, 1964).

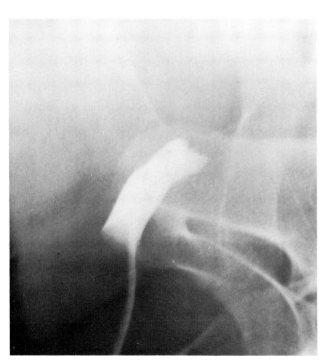

FIG. 2.26 Normal vaginogram. A balloon catheter has been inserted into the lower part of the vagina, and contrast medium has been injected.

2. Congenital or acquired abnormalities of the vagina, such as diverticula (Coe, 1963).

3. Reflux of contrast medium up a vaginal ectopic ureter (Katzen & Trachtman, 1954).

REFERENCES

Hysterosalpingography

AARON J. B. & LEVINE W. (1954) Endometrial oil granuloma following hysterosalpingography. *Amer. J. Obst. Gynec.*, **68**, 1594–1597.

ABBAS R. H. (1954) The value of hysterosalpingography in infertility. *J. Obst. Gynaec. Br. Emp.*, **61**, 268–269.

ALTEMUS R., CHARLES D. & YODER V. E. (1967) Conventional hysterosalpingography used in the evaluation of sterility problems. *Fertil. Steril.*, **18**, 713–718.

ARNET N. L. & ELKIN M. (1967) Hysterosalpingography. *Radiol. Clin. N. Amer.*, **5**, 105–120.

ASPLUND J. (1952) The uterine cervix and isthmus under normal and pathological conditions. *Acta Radiol. Suppl.* 91.

BARNETT E. & BEWLEY D. K. (1954) Ovarian radiation during hysterosalpingography. *J. Fac. Radiol.*, **6**, 186–188.

BECKER M. S., MARBACK A. H. & SCHINFELD L. H. (1955) Intestinal obstruction following the use of a water soluble contrast medium (Medopaque-H) in hysterosalpingography. *Amer. J. Obst. Gynec.*, **69**, 917–921.

BEHRMAN S. J. & POPPY J. H. (1957) Hysterosalpingography. *Canad. Med. Ass. J.*, **77**, 938–950.

BERGMAN F., GORTON G., NORMAN O. & SJÖSTEDT S. (1953) Foreign body granulomas following hysterosalpingography with a contrast medium containing carboxymethylcellulose. *Acta Radiol.*, **43**, 17–29.

BLIGH A. S. & WILLIAMS E. O. (1956) The effect of the full bladder in hysterosalpingography. *Brit. J. Radiol.*, **29**, 99–102.

BRANTLEY W. M., del VALLE R. A., AABY G. W. & SCHOENBUCHER A. K. (1960) Rupture of a silent pyosalpinx following a hysterosalpingogram. *Obst. Gynec.*, **16**, 483–485.

CALANDRA D., GLUCK J. C. & CALANDRA J. (1959) Hysterosalpingography and colpohysterosalpingography. New techniques and modifications. *Obst. Gynec.*, **13**, 563–567.

CARY W. H. (1914) Note on determination of patency of Fallopian tubes by the use of collargol and X-ray shadow. *Amer. J. Obst.*, **69**, 452–464.

CATALANO D. (1966) Hysterosalpingography with Conray 60 per cent and a vacuum uterine cannula. *Amer. J. Roentgenol.*, **98**, 244–247.

CHUANG J. T., HEWETT W. J. & HESHCHYSHYN M. (1971) Death after hysterosalpingography in choriocarcinoma with pelvic abscess. *Obst. Gynec.*, **37**, 543–545.

CLITHEROE H. J. (1964) Etiology of primary dysmenorrhoea. *Obst. Gynec. Survey.*, **19**, 649–659.

DAVIDS A. M. & WEINER I. (1950) The effects of sedation on Fallopian tube motility. *Amer. J. Obst. Gynec.*, **59**, 673–678.

DEAK P., FRIED L. & BÄDER A. (1958) Double contrast method for examination of the uterine cavity. *Fortschr. a. d. Geb. d. Röntgenstrahlen*, **88**, 422–426.

DIETZ W. (1956) Comparative measurements of dose to the ovary during pelvic radiography during fluoroscopy of the small pelvis under 'normal' conditions and with image intensification. *Fortschr. a. d. Geb. d. Röntgenstrahlen*, **85**, 456–459.

DRUNKMAN I. A. & ROZIN S. (1951) Uterovenous and utero-lymphatic intravasation in hysterosalpingography. *J. Obst. Gynaec. Br. Emp.*, **58**, 73–78.

DUTTON W. A. W. & STAPLETON J. G. (1963) The use of hysterosalpingography in the diagnosis of infertility and other gynaecological conditions. *Canad. Med. Ass. J.*, **89**, 1159–1164.

EKENGREN K. & RYDEN A. B. V. (1954) The diagnostic value of hysterosalpingography in tubal pregnancy. *Acta Radiol.*, **41**, 247–155.

ELLIOTT G. B., BRODY H. & ELLIOTT K. A. (1965) Implications of 'lipoid salpingitis'. *Fertil. Steril.*, **16**, 541–548.

ERBSLÖH J. (1949) Radiological demonstration of the lymphatic system of the uterus. *Schweiz med. Wschr.*, **79**, 78–79.

ERBSLÖH J. (1959) Double contrast method in hysterography with propyliodone. *Fortschr. a. d. Geb. d. Röntgenstrahlen*, **91**, 249–252.

FARIS A. M. & McMURRAY A. (1947) Uterosalpingography. Report of a fatality. *Texas State Med. J.*, **42**, 592–597.

FISHER M. S. (1966) Lymphangiogram following hysterosalpingography. *Amer. J. Roentgenol.*, **98**, 233–235.

FORSDIKE S. (1925) The investigation of the uterus and Fallopian tubes by air and opaque bodies in sterility. *Proc. Roy. Soc. Med.*, **18**, 77–81.

FREEDMAN H. L., TOFEEN C. H., FRIEDMAN H. & PINCK R. L. (1959). Hypaque as a contrast medium for hysterosalpingography. *Fertil. Steril.*, **10**, 403–408.

FREETH D. (1952) Hysterosalpingography in female infertility and a comparison of Lipiodol and Viskiosol Six. *Lancet*, **1**, 15–19.

FULLENLOVE T. M. (1973) Improvement of the cup used with the Malmström Thoren vacuum uterine cannula in uterosalpingography. *Amer. J. Roentgenol.*, **119**, 852–853.

GERLOCK A. J. & HOOSER C. W. (1976) Oviduct response to glucagon during hysterosalpingography. *Radiology*, **119**, 727–728.

GRIFFITHS H. J. L. (1969) A clinical and radiological evaluation comparing the use of two contrast media in hysterosalpingography – Salpix and Urografin. *Brit. J. Radiol.*, **42**, 835–837.

GROSSMAN M. (1946) Pulmonary oil embolism. *Brit. J. Radiol.*, **19**, 178–180.

HENRY G. W. & HUNTER R. G. (1960) Hysterosalpingography with water soluble medium (Salpix). *Amer. J. Roentgenol.*, **84**, 924–928.

HEUSER C. (1925) Lipiodol in the diagnosis of pregnancy. *Lancet*, **2**, 1111–1112.

HIPONA F. A. & DITCHEK T. (1966) Uterine lymphogram following hysterosalpingography. *Amer. J. Roentgenol.*, **98**, 236–238.

HUEPER W. C. (1957) Experimental carcinogenic studies in macromolecular chemicals. *Cancer*, **10**, 8–18.

HUNTER R. G., HENRY G. W. & HEINICKE R. M. (1957) The action of papain and bromelain on the uterus. *Amer. J. Obst. Gynec.*, **73**, 867–880.

INGERSOLL F. M. & ROBBINS L. L. (1947) Oil embolism following hysterosalpingography. *Amer. J. Obst. Gynec.*, **53**, 307–311.

JARCHO J. (1929) Uterosalpingography. *Amer. J. Surg.*, **6**, 693–719.

JAROSCHKA K. (1926) On salpingography. *Zbl. Gynäk.*, **50**, 25–42.

JEFFERIS D. & SAMUEL E. (1946) Pelvigraphy. *Brit. J. Radiol.*, **19**, 462–468.

JORDAN J. A., EDWARDS R. L., PEARSON J. & MASKERY P. J. K. (1971) Laparoscopic sterilization and follow-up hysterosalpingogram. *J. Obst. Gynaec. Br. Cwth.*, **78**, 460–466.

KANTOR H. I., KAMHOLZ J. H. & SMITH A. L. (1956) Foreign body granulomas following the use of Salpix. *Obst. Gynec.*, **7**, 171–174.

KENNEDY W. T. (1923) Radiography of closed Fallopian tubes to determine location of obstructions. *Amer. J. Obst. Gynec.*, **6**, 12–23.

KIKA K. (1954) A clinical analysis of the 'angiograms' found in the course of hysterosalpingography with special reference to tuberculosis of the female genitals. *Amer. J. Obst. Gynec.*, **67**, 56–63.

KJELLMAN L. (1953) A new instrument for hysterosalpingography. *Acta Radiol.*, **40**, 35–38.

KOHANE S. & SCHWARZ Z. (1961) The diagnostic value of routine hysterography in cases of metrorrhagia. *J. Obst. Gynaec. Br. Cwth.*, **68**, 320–326.

McNABB R. W. (1959) The technique and use of Urografin as a contrast medium in hysterosalpingography. *J. Fac. Radiol.*, **10**, 108–110.

MALSTRÖM T. (1961) A vacuum uterine cannula. *Obst. Gynec.*, **18**, 773–776.

MEASDAY B. (1960) An analysis of the complications of hysterosalpingography. *J. Obst. Gynaec. Br. Emp.*, **67**, 663–667.

NEUSTAEDTER T., EHRLICH D. E., du BOIS J. C. & BLALOCK G. R. (1933) A new contrast medium for use in uterosalpingography. *Radiology*, **21**, 568–572.

NIELSEN P. H. (1946) Injuries caused by hysterosalpingography. *Acta Obst. Gynec. Scandinav.*, **26**, 565–597.

PAGE E. P. (1968) Use of isoxsuprine in uterosalpingography and uterotubal insufflation. *Amer. J. Obst. Gynec.*, **110**, 358–364.

POLAK P. (1920) In discussion. *J. Amer. Med. Assoc.*, **75**, 666.

PONTIFEX G., TRICHOPOULOS D. & KARPATHIOS S. (1972) Hysterosalpingography in the diagnosis of infertility (statistical analysis of 3437 cases). *Fertil. Steril.*, **23**, 829–833.

REISS H. E. & GROSSMAN M. (1958) Experience with new contrast media for hysterosalpingography. *J. Obst. Gynaec. Br. Emp.*, **65**, 782–787.

RINDFLEISH W. (1910) Derstellung der cavum uteri. *Berlin Klin. Wschr.*, **47**, 780–782.

ROBINS S. A. & SHAPIRA A. A. (1931) The value of hysterosalpingography. A study of 1000 cases. *New Engl. J. Med.*, **205**, 380–395.

ROYALS J. L., PRICE C. N. & TITUS P. (1950) Hysterosalpingography – its dangers and their prevention. *Postgrad. Med.*, **8**, 363–370.

RUBIN I. C. (1914) Roentgen dianostik der uterus tumoren mit hilfe von intrauterinen collangolinjectionen. *Zbl. Gynäk.*, **38**, 658.

RUBIN I. C. (1928) Diagnostic use of intrauterine iodized oil combined with the X-rays as compared to peruterine CO_2 insufflation. *Radiology*, **11**, 115–125.

RUBIN I. C. (1941) A new soluble viscous contrast medium for hysterosalpingography. *J. Mount Sinai Hosp.*, **7**, 479–485.

RUBIN I. C. & BENDICK A. J. (1926) Uterotubal roentgenography with Lipiodol. *Amer. J. Roentgenol.*, **16**, 251–256.

RUBIN I. C., MYLLER E. & HARTMAN C. G. (1953) Salpix. A new approach to the ideal radiopaque medium for hysterosalpingography. *Fertil. Steril.*, **14**, 357–370.

SANDLER B. (1956) Biligrafin for hysterosalpingography. *Lancet*, **2**, 896.

SCILA P., GRÖNROOS M., KAVPPILA O. & PYKÖNEN L. (1962) Water soluble, viscosized water soluble and iodized oily contrast media in hysterosalpingography. Comparative studies. *Acta Radiol. Suppl. 218*.

SEEGAR JONES G. E. & WOODRUFF J. D. (1960) Effect of a radiation opaque, water soluble medium on the histopathology of the endometrium. *Amer. J. Obst. Gynec.*, **80**, 337–340.

SEIBERT E. (1953) Relaxant effect of dihydroergotamine (Sandoz) and hydergine in hysterosalpingography. *Gynecologica*, **135**, 172–176.

SHEACH J. M. (1959) Hysterosalpingography. A survey of some opaque media. *J. Fac. Radiol.*, **10**, 103–107.

SICARD J. A. & FORESTIER J. (1922) General method of radiological exploration by iodized oil (Lipiodol). *Bull. Soc. Chirurgiens Paris*, **46**, 463–469.

SIEGLER A. M. (1967) Dangers of hysterosalpingography. *Obst. Gynec. Survey*, **22**, 284–308.

SLATER S., PAZ-CARRANZU J., SOLOMONS E., PEALMUTTER C. (1959) Effect of hysterosalpingography on assay of thyroid function. *Fertil Steril.*, **10**, 144–149.

SLEZAK P. & TILLINGER K. G. (1968) The occurrence and significance of a double outlined uterine cavity in the hysterographic picture. *Radiology*, **90**, 756–760.

SLEZAK P. & TILLINGER K. G. (1973a) The significance of the spiculated outline of the uterine cavity in hysterography. *Radiology*, **107**, 527–531.

SLEZAK P. & TILLINGER K. G. (1973b) Broad longitudinal

folds in the uterine cavity at hysterography. *Radiology*, **106**, 87–90.

SLEZAK P. & TILLINGER K. G. (1975) Hysterographic evidence of polypoid filling defects in the uterine cavity. *Radiology*, **115**, 79–83.

SLEZAK P. & TILLINGER K. G. (1976) The incidence and clinical importance of hysterographic evidence of cavities in the uterine wall. *Radiology*, **118**, 581–586.

SMITHAM J. H. (1959) A viscous solution of sodium acetrizoate as a medium for hysterosalpingography. *Brit. J. Radiol.*, **32**, 193–197.

STEWART A., WEBB J. & HEWITT D. (1958) A survey of childhood malignancies. *Brit. Med. J.*, **1**, 1495–1508.

STALLWORTHY J. (1948) Facts and fantasy in the studies of female infertility. *J. Obst. Gynaec. Brit. Emp.*, **55**, 171–180.

SWEENEY W. J. (1958) Hysterosalpingography. II Postoperative hysterograms. *Obst. Gynec.*, **12**, 83–90.

SWICK M. (1929) Hysterosalpingography with Uroselectan. *Klin. Wschr.*, **8**, 2087–2092.

TEILUM G. & MADSEN V. (1950). Endometriosis ovarii et peritonaei caused by hysterosalpingography. *J. Obst. Gynaec. Br. Emp.*, **57**, 10–16.

THOMAS H. H. & DUNN D. (1956) Salpix as a medium in hysterosalpingography. *Fertil. Steril.*, **7**, 155–165.

TITUS P., TAFEL R. E., McCLELLAN R. H. & MESSER F. C. (1938) A new nonirritating opaque medium for uterosalpingography. *Amer. J. Obst. Gynec.*, **36**, 881–898.

WEXLER D. J., BIMBERGER C. H. & KURZRAK L. (1949) Hysterography in the diagnosis of uterine bleeding. *Amer. J. Surg.*, **77**, 755–760.

WILLIAMS E. & REYNOLDS R. (1925) A method of determining the patency of the Fallopian tubes by X-rays. *Brit. Med. J.*, **1**, 691–692.

WITWER E. R., CASHMAN H. P. & LEUCUTIA T. (1930) The present status of hysterosalpingography. *Amer. J. Roentgenol.*, **23**, 125–159.

WOLTZ J. H. E., BRADFORD W. Z., BRADFORD W. B. & McCOY J. B. (1958) Complications of hysterosalpingography. *Amer. J. Obst. Gynec.*, **76**, 736–741.

WRIGHT J. T. (1961) A new method of hysterosalpingography. *Brit. J. Radiol.*, **34**, 465–467.

Pelvic pneumography

ANSARI A. H. (1970) The cul-de-sac approach to induction of pneumoperitoneum for pelvic laparoscopy and pneumography. *Fertil. Steril.*, **21**, 599–605.

BRASCHO D. J. (1970) Use of pelvic pneumography in planning radiotherapy of endometrial carcinoma. *Radiology*, **97**, 113–120.

GOETZ O. (1918). New method of roentgendiagnosis by pneumoperitoneum. *Munchen. Med. Wschr.*, **46**, 1276.

KREEL L., GINSBERG J. & GREEN M. F. (1969) Gynaecography in premature ovarian failure and ovarian dysgenesis. *Brit. Med. J.*, **1**, 682–686.

LEA THOMAS M., PRUNTY F. T. G. & SPATHIS G. S. (1968) Gynaecography in primary amenorrhoea. *J. Obst. Gynaec. Br. Cwth.*, **75**, 652–658.

LUNDERQUIST A. (1968) Pneumopelvigraphy in the early diagnosis of intersexuality. *Amer. J. Roentgenol.*, **103**, 202–209.

SALA J. M., KEATS T. E. & DOLAN K. D. (1967) The pelvic pneumogram in carcinoma of the cervix. *Radiology*, **78**, 274–276.

STEIN I. F. (1937) Why pneumoperitoneum? *Radiology*, **28**, 391–398.

STEVENS G. M. (1967) Pelvic pneumography in the assessment of infertility. *Radiol. Clin. N. Amer.*, **5**, 87–103.

WEBER E. (1918) Concerning the significance of the introduction of oxygen or air into the peritoneal cavity for experimental and diagnostic roentgenology. *Fortschr. a. d. Geb. d. Röntgenstrahlen*, **20**, 453–455.

WEIGEN J. F. & STEVENS G. M. (1967) Pelvic pneumography in the diagnosis of polycystic disease of the ovary, including Stein-Leventhal syndrome. *Amer. J. Roentgenol.*, **100**, 680–687.

Vaginography

COE F. O. (1963) Vaginography. *Amer. J. Roentgenol.*, **90**, 721–722.

KATZEN P. & TRACHTMAN B. (1954) Diagnosis of vaginal ectopic ureter by vaginogram. *J. Urol.*, **72**, 808–811.

WOLFSON J. J. (1964) Vaginography for demonstration of ureterovaginal, vesicovaginal and rectovaginal fistulas, with case reports. *Radiology*, **83**, 438–444.

CHAPTER 3

Radiological Techniques III: Gastrointestinal and Urinary Tract Radiology in Relation to Gynaecology

BARIUM MEAL AND SMALL BOWEL FOLLOW-THROUGH

Gastric carcinoma may rarely metastasize to the ovaries, presumably by transcoelomic spread, giving rise to Krukenberg tumours (Figs 3.1 and 3.2 and see Chapter 8).

Fistulae between the small bowel and the vagina are uncommon and may be associated with appendicectomy, pelvic abscess, injury to the small intestine, and foreign bodies left at pelvic surgery (Fig. 3.3).

Segments of small intestine may be distorted and narrowed by secondary peritoneal spread from ovarian and uterine carcinoma. These changes are invariably accompanied by ascites. The distal small intestine may be obstructed by strictures secondary to pelvic radiotherapy, an uncommon complication nowadays, or by adhesions from pelvic surgery, inflammatory disease and endometriosis.

BARIUM ENEMA

The barium enema may reflect the secondary effects of some gynaecological conditions on the large bowel:

Evaluation of large pelvic masses (Bryk, 1967)

When the uterus is markedly enlarged by fibroids, it may be deviated inferiorly by its attachment to intrapelvic structures tending to cause compression of the superior aspect of the distal sigmoid colon. In general, the sigmoid colon may be either elevated or depressed by the fibroid uterus (Fig. 3.4). Benign ovarian masses, being mobile and often in the abdomen, tend not to affect the rectum

or distal sigmoid segment but may compress the sigmoid colon anteriorly at pelvic brim level (Fig. 3.5). Kabakian & Massabri (1973) have stressed the importance of the postevacuation film in the evaluation of pelvic masses. During barium filling, there is a tendency for the sigmoid colon to rise as it uncoils with distension and to descend and drape the pelvic mass after colonic emptying. The effect of an extrinsic mass on the sigmoid mucosa can then be plainly seen.

Assessment of spread of pelvic malignant disease
(Marshak, 1947)

It is not uncommon for carcinoma of the ovary to invade the rectosigmoid, causing mucosal destruction as well as stenosis which may eventually lead to severe obstruction (Chapter 8).

When pelvic spread from carcinoma of the cervix affects the distal large bowel, it most frequently presents on barium enema as a smooth compression with an intact mucosa but with fixation of the constricted segment. However, this appearance may also be found in pelvic inflammatory disease.

Large vaginal carcinomas may invade the rectum, although this is readily appreciated by direct inspection.

Diverticular disease (Bolz, 1968)

Diverticulitis may clinically be a diagnostic problem in gynaecology and can mimic pelvic inflammatory disease, especially tubo-ovarian abscesses. Sigmoidouterine (see Fig. 6.5) and sigmoidovaginal fistulae (Fig. 3.6, and see Fig. 6.6 and 6.7) are possible sequelae of diverticular disease.

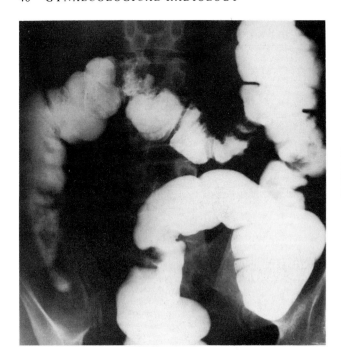

FIG. 3.1 Carcinoma of stomach with Krukenberg tumours to both ovaries. Barium enema shows peritoneal metastasis involving transverse segment of colon, and a nodule in sigmoid colon from direct invasion by ovarian metastasis.

FIG. 3.2 Krukenberg tumours in both ovaries from carcinoma of the stomach. Direct spread of tumour from ovary has caused stricture of sigmoid colon.

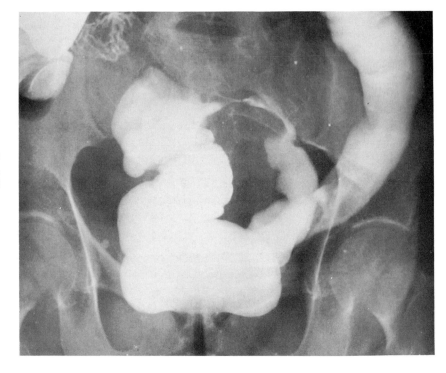

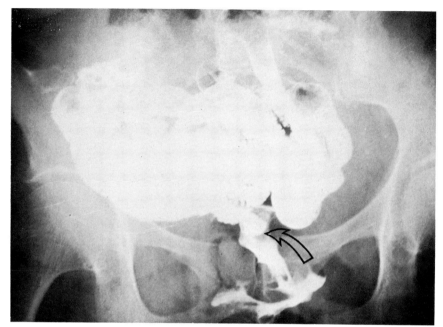

FIG. 3.3 Fistula (arrow) between small intestine and vagina shown on barium follow-through examination. This followed radiotherapy in a case of cervical carcinoma.

FIG. 3.4 Elevation of proximal part of sigmoid segment with compression of distal portion, caused by fibroid uterus.

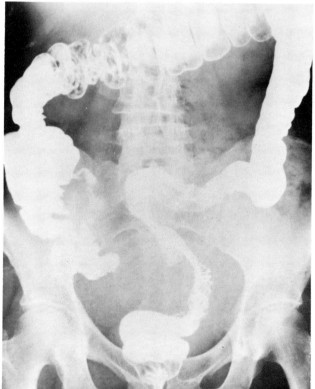

FIG. 3.5 Elevation of the sigmoid segment and compression at pelvic brim level by an ovarian mass.

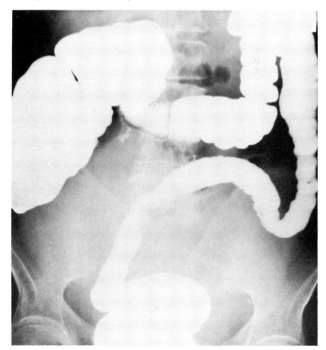

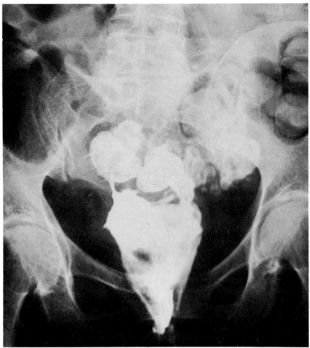

FIG. 3.6 Barium enema. Sigmoido-vaginal fistula due to diverticular disease.

Colonic endometriosis

See Chapter 10

INTRAVENOUS UROGRAPHY

Intravenous urography is an important and often under-emphasized diagnostic tool in the assessment of many gynaecological conditions. The close association of the genital and urinary system will be stressed in subsequent chapters. The whole of the urinary tract must be well shown, in particular good demonstration of the ureters is of paramount importance. In most cases, 50 ml of Conray 420 is an adequate dose of contrast medium, although 100 ml should be given when ureteral obstruction or a urinary fistula is suspected, when abdominal compression cannot be applied or in the presence of renal failure. Compression is contraindicated when a very large mass lesion arises from the pelvic cavity and after recent abdominal surgery. Oblique or lateral views of the pelvis should be taken when damage to the bladder or a urinary fistula is suspected.

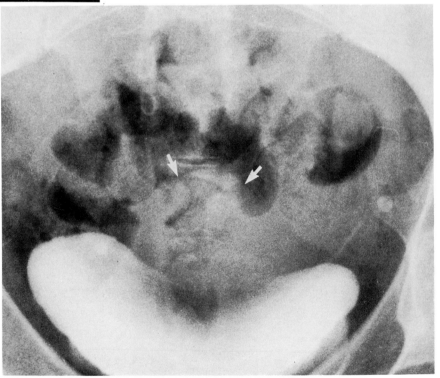

FIG. 3.7 Intravenous urography showing normal indentation of bladder by uterus (arrows).

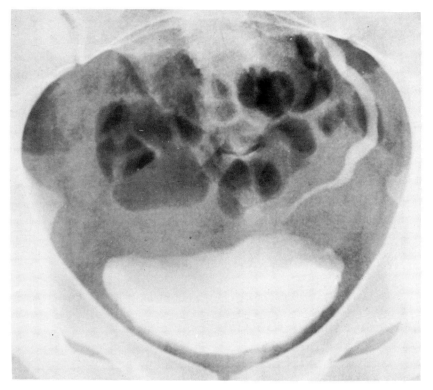

FIG. 3.8 Intravenous urography showing lobulated indentation of dome of bladder by fibroid uterus.

Three-quarters of premenopausal women show a concave uterine impression on the upper border of the bladder (Marr & Portmann, 1944) (Fig. 3.7). The absence of the sign in this age group is due to uterine retroversion, an immature uterus or a very distended bladder. A uterine impression on the bladder is seen in only a quarter of post-menopausal women and is exceptional before the menarche. Fibroids may compress the bladder (see Fig. 7.15) or give a lobulated impression on its dome (Fig. 3.8), while a benign ovarian mass will tend to give a smooth but perhaps eccentric indentation (Fig. 3.9). An extrapelvic extension of a fibroid uterus, or a large ovarian mass, may, on occasion, apparently pull the uterus away from the bladder which then has a smooth upward convexity to its dome (Bryk, 1966). Pelvic adhesions may cause tenting or an irregular bladder contour.

High dose infusion urography causes opacification of the normal uterus by contrast accumulation in about 6%

of women (Birnholz, 1972). The reason is not clear, but this passive accumulation of contrast medium in the myometrium may be related to physiological premenstrual uterine hyperaemia. A diffuse opacification of contrast medium was seen by Phillips *et al.* (1974) in uterine fibroids in 80% of cases, and as a thin curvilinear rim of contrast density in the wall of most ovarian cystic lesions (see Fig. 8.3). The effect may be most apparent on tomography after the end of the infusion (Love *et al.*, 1974).

Intravenous urography is useful in the following circumstances:

1. In the presence of *large uterine and ovarian masses,* the ureters may be deviated or compressed, possibly with associated hydronephrosis (Fig. 3.10). There is often compression of the bladder.

2. *Before and after gynaecological surgery* (Chapter 11). A prior knowledge of the position of the ureters, which may be deviated due to the underlying pelvic

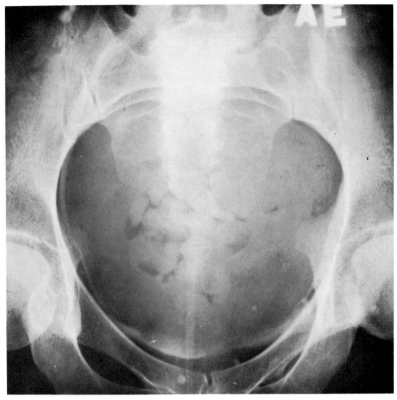

FIG. 3.9 Intravenous urography showing large ovarian cyst causing lateral displacement of pelvic portion of ureters and marked indentation of bladder.

pathology, will help to prevent inadvertent ureteral damage during the operation. There may be some congenital anomaly of the ureters, particularly a duplex system, ignorance of which could lead to their injury at surgery. Also, if symptoms referable to the urinary tract develop after surgery, preoperative urography provides a useful baseline in the postoperative assessment of nonfunction of a kidney or obstruction of a ureter. Roden *et al.* (1961) found an incidence of previously unsuspected significant urinary tract abnormalities in 22% of 455 patients who had a wide range of gynaecological abnormalities. A third of these patients had hydronephrosis and/or hydroureter, while urinary calculi, congenital abnormalities and chronic pyelonephritis were found in others. Suspected damage to the urinary tract during a gynaecological operation of course provides a definite indication for urography (Whitehouse, 1977).

3. In cases of *uterine malignancy*, unsuspected neoplastic involvement of the urinary tract may be revealed and a base line appearance is provided for comparison with post-treatment urography. In the series of Stander *et al.* (1961), urinary tract dilatation or non-functioning kidneys were found on urography in 12.7% of cases of cervical carcinoma prior to treatment. Urinary tract complications of radiotherapy and surgery in uterine cancer and their urographic appearances are discussed in Chapter 11.

4. Urography is indicated when there is extensive pelvic *endometriosis* or when surgery is contemplated in endometriosis. Over 40% of cases of pelvic endometriosis are associated with urinary tract dilatation (Klempner, 1952; Long & Montgomery, 1952). The aftermath of pelvic inflammatory disease may involve the urinary tract in adhesions.

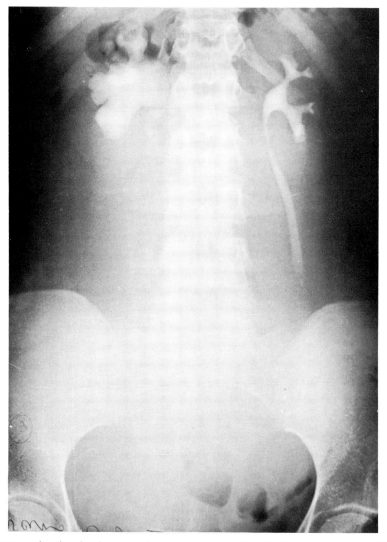

FIG. 3.10   Intravenous urography showing huge ovarian cyst causing right-sided hydronephrosis and lateral deviation of left ureter.

5. Ureteric obstruction is occasionally present in cases of severe *uterine prolapse* (Chapter 12).

6. *Urinary tract symptoms* such as haematuria and loin pain or recurrent urinary infection.

7. Severe *congenital abnormalities of the genital tract* are associated with a 25% incidence of urinary tract anomalies. Ipsilateral absence of a kidney is an especially common association with absence of a Fallopian tube and ovary.

URETHROGRAPHY

Retrograde urethrography is mainly used to delineate urethral diverticula or strictures. The simplest method is to inject contrast medium through an acorn cannula inserted within the urethral meatus, but marked leakage of contrast medium often occurs. Another method employs a No. 18 Foley catheter with a 30 ml balloon. The distal end of the catheter is occluded, side holes being made 1.5 cm proximal to the balloon, and the balloon is then passed into the bladder where it is inflated with air. Following infiltration of the urethral meatus with local anaesthesia, it is grasped on its ventral aspect by an Allis clamp and gentle traction is applied to the catheter while contrast medium is injected, the patient lying in the oblique position. The balloon prevents contrast medium from escaping into the bladder, while the clamp arrests flow through the urethral orifice (Redman & Taylor, 1972). Davis & Cian (1956) also use a Foley catheter with the balloon against the bladder base, but with the modification of a sliding balloon on the catheter. This proximal balloon is advanced to the meatus and is then inflated to prevent leakage.

Alternatively, a vacuum cannula, as in hysterography, may be used for retrograde urethrography with less risk of spillage of the contrast medium (Becker & Gregione, 1968). The acorn tip is placed within the urethral meatus while a plastic cup (23 or 30 mm outside diameter) is pressed against the periurethral soft tissues. When an air-tight seal had been established, air is extracted from the cup, and contrast medium is injected through the cannula.

CYSTOGRAPHY

The bladder is usually filled with contrast medium via a urethral catheter. A strict aseptic technique is necessary to prevent the introduction of infection into the bladder. It is preferable to avoid the investigation during an acute urinary tract infection, and an antibiotic cover is indicated when there is a history of recurrent urinary infection. The bladder is distended, under screening control, with a suitable water soluble contrast medium such as Retro-Conray, Hypaque 25% or Urografin 150.

Cystography is a dynamic procedure which is useful in demonstrating the peripheral control of micturition and the ability of the bladder to contract. Abnormalities of the bladder neck and urethra may be shown by this method. Vesicoureteral reflux and vesicovaginal fistulae are other abnormalities demonstrated by cystography. Cine radiography, a 110 mm radiographic camera and videotape are the methods of choice for recording the micturition process and its abnormalities. If these are not available, then standard radiographs have to suffice. The bladder neck and urethra are best shown in a position just short of the lateral in order that they are not obscured by overlying femoral heads.

Modifications of this basic technique in the investigation of stress incontinence are discussed in a later chapter.

REFERENCES

Barium enema

BOLZ F. F. (1968) Diverticulitis as a diagnostic problem in gynaecology. *Amer. J. Roentgenol.*, **101**, 372–376.

BRYK D. (1967) Barium enema examination in the evaluation of large pelvic masses. *Amer. J. Roentgenol.*, **101**, 970–977.

KABAKIAN H. A. & MASSABRI S. R. (1973) The value of the postevacuation view of the colon in the detection of pelvic pathology. *Amer. J. Roentgenol.*, **119**, 393–403.

MARSHAK R. H. (1947) Extrinsic lesions affecting the rectosigmoid. *Amer. J. Roentgenol.*, **58**, 439–450.

Urography

BIRNHOLZ J. C. (1972) Uterine opacification during excretion urography. *Radiology*, **105**, 303–307.

BRYK D. (1966) Roentgen evaluation of large uterine and ovarian masses. *Obst. Gynec.*, **28**, 630–636.

KLEMPNER E. (1952) Gynecological lesions and ureterohydronephrosis. *Amer. J. Obst. Gynec.*, **64**, 1232–1241.

LONG J. P. & MONTGOMERY J. B. (1952) The incidence of ureteral obstruction in benign and malignant gynecological lesions. *Amer. J. Obst. Gynec.*, **59**, 552–562.

MARR J. T. & PORTMANN V. V. (1944) Incidental findings in urograms concerning the uterus. *Amer. J. Roentgenol.*, **51**, 426–433.

PHILLIPS J. C., EASTERLY J. E. & LANGSTON J. W. (1974) Contrast enhancement of pelvo-abdominal masses: The rim sign. *Radiology*, **112**, 17–21.

RODEN J. S., HAUGEN H. M., HALL D. G. & GREENBENZ P. A. (1961) The value of intravenous pyelography prior to elective gynecologic operations. *Amer. J. Obst. Gynec.*, **82**, 568–571.

STANDER R. W., RHAMY R. K., HENDERSON W. P., LANSFORD K. G. & PEARCY M. (1961) The intravenous pyelogram and carcinoma of the cervix. *Obst. Gynec.*, **17**, 26–29.

LOVE L., MELAMED M., COOPER R. A., MONCADA R. & SCHWARTZ H. (1974) Infusion tomography of the female pelvis. *Amer. J. Roentgenol.*, **122**, 299–307.

WHITEHOUSE G. H. (1977) The radiology of urinary tract abnormalities associated with hysterectomy. *Clin. Radiol.*, **28**, 201–210.

Urethrography

BECKER J. A. & GREGIONE A. (1968) Retrograde urethrography. *J. Urol.*, **100**, 92–93.

DAVIS H. J. & CIAN L. G. (1956) Positive pressure urethrography: A new diagnostic method. *J. Urol.*, **75**, 753–757.

REDMAN J. F. & TAYLOR J. N. (1972) A technique for urethrograms in female patients. *J. Urol.*, **108**, 91–92.

CHAPTER 4

Radiological Techniques IV: Angiography

ARTERIOGRAPHY

Over the last twenty years, pelvic arteriography has been used to a varying extent in the diagnosis and subsequent management of female pelvic mass lesions. Lang in 1967 claimed that pelvic arteriography was the single most important advance towards accurate preoperative diagnosis in the assessment of pelvic tumours, although he has recently considered that this technique has been superseded by computerized axial tomography and ultrasonography (Lang, 1979). However, he still sees a place for arteriography in the identification of residual or recurrent neoplastic pelvic disease after treatment, when the normal anatomy has been distorted.

Various arteriographic methods have been used in gynaecological diagnosis.

Aortography

The rectosigmoid is cleansed by purgation before the procedure. The tip of a 60 cm long PE205 Teflon catheter with several side holes is inserted just above the aortic bifurcation, having been introduced from one of the femoral arteries using the Seldinger technique. If the catheter tip is inserted at the level of the third lumbar vertebra, there is a chance of delineating the ovarian arteries. Usually 30 ml of Conray 280, Urografin 325 or Hypaque 45 are injected. Lang (1967) used an injection phase of three seconds or longer in order to give a pulsed flow of contrast medium, which he claims will give optimal visualization of genital tract tumours. Radiographs are exposed towards the end of the contrast medium injection at a rate of 4 per second for 3 seconds and then one per second for up to 12 or 15 seconds. Generally the run is made with the patient supine, although oblique views may occasionally be required to delineate the uterine arteries to better effect. Bilateral compression of the thighs is sometimes applied in an attempt to improve the filling of pelvic arteries with contrast medium.

Common iliac arteriography

This has no advantage over aortography and has the disadvantage of requiring bilateral femoral artery puncture. Contrast medium is injected simultaneously through two straight catheters, which lie within the right and left common iliac arteries.

Internal iliac arteriography

The right and left internal iliac arteries are selectively catheterized, using catheters with acutely flexed tips. Onnis *et al.* (1967) prefer a yellow Odman catheter and a PE205 movable core guide wire for entry into the internal iliac artery. Although bilateral femoral punctures are necessary, the method has the advantage of causing less confusion by not opacifying vessels which supply structures other than the pelvic organs. A large pelvic tumour may cause deviation of the internal iliac artery and thus prevent its selective catheterization. 15–20 ml of contrast medium are injected into each of the internal iliac arteries by firm hand injections, or from one syringe through a Y connection. Lawson (1965) has described a technique of transgluteal internal iliac artery catheterization, but the method is difficult and has no advantage over the Seldinger technique.

Vecchietti (1952) developed a technique of direct transvaginal cannulation of the uterine artery at the junction of its parametrial and marginal segments. The method is only of historical interest, although he claimed to obtain good arteriographic demonstration.

Elaborations on pelvic arteriography include its combination with hysterosalpingography, negative contrast cystography, or pelvic pneumography to better demonstrate the relation of vessels to the pelvic organs.

Ovarian arteriography

The ovarian arteries may be seen in 20% of aortograms, but this incidence rises to 63% when aortic compression is applied during aortography (Borell & Fernstrom, 1954). Following aortography, with the catheter tip at renal artery level, the ovarian arteries may be selectively catheterized using a BD RPX054 catheter tapered to a 035 wire and shaped so that the diameter of the curve of the catheter tip slightly exceeds the aortic diameter. 4–15 ml of Conray 280 are injected by hand over 3–6 seconds, and serial films taken over 15 seconds (Frates, 1969).

Pelvic arterial anatomy

UTERINE ARTERIES

Usually the uterine artery arises separately from the internal iliac artery, immediately above the origin of the superior gluteal artery, but occasionally shares a common origin with either the internal pudendal artery or the vaginal artery. The uterine artery is divided into three segments. The first part runs close to the pelvic wall, but its point of origin is generally superimposed on other arteries and is not clearly visible on arteriography. The second part of the uterine artery courses medially to the level of the cervix, where it then continues as the third part which ascends along the lateral margin of the uterus as far as the fundus before dividing into its terminal branches. A ureteral branch arises from the transverse second part of the uterine artery, usually 1.5 cm lateral to the uterus, and another branch arises just medial to where it crosses the ureter, and supplies the cervix and upper vagina. This latter branch is especially useful in the assessment of cervical carcinoma (Lang, 1967). Many branches arise perpendicular to the ascending third portion of the uterine artery, supply the uterus, and anastomose with corresponding branches from the contralateral

side. Just below the level of the uterine cornu, the third part of the uterine artery divides into three vessels; a branch which runs laterally, and then upwards before turning medially to supply the uterine fundus; a branch running laterally to supply a variable length of the Fallopian tube, usually its medial two thirds, and anastomoses with the corresponding branch of the ovarian artery; a branch coursing along the ovarian ligament to the mesovarium, giving off small branches to the ovary.

While the size of the uterine arteries is constant through the phase of the menstrual cycle, the small branches which directly supply the uterus appear most numerous in the secretory phase, and during menstruation. Between the tenth and sixteenth day of a twenty-eight day cycle, these arteries are fewer in number and are widely separated. This apparent paucity of intramural blood vessels around the time of ovulation is thought to be due to oedema of the uterine wall (Borell et al., 1953). The width of the uterine arteries decreases in size after the menopause, and is associated with shrinkage of uterine size.

OVARIAN ARTERIES

The ovarian arteries are usually a single pair of vessels, typically arising from the aorta below the level of the renal arteries. However, in a quarter of cases, one ovarian artery, but rarely both, arises from a renal artery, usually on the right side. In 19% of women, there are three or four ovarian arteries, although these usually then arise from the aorta (Frates, 1969). The ovarian artery pursues a tortuous downward course, and divides into three branches after entering the pelvic cavity. One terminal branch runs to the fimbrial end of the Fallopian tube, another supplies the lateral third of the Fallopian tube and anastomoses with the first branch as well as with the tubal branch of the uterine artery, while the main terminal branch supplies the lateral part of the ovary. The normal width of the ovary artery is 1–5 mm (Borell & Fernstrom, 1954).

Indications for arteriography

UTERINE FIBROIDS

There are arteriographic signs which suggest the presence of fibroids (see Fig. 7.16), although arteriography is rarely used in this condition. However, arteriography is of diagnostic help when sarcomatous changes are suspected (Lang, 1967).

CARCINOMA OF THE CERVIX

Arteriographic signs may be subtle and are not always reliable, although the investigation may enable a more accurate staging of the tumour to be made, and provides a useful means of diagnosing tumour recurrence after therapy (see Fig. 7.20). Tumours may not be recognized by angiography unless they are at least 1–2 cm in diameter.

CARCINOMA OF THE ENDOMETRIUM

This may be demonstrated by arteriography (Chapter 7).

TROPHOBLASTIC TUMOURS

The most commonly used application of arteriography in gynaecology is in cases of trophoblastic tumour (see Figs 7.30 and 7.31). Usually aortography is used, but it is claimed that selective internal iliac and ovarian artery studies give improved delineation of the tumour vascularity.

OVARIAN TUMOURS

Ovarian tumours derive their blood supply from the adnexal branch of the uterine artery and from the ovarian artery, and may have an abnormal vascularity (see Fig. 8.17). The course of the uterine artery may be altered by ovarian mass lesions.

TUBAL PREGNANCY

Ozarus (1959) claims that tubal pregnancy may be diagnosed by arteriography in 70% of cases, but the method is generally little used.

GENERAL DIFFERENTIATION OF A PELVIC MASS

The differentiation of a pelvic mass lesion into an inflammatory or neoplastic origin may sometimes be made on angiographic studies, but the appearances may be misleading or impossible to differentiate.

CYTOTOXIC DRUGS

Prior to continuous infusion of cytotoxic drugs in carcinoma of the cervix, uterine body and vagina, selective internal iliac arteriography has been used to determine catheter placement and the blood supply of the tumour (Zeit et al., 1960).

UTERINE HAEMORRHAGE

Arteriography has been little used in this context, but may identify the bleeding site by the delineation of a focal abnormality, such as a uterine arteriovenous malformation (Bottomley & Whitehouse, 1975). Transcatheter embolization of the anterior division of the internal iliac artery has been successfully used in the treatment of haemorrhage from advanced or recurrent carcinoma of the cervix (Lang, 1979).

VENOGRAPHY

Pelvic iliac venography may be performed by injecting contrast medium simultaneously through needles inserted into both femoral veins, or through short venous catheters whose tips lie in the external iliac veins (Bartley, 1958). An alternative is intraosseous venography via the greater trochanters of both femora (Wise et al., 1963), but necessitates a general anaesthetic and may be associated with local bone complications.

Intraosseous pubic venography

Intraosseous pubic venography from the anterior aspect of the body of the pubis gives a demonstration of the venous drainage of the pelvic organs. A hand injection of 20 ml of contrast medium (Conray 280 or Hypaque 45) is made, and radiographs are taken every two seconds. This method was first used by Topalanski-Sierra (1958). Lea Thomas et al. (1967) have demonstrated the venous connections of vulval varices with this technique.

Ovarian venography

The left ovarian vein opens into the left renal vein, and the right ovarian vein drains into the inferior vena cava below the level of the renal veins. The injection of a large bolus of contrast medium through a catheter in the left renal vein will result in delineation of the left ovarian vein. Valves are usually present in the ovarian vein, and if these are absent or incompetent there will be extensive delineation of the left ovarian vein. The diameter of the left ovarian vein is at least 9 or 10 mm in diameter (Ahlberg et al., 1965) and, generally with multiparity, the ovarian vein becomes sufficiently wide so that the valves become incompetent. This retrograde passage of contrast medium is, therefore, not necessarily indicative of pathological change, but may exist when there is a varicocoele of the broad ligament (Chidekel, 1968), when the left ovarian vein may be so dilated as to cause an extrinsive non-obstructing impression upon the left ureter at the level of the third or fourth lumbar vertebra (Bartley &

Chidekel, 1968). A varicocoele of the broad ligament may also be demonstrated by injecting contrast medium through catheters inserted from the femoral veins with their tips lying at the bifurcation of both common iliac veins, during inferior vena cava compression (Helender & Lindblom, 1960).

Pelvic venous anatomy

The uterine, vaginal and vesical veins originate in venous plexuses and are tributaries of the internal iliac vein, which in turn passes upward behind and slightly medial to the internal iliac artery, and joins with the external iliac vein to form the common iliac vein. The uterine plexuses lie along the lateral margins and cornua of the uterus between the two layers of the broad ligament. A pair of uterine veins arise from the lower parts of plexuses, at the level of the external os of the uterus. The vaginal plexuses lie along the sides of the vagina, and are drained by the vaginal veins. Several vesical veins leave the vesical plexus which envelopes the lower part of the bladder. There are communications between the uterine, vaginal and vesical plexuses.

The ovarian veins arise from the ovarian plexuses, which are situated in the broad ligaments, in close association with the ovaries and Fallopian tubes.

Indications

Venography is used to demonstrate the extent of known neoplastic disease of the female genital tract, and its effect on the venous system of the pelvis and inferior vena cava. In a gynaecological context thrombosis of the pelvic veins may arise secondary to genital tract cancer or following pelvic surgery. The following features may be seen in the iliac veins or the inferior vena cava: (1) Complete obstruction to flow of contrast medium within one of the major veins, secondary to neoplastic spread, thrombosis or surgical ligation. (2) Narrowing of the vein, due either to adherent mural thrombus or to extrinsic compression. (3) The presence of an intra or extra pelvic collateral venous circulation secondary to obstruction. In the case of obstruction of the external or common iliac veins, contrast medium is shunted across to the opposite side of the pelvis via the presacral plexus or by perineal veins and ascends the contralateral iliac veins. When the common iliac vein is extensively occluded, large abdominal and pelvic collateral veins open up. Obstruction to both common iliac veins or to the inferior vena cava will initiate a collateral venous return through the vertebral plexus. Unless the collateral channels are occluded, iliac vein obstruction will not cause leg oedema. (4) Stasis, secondary to obstruction. Dilatation of the corresponding femoral, saphenous or internal iliac veins, with reflex of contrast medium down these vessels, may be seen.

These changes may be due to venous obstruction by lymph nodes which contain metastases, as well as by direct invasion and compression from the primary tumour. Before the advent of lymphography, venography was used to provide a crude and very inaccurate method of determining neoplastic lymph node masses in genital carcinoma. To some extent, lymphography and venography are complementary procedures.

Smith & Bosniak (1974) have used iliac venography to determine whether or not ureteral obstruction, in the presence of pelvic malignant disease, is due to neoplastic involvement or to a benign cause. Iliac vein occlusion tended to be associated with obstruction of the closely situated ureter by the neoplastic process.

UTERINE PHLEBOGRAPHY

The object of direct uterine phlebography is to inject water-soluble contrast medium into the myometrium of the uterine fundus, with subsequent delineation of the uterine and pelvic venous system. The technique was first used by Guilhem & Baux in 1954.

Method

The patient is placed in the lithotomy position, a vaginal speculum is inserted, the uterus is sounded, and the arterior cervical lip is grasped with a tenaculum. The injection cannula lies within a metal tube which allows the cannula to project for up to 4 mm beyond its end. The tip of the metal tube is introduced into the uterus so that it abuts on the fundus, and the cannula is pushed forward beyond the end of the tube. The cannula tip then lies within the myometrium. Alternatively, two separate systems may be used, each cannula being inserted to either side of the midline of the uterine fundus (Hammen, 1965).

Correct positioning is ensured by the injection of 5 ml of water-soluble contrast medium through the cannula, under screen control. When the cannula implantation is satisfactory, 500 units of hyaluronidase is then injected,

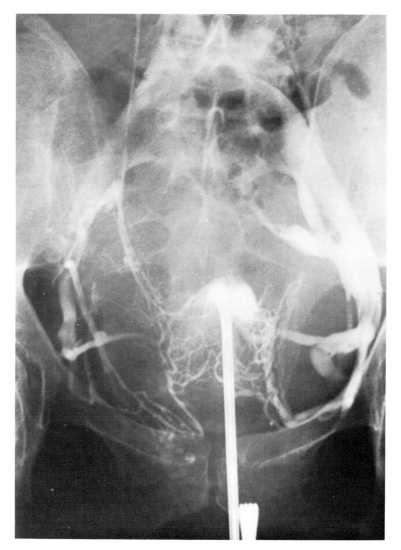

Fig. 4.1 Uterine phlebogram. Multiple intramural venous radicles connect with uterine veins which run transversely across the pelvic into the internal iliac veins. The common iliac veins and the ovarian veins are also demonstrated. The left-sided pelvic veins are larger than the right. The patient was subsequently shown to have endometriosis of the left ovary. Courtesy of Dr David Trapnell.

followed within five minutes by 20 ml of Urografin 370 injected over less than twenty seconds. A radiograph of the pelvic region is taken immediately at the end of the contrast injection, and at twenty second intervals up to one minute.

By this method it should be possible to demonstrate the intrauterine, uterovaginal and both ovarian venous plexi (Fig. 4.1). Better filling of the pelvic venous system is obtained if rubber balloons, as used in ureteric compression during intravenous urography, are applied to the inferior vena cava and perhaps the right ovarian vein (Kauppila et al., 1971). Injection through a single cannula, which has been inserted to one side of the midline, will predispose to asymmetrical filling of the pelvic venous

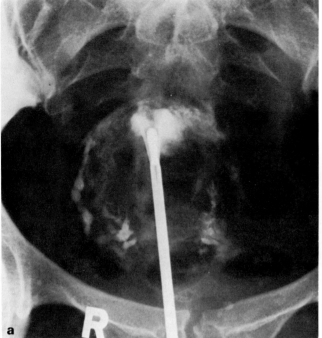

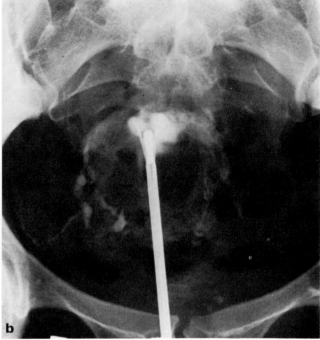

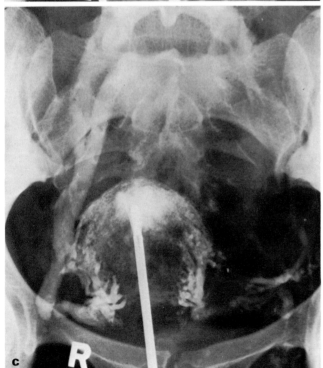

FIG. 4.2 Uterine phlebogram (a) at end of injection, (b) 1 minute later, (c) 2 minutes after injection. Varicocoele of right uterine vein, with dilatation and stasis of contrast medium within this vein and its radicles. Patient complained of persistent obscure right iliac fossa pain. Courtesy of Dr David Trapnell.

system. If there is non-filling of one of the ovarian plexuses, it will often be delineated if the injection is repeated with the patient tilted 45° towards that side. Uterine phlebography is contraindicated during menstruation and if there is a history of recent pelvic inflammatory disease. The injection of contrast medium may cause a variable amount of pain in the lower abdomen or lumbar region, but may be prevented by a previous injection of Buscopan (Murray & Comparato, 1968).

Applications

The main indication for intrauterine phlebography is the demonstration of a suspected pelvic varicocoele. When this is the case, contrast medium may remain in a dilated venous drainage system for up to twenty seconds after the end of injection. The uterine and ovarian veins are found to be dilated and turtuous in the presence of pelvic varicocoele. Both varicocoele (Fig. 4.2) and pelvic congestion will show a prominence and dilatation of the intramural uterine venous network and ovarian plexuses as well as a delay in the passage of contrast medium (Murray & Comparato, 1968). There is often a slow passage of contrast medium in the presence of chronic cervicitis, a finding which is reversed by treatment, and in uterine prolapse, pelvic inflammatory disease and extrauterine endometriosis. Uterine fibroids may be associated with a circular distortion of the uterine venous plexuses, an irregular distribution of opacified veins, and a paucity of these vessels.

LYMPHOGRAPHY

Lymphography has significantly altered the assessment and management of pelvic malignancy. The technique, interpretation and application of lymphography are fully described in some standard works, such as that by Fuchs *et al.* (1969).

The lymphatic drainage of the female genital tract has been excellently described by Nelson *et al.* (1964) and by Jackson (1969). Although the inguinal, iliac and para-aortic lymph nodes are accurately delineated by ascending lymphography, the main short-coming of the technique in gynaecological practice is failure to reliably delineate the hypogastric, paracervical, obturator and presacral lymph nodes. This is offset by the knowledge that these lymph nodes are likely to be included in the portal of radiation treatment. The method is exceedingly useful in detecting tumour spread or recurrence outside the pelvic cavity (see Fig. 7.17). An angled projection of the pelvic inlet has been claimed by Lee *et al.* (1971) to give some separation of the overlapping iliac lymph nodes, and therefore a better demonstration of their architecture.

Lymphography should be performed with careful monitoring of lymph node filling in the presence of known pelvic malignancy, there being a risk of oil embolism when lymphatic involvement is extensive or when radiotherapy has been given.

Applications

DETECTION OF METASTASES TO LYMPH NODES

In particular, lymphography has a place in the assessment of lymphatic metastases from carcinoma of the vulva, vagina, uterine cervix and body and ovaries. Metastases may cause lymph nodes to be enlarged or to remain of normal size. Early lesions tend to be located at the periphery of the node and give it a 'moth eaten' configuration. Extensive involvement may give the opacified lymph node a fragmented appearance, total replacement of a node, or clumping of adjacent involved nodes (see Fig. 7.17). The lymph channels supplying extensively involved nodes may be dilated or show persistant opacification with contrast medium and collateral lymphatic channels may be seen to circumvent involved nodes. A pelvic mass lesion may cause displacement of lymphatic structures. Benign lesions such as a tubo-ovarian abscess, extensive endometriosis or pelvic fibrosis may cause lymphatic deviation, while a freely mobile lesion, such as an ovarian cyst, will cause no change in the lymphatic pattern (Hahn *et al.*, 1963).

A preoperative lymphographic assessment will assist in determining the feasibility and extent of a proposed surgical procedure in pelvic malignancy, and the completeness of the dissection may be determined after the operation. Cervical carcinoma can be staged with a diagnostic error of 15% (Fuchs *et al.*, 1969), and positive nodes are demonstrated by lymphography in 12–33% of clinical stage I and II carcinomas of the cervix.

Chlorophyll has been added to the contrast medium, and the subsequent green staining of the lymph nodes was originally claimed to facilitate their more complete removal during radical pelvic surgery for carcinoma of the cervix, and also in groin dissection for carcinoma of the vulva (Averette *et al.*, 1963). However, at operation the nodes are often still obscured by surrounding fatty tissue, and the chlorophyll in association with prolonged severe tissue reaction and stasis of contrast medium in lymph vessels which will obscure lymph nodes (Lemmon *et al.*, 1966).

Accurate portal placement may be made in the radiation treatment of lymph node involvement. Successful radiotherapy to malignant lymph nodes will render them small but well defined, with fairly uniform opacification. Contrast medium will remain in the lymph nodes for a variable length of time, between six weeks and two years so that the disease process and its response to therapy may be followed.

After pelvic surgery, lymphography may demonstrate lymphocyst formation. This is a collection of lymphatic fluid in the pelvic retroperitoneal space which may follow the division of afferent lymphatic vessels during pelvic clearance, resulting in extravasation of contrast medium during lymphography. The interruption of the lymphatic pathways and the compression of pelvic veins by the lymph collection may cause leg oedema, often the presenting feature of this condition.

MODIFIED FORMS OF LYMPHOGRAPHY

Because of the failure of ascending lymphography to show the internal pelvic lymphatic chains, attempts have been made to delineate these hypogastric, presacral, obturator and paracervical lymph nodes. Patillo *et al.* (1964) have injected Lipiodol into the parametrium and Howett & Greenberg (1966) have directly injected the cervix. However, opacification of the central pelvic nodes was inconsistent.

RELATION OF LYMPHOGRAPHY TO OTHER DIAGNOSTIC PROCEDURES

Baum *et al.* (1963) found that 60% of patients with pelvic and abdominal metastases demonstrated by lymphography had associated abnormality on inferior vena cavography and/or intravenous urography. Even large lymph node masses may not cause any impression on the inferior vena cava or on the iliac veins. Metastatic mass lesions up to 8 cm in diameter may fail to cause obvious ureteral displacement.

REFERENCES

Angiography

BORELL U., FERNSTROM I. & WESTMAN A. (1953) Hormonal influence on the uterine arteries. *Acta Obstet. Gynec. Scand.*, **32**, 271–284.

BORELL U. & FERNSTROM I. (1954) The ovarian artery. *Acta Radiol.*, **42**, 253–265.

BOTTOMLEY J. P. & WHITEHOUSE G. H. (1975) Congenital arteriovenous malformations of the uterus demonstrated by angiography. *Acta Radiol. (Diag.)*, **16**, 43–48.

BRIET A. (1967) *Angiography of Uterine Tumours and their Recurrences.* George Thieme, Stuttgart, Germany

FRATES R. E. (1969) Selective angiography of the ovarian artery. *Radiology*, **92**, 1014–1019.

LANG E. K. (1967) Arteriography in gynecology. *Radiol. Clin. N. Amer.*, **5**, 133–149.

LANG E. K. (1979) Current and future applications of angiography in the abdomen. *Radiol. Clin. N. Amer.*, **17**, 55–76.

LAWSON R. L. (1965) Transgluteal-hypogastric arterial catheterization. *Cancer*, **18**, 893.

ONNIS A., MARSILLETTI G. C., DE SALVIA D. & BEVILACQUA L. (1967) Percutaneous selective catheterization of the hypogastric artery and its branches. *Amer. J. Obst. Gynec.*, **98**, 966–975.

OZARUS H. (1959) Diagnostic value of pelvic arteriography in tubal pregnancy. *Acta Radiol. Scandinav.*, **51**, 257–265.

VECCHIETTI G. (1952) Prime ricerche de angiografia pelvica nella donna. *Minerva. Ginec.*, **4**, 47–54.

ZEIT P. R., HUGES C. R., CAHILL J. J. & HAMILTON J. G. (1960) Hypogastric arteriography prior to continuous infusion of malignant tumours of uterine cervix and vagina. *Cleveland Clin. Quart.*, **27**, 119–124.

Venography

AHLBERG N. E., BARTLEY O. & CHIDEKEL N. (1965) Retrograde contrast filling on the left gonadal vein. *Acta Radiol. (Diag.)*, **3**, 385–392.

AHLBERG N. E., BARTLEY O. & CHIDEKEL N. (1965) Circumference of the left gonadal vein. *Acta Radiol. (Diag.)*, **3**, 503–512.

BARTLEY O. & CHIDEKEL N. (1968) Venography in the diagnosis of pelvic tumours. *Acta Radiol. Scandinav.*, **49**, 169–186.

BARTLEY O. & CHIDEKEL N. (1968) Ureteric imprint caused by the left gonadal vein. *Acta Radiol. (Diag.)*, **7**, 212–218.

CHIDEKEL N. (1968) Female pelvic veins demonstrated by selective renal phlebography with particular reference to pelvic varicosities. *Acta Radiol. (Diag.)*, **7**, 193–211.

HELENDER C. G. & Lindblom A. (1960) Varicocoele of the broad ligament. *Acta Radiol.*, **53**, 97–104.

LEA THOMAS M., FLETCHER E. W. L., ANDRESS M. R. & COCKETT F. B. (1967) The venous connections of vulval varices. *Clin. Radiol.*, **18**, 313–317.

SMITH T. R. & BOSNIAK M. A. (1974) Evaluation of ureteral obstruction in the bony pelvic with iliac vein venography. *Amer. J. Roentgenol.*, **120**, 124–129.

TOPALANSKI-SIERRA R. (1958) Pelvic phlebography. *Amer. J. Obst. Gynec.*, **76**, 44–52.

WISE R. E., SALZMAN F. A., JOHNSTON D. O. & SIBER R. J. (1963) Intraosseous venography in pelvic malignancy. *Amer. J. Roentgenol.*, **90**, 373–385.

Uterine phlebography

GUILHEM P. & BAUX R. (1954) *Le phlebographic pelvienne par voies veineuse osseuse et uterine.* Massan et Cie, Paris.

HAMMEN R. (1965) The technique of pelvic phlebography. *Acta Obstet. et Gynec. Scandinav.*, **44**, 370–374.

KAUPPILA A., JARVINEN P. A. & VUORINEN P. B. (1971) Improved visualization in uterine phlebography. *Brit. J. Radiol.*, **44**, 285–289.

MURRAY E. & COMPARATO M. R. (1968) Uterine phlebography. *Amer. J. Obst. Gynec.*, **102**, 1088–1093.

Lymphography

AVERETTE H. E., VIAMONTE M. I. & FERGUSON J. G. (1963) Lymphangioadenography as a guide to lymphadenectomy *Obst. Gynec.*, **21**, 682–686.

BAUM S., BRON K. M., WEXLER L. & ABRAMS H. L. (1963) Lymphangiography, cavography and urography. *Radiology*, **81**, 207–218.

FUCHS W. A., DAVIDSON J. W. & FISCHER H. W. (1969) *Lymphography in Cancer*. Springer-Verlag, New York.

HAHN G. A., WALLACE S., JACKSON L. & DODD G. (1963) Lymphangiography in gynaecology. *Amer. J. Obst. Gynec.*, **85**, 754–771.

HOWETT M. & GREENBERG A. J. (1966) Direct lymphangioadenography of the uterine cervix. *Obst. Gynec.*, **27**, 392–398.

JACKSON R. J. A. (1969) Topography of the ileopelvic lymph nodes. *Amer. J. Obst. Gynec.*, **104**, 1118–1123.

LEE K. G., HODES P. J. & LIN S. R. (1971) The value of the inlet and outlet views of the pelvis in lymphography. *Radiology*, **111**, 297–300.

LEMMON W. T. JR., KETCHAM A. S., MACHOWRY J. D. & HERDT J. (1966) Surgical applications of Ethiodol with chlorophyll in lymphangiography. Histopathologic, radiographic and clinical disadvantages in 36 cases. *Ann. Surg.*, **164**, 114–122.

NELSON J. H., MASTERSON J. G., HERMAN P. G. & BENNINGHOF D. L. (1964) Anatomy of the female pelvic and aortic lymphatic systems demonstrated by lymphography. *Amer. J. Obst. Gynec.*, **88**, 460–469.

PATILLO R. A., FOLEY D. V. & MATTINGLEY R. F. (1964) Internal pelvic lymphography. *Amer. J. Obst. Gynec.*, **88**, 110–122.

CHAPTER 5

Congenital Abnormalities of the Female Genital Tract

EMBRYOLOGY

In the third week after conception, the embryonic mesoderm becomes arranged into three parts either side of the axial line: paraxial mesoderm, the intermediate cell mass and lateral plate mesoderm. By the seventh week, the genital ridge arises on the inner aspect of the intermediate cell mass. The ovary develops from the elongated vertical prominence of the genital ridge, and becomes attached to the intermediate cell mass by a mesentery, the mesovarium, and will in time migrate caudally from the lumbar region to the pelvis.

Renal elements develop during the fourth week in the intermediate cell mass, which is then termed the nephrogenic cord. The tubules of the pronephros are formed in the cervical portion of the nephrogenic cord and then rapidly degenerate, but give rise to the pronephric duct which grows caudally to join the endodermal cloaca. The mesonephros subsequently develops in the thoracic and upper lumbar portion of the nephrogenic cord, and the mesonephric tubules communicate with the pronephric duct which is then renamed the mesonephric or Wolffian duct. Most mesonephric tubules disappear in the sixth week, except for some in the region of the developing gonad. Those level with the upper part of the gonad become the ductuli aberrantes superiores and part of the epoophoron in the female, while the mesonephric tubules adjacent to the lower part of the gonad form the ductuli aberrantes inferiores and the paroophoron. The metanephric tubules arise from the caudal part of the nephrogenic cord; while the collecting tubules, calyces, pelvis and ureter develop from the ureteral bud, which grows out

from the Wolffian duct near its junction with the urogenital part of the cloaca. The metanephros, or definitive kidney, ascends from the sacral region as the gonad migrates downwards. The caudal portion of the Wolffian duct expands, and both it and the ureter come to open separately into the urogenital sinus, the lower ends of the ureters forming the trigonal area which separates the orifices of the ureters from those of the Wolffian ducts.

At about six weeks of gestation, the paramesonephric or Müllerian ducts form as invaginations of coelomic epithelium into the lateral sides of the nephrogenic cords at the level of the mesonephros. By the ninth week, each Müllerian duct has grown down to the pelvic region, running lateral to the immediately adjacent corresponding Wolffian duct. The Müllerian ducts then turn medially in the pelvic region, crossing in front of the Wolffian ducts, and then unite with each other in the mid line and within the urogenital septum between the urogenital sinus and the rectum. Initially, the lumina of the fused Müllerian ducts are separated by a septum, but this normally disappears by the tenth or eleventh weeks to form the uterovaginal canal which is by then in contact with the posterior wall of the urogenital sinus. The cranial, unfused portions of the Müllerian ducts become the Fallopian tubes, while the uterovaginal canal becomes the uterus and upper part of the vagina. The distal portion of the vagina arises from paired endodermal protrusions, the sinovaginal bulbs, of the urogenital sinus. These sinovaginal bulbs merge with the vaginal portion of the uterovaginal canal. The urogenital sinus is initially tubular, but becomes wider and shorter as the embryo grows, with the urethral and vaginal orifices descending caudally to open into the vestibule. Disintegration of the thin septum, or hymen, which separates the uterovaginal canal from the urogenital sinus, is the eventual normal occurrence.

The Wolffian system regresses as the Müllerian system develops, and is represented as vestigial remnants in the adult female. Remains of the Wolffian duct may form paraovarian cysts in the mesovarium or, occasionally, cysts within the broad ligaments. Sometimes the Wolffian duct persists as Gartner's duct, which is incorporated into the anterolateral part of the vaginal wall, and gives rise to cystic swellings. Gartner's duct may rarely open into the vagina.

Development of the Müllerian system may be impaired at various stages to produce a wide spectrum of genital tract anomalies, some of which are relatively common while others are very rare.

UTERINE HYPOPLASIA

Agenesis of the uterus is a very rare condition, usually associated with other severe anomalies of the genitourinary tract. The severely hypoplastic 'fetal' uterus is also often seen in conjunction with other abnormalities, such as absence of the vagina, the uterus being represented by only a solid knob of mainly fibrous tissue. The infantile uterus is shown by hysterography to have a small body and a relatively long cervical canal which is either tubular or conical in shape (Fig. 5.1). In the normal adult state the ratio of length of cervical canal to uterine body, as demonstrated by hysterography, is about 1:2. In the immature or hypoplastic uterus, there is reversal of this ratio. Normally, these proportions persist until the age of ten years with rapid development to the adult length during puberty (Meaker, 1940).

A less severe abnormality than the infantile uterus is the pubescent uterus in which the cervical canal is the same length as the uterine body cavity (Fig. 5.2). There are many cases in which the uterus may be defined as the 'small adult type' in which a small capacity uterine cavity is delineated by hysterosalpingography, with a slender cervical canal and perhaps relatively long tubes (Fig. 5.3).

The hypoplastic type of uterus is found in about 8% of cases of primary infertility (Reenkola, 1949; Pontifex et al., 1972). Conception occasionally occurs with an immature uterus, but there is often an early miscarriage.

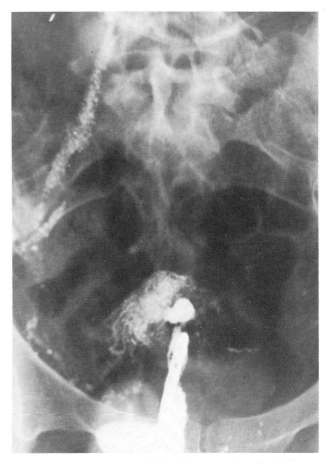

Fig. 5.1   Hysterogram of infantile uterus. Small globular uterine cavity with relatively long conical cervical canal. Lipiodol has been used and there is intravasation of contrast medium with subsequent delineation of the uterine and iliac veins.

Other uterine abnormalities are sometimes associated with hypoplasia, such as bicornuate or arcuate deformities (Fig. 5.4). The hypoplastic uterus may also be in acute anteflexion or retroflexion. Intravasation of contrast medium may occur despite the presence of patent Fallopian tubes, as in Fig. 5.1 (Foda et al., 1962).

FAILURE OF MÜLLERIAN DUCT FUSION

The paired nature of the original Müllerian duct system may persist in part or in toto to give a spectrum of

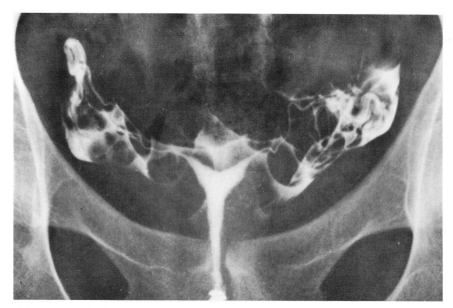

FIG. 5.2 Hysterosalpingogram of pubescent uterus. The cervical canal is almost equal in length to the uterine body. The Fallopian tubes appear disproportionately long.

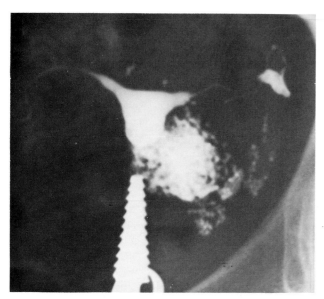

FIG. 5.3 Hysterosalpingogram of 'small adult type' of uterus. The cervical canal is slender, and there is a fairly small uterine cavity.

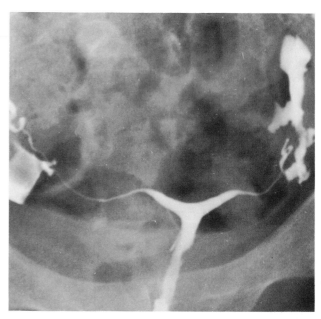

FIG. 5.4 Hysterosalpingogram of hypoplastic uterus with arcuate configuration.

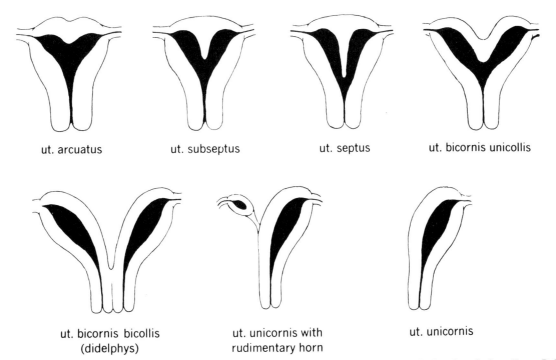

FIG. 5.5 The variety of appearances which may result from varying degrees of failure of Müllerian duct fusion. From Behrman S. J. and Gosling J. R. G. (1966) *Fundamentals of Gynaecology*, 2nd Edition. Oxford, Oxford University Press.

hysterographic appearances ranging from total failure of fusion, the uterus didelphys with a septate vagina, to the slight deformity of the arcuate uterus (Fig. 5.5).

Uterus didelphys consists of duplication of the vagina, cervix and uterus (Fig. 5.6), while the *uterus bicornis bicollis* has two separate uterine horns each with its own cervix but a single vaginal canal (Fig. 5.7). Uterus didelphys may occasionally be associated with primary infertility, abortion and obstructed labour. Brody (1954) has reported twin pregnancies involving both uterine horns.

In the *bicornuate uterus*, there are two separate uterine horns which are jointed above the cervix. Typically (Fig. 5.8), the two horns opacified on hysterography are separated by a wide obtuse angle. When this angle between the horns is acute, differentiation between a bicornuate and a septate uterus may be difficult. A bicornuate uterus is the more likely possibility when the point of cleavage lies in the isthmus, but the uterus may be bicornuate or subseptate in type when separation is at

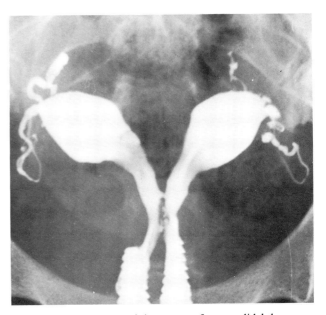

FIG. 5.6 Hysterosalpingogram of uterus didelphys.

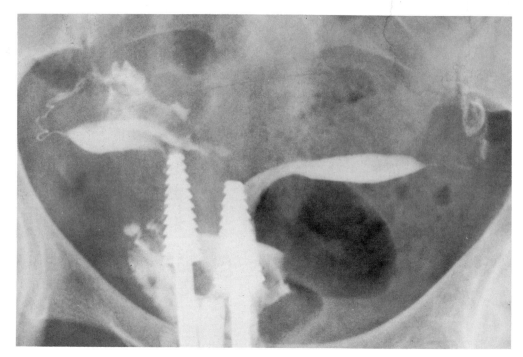

FIG. 5.7   Hysterosalpingogram of uterus bicornis bicollis.

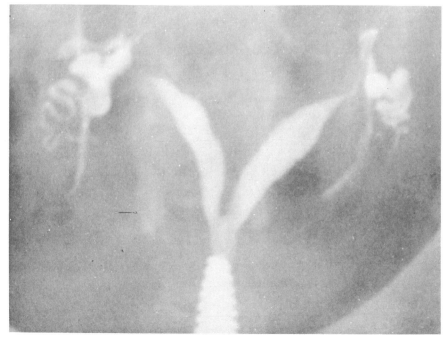

FIG. 5.8   Hysterosalpingogram of bicornuate uterus shows the low point of cleavage of uterine horns.

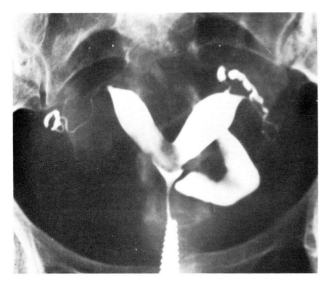

FIG. 5.9 Hysterosalpingogram of bicornuate uterus shows wide separation of uterine horns, with high cleavage point.

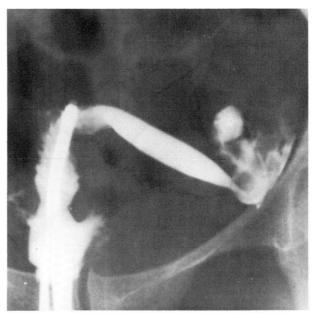

FIG. 5.10 Bicornuate uterus with nonfilling of rudimentary right horn, the presence of which was proven at subsequent Caesarean section.

a higher level (Fig. 5.9). Convexity of the lateral borders of the opacified bifid uterine cavity suggests a bicornuate uterus, as the lateral borders of a subseptate uterus tend to be fairly straight, but this is not an invariable rule. The differentiation between the subseptate and bicornuate uterus may be made by pelvic pneumography, the uterine fundus being intact in the former and obviously bifid in the latter.

Pontifex *et al.* (1972) found a bicornuate uterus in 3% of cases of primary infertility. Malpositioning of the fetus, retained placenta, subinvolution and inco-ordinate uterine action may be especially prevalent with bicornuate uteri. Habitual abortion is associated with the bicornuate uterus, and is considered by Foda *et al.* (1962) to be due to co-existent isthmic incompetence rather than to the bicornuate state *per se*.

A *unicornuate uterus* represents failure of development of one half of the uterus from a Müllerian duct. However, the development of one horn may be greatly impaired rather than totally absent, giving a *rudimentary horn*. This rudimentary horn communicates with the uterine cavity or cervix in only 20% of cases, and therefore will usually not be delineated on hysterography (Fig. 5.10). Despite the failure of communication of the horns, 80% of reported cases of pregnancy in rudimentary horns have occurred in these so-called isolated horns, presum-

ably due to the transperitoneal migration of sperm (Rolen *et al.*, 1966). There is a risk that the rudimentary horn may rupture in pregnancy. Most rudimentary horns are on the right side, and junction may occur with the body or fundus of the other horn or with the cervix. Foda *et al.* (1962) have observed that when attachment of the rudimentary horn is at a high level on the developed horn, the latter has a much more central position in the pelvic cavity than a true unicornuate uterus. Rarely, haematometra in a rudimentary horn may be the cause of a pelvic mass in adolescent girls (Willows & Wall, 1959).

The *septate uterus* has a normal external appearance, except for an occasional slight depression in the fundus. Internally, the septum is usually thin, divides the uterine cavity into two compartments, and extends down to the isthmus (Fig. 5.11). It is an uncommon anomaly, accounting for only 6% of significant congenital uterine abnormalities (Hay, 1958).

The *subseptate uterus* (Fig. 5.12) is a commoner anomaly than the full septate type, and the level of separation by the septum lies higher within the body of the uterus. Unlike the septate type, in which hypertrophy

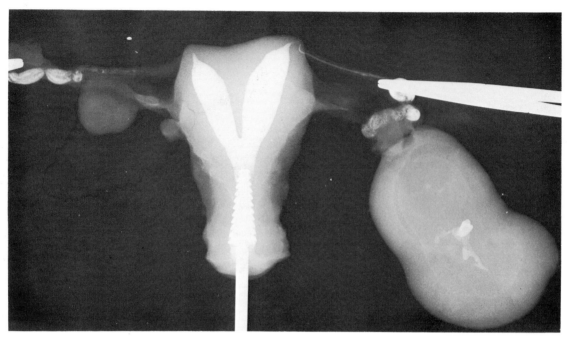

FIG. 5.11   Hysterography on excised specimen of uterus and adnexa shows a septate uterus. A teratoma of the left ovary is also present.

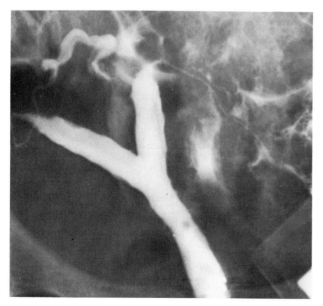

FIG. 5.12   Subseptate uterus, shown by hysterosalpingography. The septum is wide. Note the straight lateral borders to the uterine cavity.

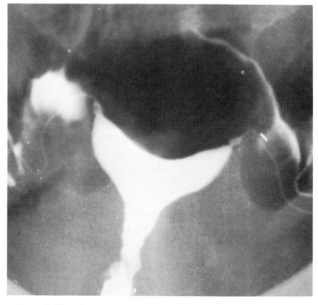

FIG. 5.13   Arcuate uterus, shown by hysterosalpingography. Rounded indentation of uterine fundus.

of one half of the uterus may cause obstruction to the delivery of a fetus situated in the other half, the sub-septate type does not usually cause dystocia although it may be responsible for an oblique or transverse lie (Jarcho, 1946).

An *arcuate uterus* is one of the commonest types of malformation, and shows a rounded indentation of the fundal contour on hysterography (Fig. 5.13). A corresponding concavity is also present on the external aspect of the fundus. Slight fundal concavity on hysterography may be regarded as a normal variant, while an arcuate uterus may be diagnosed when the concavity is at least one fifth of the height of the opacified uterine body (Reenkola, 1949). A fundal fibroid may exactly mimic the appearances of an arcuate uterus on hysterography.

The hand-foot-uterus syndrome (Stern *et al.*, 1970; Poznanski *et al.*, 1970). Disorders of Müllerian duct fusion, namely bicornuate uterus, and uterus didelphys with septate vagina, have been described in association with various abnormalities of the hands and feet. A short first metacarpal bone, with a prominent pseudoepiphysis at its distal end, a small pointed distal phalanx to the thumb, and clinodactyly with shortening of the middle phalanx of the little finger, are found in the hand. Carpal fusion and a prominent ulnar styloid process are seen in the wrist. The feet show tarsal abnormalities and a short first metatarsal with a hypoplastic distal phalangeal tuft in the hallux, and fusion of all distal interphalangeal joints. The syndrome is inherited as an autosomal dominant with full penetrance and variable expression.

Urinary tract abnormalities associated with anomalies of Müllerian duct fusion

Unicornuate uterus, with or without a rudimentary horn, is associated with a high incidence of urinary tract abnormalities (Fig. 5.14). Unilateral renal agenesis, and renal ectopia on the same side as the deficient uterine horn are especially common (Schumacker, 1938). Woolfe & Allen (1953) consider that urinary tract abnormalities are invariably found in the presence of a unicornuate uterus. Renal agenesis and ectopia may also be found in cases of bicornuate uterus (Muller, 1968), although other urinary tract abnormalities are sometimes seen (Fig. 5.15). The frequency of associated urinary tract abnormalities warrants urographic investigation in cases of severe genital malformation.

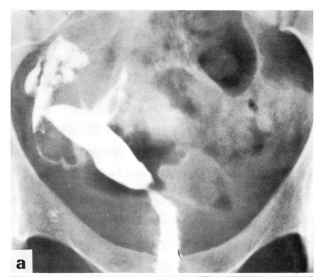

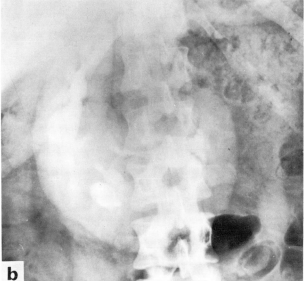

FIG. 5.14   (a) Unicornate uterus, hysterosalpingogram. (b) Fused kidney (horseshoe type) on intravenous urography.

CONGENITAL ABNORMALITIES OF THE VAGINA

Vaginal aplasia

Congenital absence of the vagina is rarely an isolated anomaly. Bryan *et al.* (1949) found that only four of

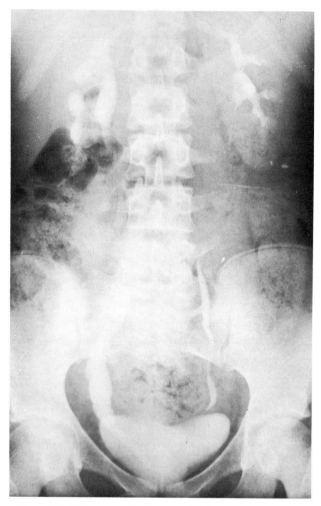

FIG. 5.15 This patient had uterus didelphys with a septate vagina. Intravenous urography showed an ectopic right ureteral orifice situated low and median in the bladder, with low ureteral obstruction.

twenty-six cases of vaginal aplasia had normal Fallopian tubes, ovaries and uterus; six cases had no uterus and ten patients had severe uterine abnormalities ranging from hypoplasia to bicornuate and unicornuate uterus. Haematosalpinx and endometriosis were frequent findings. Miller & Stout (1957) found a uterus in only a quarter of cases of vaginal aplasia, and noted that the uterus was invariably rudimentary when present. In the series of Thompson et al. (1957), a uterus was present in only two of thirty cases, and it was noted that the Fallopian tubes may be rudimentary and contain either blood or endometriosis.

Armstrong & Schreiber (1971) described the use of pelvic pneumography in the assessment of the internal genital organs in the presence of vaginal aplasia, although they noted that the uterus and adnexa may be incorrectly deemed as absent on this investigation when they have an infraperitoneal situation. Spasov et al. (1976) found no recognizable uterus in eleven of twelve patients with vaginal aplasia who underwent pelvic pneumography, but discovered two small soft tissue masses close to the bony pelvis on each side, below the ovary, which they interpreted as rudimentary bicornuate uteri.

Severe urinary tract anomalies are often associated with vaginal aplasia. Phelan et al. (1953) found renal agenesis in ten, renal ectopia in six, and mild pelviureteric obstruction in a further eight cases out of seventy-two patients with vaginal aplasia. In the series of Miller & Stout (1957), renal agenesis was found in eight of seventy-one cases.

Congenital absence of the vagina associated with a variety of other genital tract abnormalities, but normal ovarian function and female secondary sex characteristics, together with the presence of renal and skeletal anomalies and dermatoglyphic phenomena has been termed the Meyer-Rokitansky-Kuster-Hauser syndrome.

Major vertebral changes were present in 12.5% of two hundred cases of vaginal aplasia reported by Turenen & Unnerus (1967). These included wedge vertebrae, vertebral fusions, rudimentary vertebral bodies and supernumerary vertebrae.

Vaginal atresia and imperforate hymen

The atretic region is usually at the junction of the upper two-thirds and lower third of the vagina, and is due to failure in communication between the lower end of the Müllerian duct system and the urogenital sinus. In some cases, the atresia may be regarded as a failure of canalization of the vagina. An imperforate hymen will give the same clinical picture as frank vaginal atresia. These conditions may present with a lower abdominal mass either in the neonatal period or soon after the menarche. An accumulation of fluid in the vagina proximal to a congenital obstruction will give a hydrocolpos, or a hydrometrocolpos when there is also uterine distention.

The fluid is derived from cervical glands in the neonate, under the influence of maternal hormonal stimulation.

Most cases are identified in the first week of life, and the rest in the first six months (Reed & Griscom, 1973). The presence of the pelvic and abdominal mass is confirmed on plain radiographs as a dome-like soft tissue density. Intravenous urography shows bilateral hydronephrosis and hydroureter due to ureteral compression by the mass, usually of a mild or moderate degree (Fig. 5.16), in 70% of cases (Cook & Marshall, 1964). The bladder is often flattened, and displaced in a superior and anterior direction. The ureters are deviated laterally,

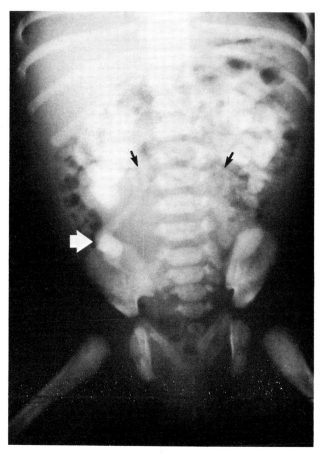

FIG. 5.16 Hydrometrocolpos in an infant. Large abdominal soft tissue mass (black arrows) with bilateral hydronephrosis and hydroureter on intravenous urography. Upward and lateral ureteral kinking (white arrow) due to distention of vaginal fornices. Courtesy of Dr Helen Carty.

especially above the pelvic brim, at which level Kafka (1966) has described upward and lateral ureteral kinking which he ascribed to distention of the adjacent vaginal fornices. The sigmoid colon may be seen on barium enema to be displaced superiorly by the mass, but severe intestinal obstruction may be due to an associated imperforate anus. Radio-opaque contrast medium injected into the vagina through a short segment of atresia or an imperforate hymen will delineate the dilated vagina (Westerhaut et al., 1964). Occasionally when there is an associated imperforate anus, gas within the pelvic mass indicates the presence of a fistula from the rectum. Cystography may sometimes reveal opacification of the vagina via a fistulous communication between bladder and vagina (Reed & Griscom, 1973). The vaginal obstruction may also be associated with a persistent urogenital sinus. McKusick et al. (1964) have shown that hydrometrocolpos with vaginal atresia may in some cases be inherited as an autosomal recessive trait, and this anomaly may be associated with polydactyly (Dundy et al., 1971).

Uterus didelphys with a longitudinal vaginal septum may be associated with a unilateral haematocolpos, and there is often renal agenesis on the same side as the vaginal occlusion (Johansen, 1972).

Haematocolpos and haematometrocolpos due to vaginal atresia or an imperforate hymen may present as an abdominal mass and amenorrhoea in teenagers. A soft tissue pelviabdominal mass is seen on abdominal radiographs and, as in the infantile group, vesical compression and ureteral obstruction are demonstrated by urography.

An incomplete *longitudinal vaginal septum* may occur as an isolated anomaly, and is a further example of failure of Müllerian duct fusion.

DISORDER OF WOLFFIAN DUCT REMNANTS

The ureters and the vestibule both develop from the Wolffian ducts, and so it is not surprising that ectopic ureters may open into the vestibule in the female. The ectopic ureter may rarely empty into the vagina, invariably on the anterior wall in the midline. Katzen & Trachtman (1954) have described the demonstration on vaginography of an ectopic ureter inserted into a vaginal fornix. Vanhoutte (1970) reported a case in which an ectopic ureter entered the apex of an apparent urethral diverticulum which was a persistent portion of the caudal part of the Wolffian duct.

Atrophic Wolffian duct remnants form Gartner's duct in the female. The majority of vaginal cysts arise from Gartner's duct, and may rarely protrude upon the bladder base when situated in the vaginal fornix (Rhamme & Derrick, 1973).

The proximal portion of Gartner's ducts may be delineated lateral to the uterus on hysterography when they communicate with the uterine cervix. The opacified duct may extend upwards to the cornua (Wepfer & Sinsky, 1958) or downwards to the level of the lower vagina (Weston, 1960).

THE PERSISTENT UROGENITAL SINUS AND INTERSEX STATES

As described earlier, the urogenital sinus arises as the confluence of urethra and internal genitalia of Müllerian duct origin. The urinary and genital tracts, as a result of persistence of the urogenital sinus, share a common passage to the exterior.

Genitography, the radiological investigation of the urogenital sinus and its structural connections, is performed by inserting a French 8 balloon catheter into the perineal orifice and injecting contrast medium after inflation of the balloon (Cremin, 1974). Alternatively, a blunt nosed syringe may be inserted into the orifice and against the perineum (Shopfner, 1967). The procedure is carried out under fluoroscopic control, with the patient in the lateral position and with the legs held firmly together. The urogenital sinus, the urethra and vagina will often be shown by this method, and sometimes there is delineation of the uterine cavity and Fallopian tubes (Tristan et al., 1956). The urogenital sinus may be probed with a soft rubber catheter to define the urethra and bladder, as well as the vagina, by the subsequent careful injection of contrast medium.

The anatomy of the urogenital tract can be defined in various intersex states by external examination and genitography. In the female pseudohermaphrodite there are ovaries and XX chromosomes, but masculinization of the external genitalia is present with often an enlarged phallus and a single perineal opening at the base of the phallus (Fig. 5.17). Congenital adrenal hyperplasia and ingestion of androgenic hormones by the mother during

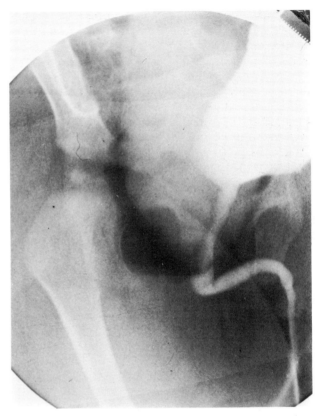

FIG. 5.17 Genitogram of pseudohermaphrodite. Female child with XX chromosomes. The mother has a suspected androgenic tumour. Orifice at base of small phallus was catheterized, and leads into a urogenital sinus via a long urethra. Contrast medium also opacifies the bladder. The vagina and uterus are delineated by air. Courtesy of Dr Helen Carty.

pregnancy are the commonest causes, although female pseudohermaphrodism may occasionally also be found as an ideopathic anomaly or in association with an imperforate anus. Genitography may be a very useful means of assessing the anatomy prior to plastic surgery. The perineal orifice is continuous with the urogenital sinus and there is a normal sized vagina, with the urethra entering the superior part of the sinus. The uterus is indicated by the cervix indenting the vagina or by actual delineation of the uterine cavity (Fig. 5.17). Precocious osseous maturation is seen in congenital adrenal hyperplasia (Levin et al., 1953).

In male pseudohermaphrodites, testes and XY chromosomes are present but there is feminization of the genitalia. There may be a blind vaginal pouch and perineal urethra, or a urogenital sinus.

True hermaphrodites have both ovaries and testes, while the majority are chromatin positive. Commonly, there is a generally male appearance to the genitalia with hypospadias and a bifid scrotum which may contain a testis or ovotestis on one side. Laparotomy is necessary in these cases, but genitography will show whether or not a vagina is present.

Pelvic pneumography has been used to delineate the internal genitalia in the pseudohermaphroditic states (McDonough & Simmons, 1971).

THE PERSISTENT CLOACA

Sometimes there is a partial or total failure of the urorectal septum to descend and divide the cloaca. Typically, a single perineal opening is found in a female infant. The retrograde injection of contrast medium through a catheter inserted into the cloaca will show communications to the rectum, vagina and urethra, and often vesicoureteric reflux (Kerlander, 1967; Cheng *et al.*, 1974). Separate catheters may be inserted into the bladder, vagina and rectum, with subsequent radiological delineation of these structures by contrast medium. Other genitourinary anomalies, such as a double vagina, hydrometra, crossed renal ectopia, and renal malrotation may be present. Cheng *et al.* suggest that AP and lateral views be taken during the 'cloacogram' as the various fistulous communications may be found at the side of the cloaca, rather than on the anterior and posterior walls. In this situation the fistulae, which are usually high in position, may be seen on one but not on the opposite lateral view.

Anorectal agenesis is much less common in the female than in the male, but is almost always associated with a communication between the rectum and vagina. There is a high incidence of sacral deformity and errors in lumbar segmentation in patients with anorectal agenesis (Berdon *et al.*, 1966). When the sacral spine is abnormal, urological abnormalities are present in over 70% of cases.

TURNER'S SYNDROME (GONADAL DYSGENESIS)

Patients with negative sex chromatin and an XO chromosome karyotype, or mosaic variations, have a virtual absence of gonads, which are represented by narrow streaks in the broad ligaments, and a fairly constant clinical pattern of sexual infantilism, primary amenorrhoea, short stature and webbed neck, with a relatively high incidence of associated congenital abnormalities.

Pelvic pneumographic appearances

The ovaries are not distinctly seen as formed structures on pelvic pneumography, but soft tissue thickening may be visible on the posterior surfaces of the broad ligaments and represent poorly developed 'streak' gonads (Alternas *et al.*, 1972). In the PA pelvic projection, the tubal ends and fimbria may be projected *en face* and appear as rounded soft tissue masses which may readily be misinterpreted as hypoplastic ovarian tissue. Oblique projections will confirm gonadal dysgenesis in these cases. The uterus is usually visible but is small in the young adult with Turner's syndrome. The uterus may be so hypoplastic as to be represented only by a slight thickening of the lateral uterine ligaments. Swahn *et al.* (1966) have demonstrated an increase in size of the uterus on pelvic pneumography following oestrogen therapy.

Skeletal abnormalities

MATURATION

Skeletal maturation in gonadal dysgenesis is abnormal from the prepubertal period onwards, with a delayed closure of epiphyses (Acheson & Zampa, 1961). Ossification centres appear at a normal time with bone age corresponding closely to chronological age until the patient reaches the age of thirteen years, epiphyseal fusion being delayed usually for three to six years and occasionally up to ten years (Kosowicz, 1965). The maturation delay is more pronounced in those parts of the skeleton in which maturation is subject to especially pronounced acceleration at puberty, namely the pelvis, hand and proximal tibia (Dalla Palma *et al.*, 1967).

BONE MINERALIZATION

While Finby & Archibald (1963) consider that younger patients have normal bone mineralization, and Preger *et al.* (1968) state that osteoporosis was found in children, both studies found that osteoporosis was a frequent and prominent occurrence after the normal age of puberty. According to Preger *et al.*, this osteoporosis does not respond to oestrogen therapy.

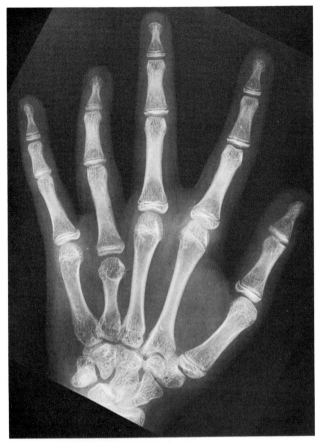

FIG. 5.18 Turner's syndrome. Short fourth metacarpal with positive 'metacarpal sign'.

ABNORMALITIES OF THE HAND AND WRIST

The 'metacarpal sign' (Archibald *et al.*, 1959) consists of shortening of the fourth metacarpal relative to the third and fifth, and is seen in most cases of gonadal dysgenesis (Fig. 5.18). The sign is evaluated by drawing a line, on a radiograph of the hand, tangential to the distal ends of the heads of the fourth and fifth metacarpals. This line will pass through the head of the third metacarpal in gonadal dysgenesis, whereas it runs distal to the head in the normal. The carpal sign is positive in other forms of growth disorders and occasionally in normal individuals.

The carpal angle

The bones of the proximal carpal row are often abnorm-

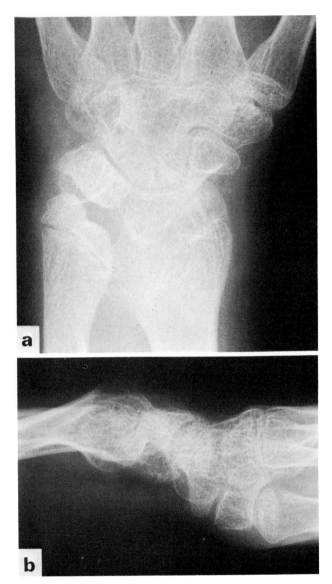

FIG. 5.19 Wrist in Turner's syndrome.
  (a) Small carpal angle with an angular configuration of proximal carpal row, and narrowing of middle of radial epiphysis. Delayed epiphyseal fusion at age of 18 years. Carpal fusion is also present.
  (b) Lateral view shows Madelung's deformity.

ally shaped, with an angular configuration in gonadal dysgenesis and do not form the normal slight arch (Fig. 5.19a). The mean angle described by the two tangents, one touching the proximal part of the scaphoid and lunate bones, and the other touching the triquetral and lunate bones is 131.5° in the normal. In gonadal dysgenesis, this carpal angle is reduced, usually to 102–117°, but never lies above the mean normal value (Kosowicz, 1962).

Phalangeal preponderance

The relative shortness of the metacarpals is contrasted to the normal length of the phalanges in gonadal dysgenesis. This is best seen in the fourth digit, but is present in all fingers. Normally, the total length of the distal and proximal phalanges of the fourth digit is equal to the length of the fourth metacarpal. In many cases of gonadal dysgenesis, the total length of these phalanges exceeds the fourth metacarpal length by 3 mm or more (Kosowicz, 1965).

Other changes are sometimes found in the wrist in gonadal dysgenesis. The distal radial metaphysis is sometimes convex towards the epiphysis, with the epiphyseal plate arched, being narrowed in its mid portion and expanded on both sides towards the metaphysis (Fig. 5.19a). In some patients there is a frank Madelung's deformity (Fig. 5.19b). The shafts of the middle and proximal phalanges are often narrowed in their mid portions, while the epiphyses of phalanges and metacarpals in patients with gonadal dysgenesis aged fifteen to twenty-two years become wider than the adjacent metaphyses and become inset into the adjacent metaphysis (Keats & Burns, 1964). Thickening of the soft tissues of the fingers may be evident (Kosowicz, 1965).

KNEES

Deformity of the medial tibial condyle resembles Blount's disease. The tibial metaphysis projects medially and becomes beak-like, while the epiphysis is tipped obliquely on its medial aspect to accommodate itself to the metaphyseal deformity (Kosowicz, 1960).

An extra ossification centre may be present on the medial aspect of the epiphysis, but soon fuses with the epiphysis. The medial femoral condyle is larger than the lateral, and extends downwards below the level of the lateral condyle.

ELBOWS

The carrying angle of the elbow is increased, with a radial tilt of the articular surface of the trochlea and buttressing of the external supracondylar ridge (Fig. 5.20). Ulnar bowing of the forearm bones may partially compensate for the increased carrying angle (Keats & Burns, 1964).

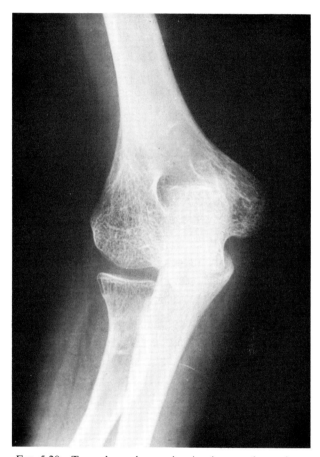

FIG. 5.20 Turner's syndrome showing increased carrying angle of elbow.

SPINE

Scheuermann's disease is not uncommon in gonadal dysgenesis (Fig. 5.21) and scoliosis and kyphosis is frequent. The lumbar vertebrae have a square shape. Hypoplasia of the atlas is common, with the posterior arch often thinner than normal and showing incomplete fusion (Finby & Archibald, 1963).

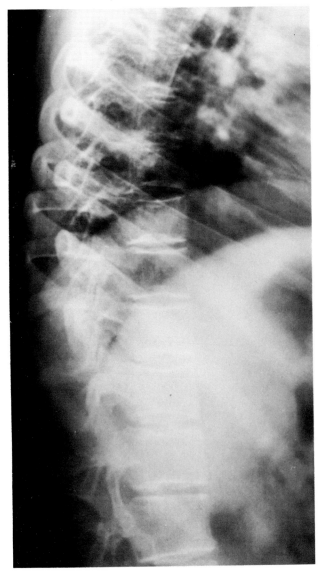

FIG. 5.21   Spine in Turner's syndrome shows osteoporosis and early change of Scheuermann's disease.

CHEST

The lateral portions of the clavicles may be thin or tapered, and the ribs may show posterior narrowing with pseudonotching (Astley, 1963).

SKULL

A small bridged sella turcica may be present, and the paranasal sinuses may show enlargement. The basal angle is sometimes increased, with basilar invagination.

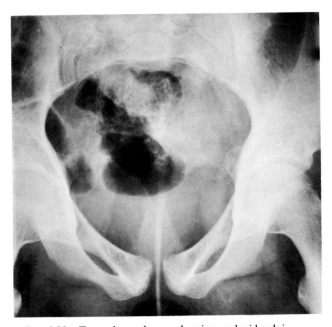

FIG. 5.22   Turner's syndrome showing android pelvis.

PELVIS AND HIPS

Many patients have an android pelvis (Fig. 5.22). The sacral ala and ilia may be small. The epiphyseal plate of the humeral neck is sometimes irregular and undulating with corresponding changes on the adjacent femoral head.

Extraskeletal abnormalities

Congenital urinary tract abnormalities are common. There is an increased incidence of rotation of the kidneys (Hung & Lopresti, 1967), horseshoe kidneys (Reveno & Palubinskas, 1966), duplication (Persky & Owens, 1971) and hydronephrosis.

Aortic coarctation is commoner in cases of gonadal dysgenesis than in the general population. Lymphoedema is sometimes found, and is due to lymphatic hypoplasia or aplasia (Benson et al., 1965).

OTHER CONGENITAL ANOMALIES OF THE OVARY

Congenital absence of the ovary has a 0.05% incidence, and is usually associated with anomalies of the Müllerian duct and metanephric systems (Igna & Darling, 1949). A functioning third ovary is also rare, and can be intra-abdominal, retroperitoneal or intraligamentous in situation. Occasionally, an ovary may be enlarged but otherwise normal. Congenital fenestrations and pouches in the broad ligaments may be associated with intestinal herniation and obstruction (Hunt, 1934; Wills, 1957).

REFERENCES

ACHESON R. M. & ZAMPA G. A. (1961) Skeletal maturation in ovarian dysgenesis and Turner's syndrome. *Lancet*, **1**, 917–920.

ALTERNAS R., CHARLES D. & STOCK R. (1972) Pelvic pneumography in adult gonadal dysgenesis. *Surg. Gynec. Obst.*, **134**, 751–754.

ARCHIBALD R. M., FINBY N. & DE VITA F. (1959) Endocrine significance of short metacarpals. *J. Clin. Endocrinol.*, **19**, 1312–1322.

ARMSTRONG M. K. & Schreiber M. H. (1971) Pelvic pneumography in congenital absence of the vagina. *Amer. J. Roentgenol.*, **112**, 607–609.

ASTLEY R. (1963) Chromosomal abnormalities in childhood, with particular reference to Turner's syndrome and mongolism. *Brit. J. Radiol.*, **36**, 2–10.

BARNETT E. (1955) The clinical value of hysterosalpingography. Part I. *J. Fac. Radiol.*, **7**, 115–129.

BENSON P. F., COUGH M. H. & POLANI P. E. (1965) Lymphangiography and chromosome studies in females with lymphoedema and possible ovarian dysgenesis. *Arch. Dis. Child.*, **40**, 27–32.

BERDON W. E., HOCHBERG B., BAKER D. H., GROSSMAN H. & SANTULLI T. V. (1966) The association of lumbosacral spine and genitourinary anomalies with imperforate anus. *Amer. J. Roentgenol.*, **98**, 181–191.

BRODY S. (1954) Double uterus with double pregnancy. *Amer. J. Obst. Gynec.*, **67**, 161–167.

BRYAN A. L., NIGRO J. A., COUNSELLER V. S. (1949) One hundred cases of congenital absence of the vagina. *Surg. Gynec. Obst.*, **88**, 79–86.

CHENG G. K., FISHER J. H., O'HARE K. G., RETIK A. B. & DARLING D. B. (1974) Anomaly of the persistent cloaca in female infants. *Amer. J. Roentgenol.*, **120**, 413–423.

COOK G. T. & MARSHALL V. F. (1964) Hydrocolpos causing urinary obstruction. *J. Urol.*, **92**, 127–132.

CREMIN B. J. (1974) Intersex states in young children. The importance of radiology in making a correct diagnosis. *Clin. Radiol.*, **25**, 63–73.

DALLA PALMA L., CARINA C., GUIST G. & BORGHI A. (1967)

Skeletal development in gonadal dysgenesis, female in genotype. *Amer. J. Roentgenol.*, **101**, 876–883.

DUNGY C. I., APTEKOV R. G. & CANN H. M. (1971) Hereditary hydrometrocolpos with polydactyly in infancy. *Pediatrics*, **47**, 138–141.

FINBY I. N. & ARCHIBALD R. M. (1963) Skeletal abnormalities associated with gonadal dysgenesis. *Amer. J. Roentgenol.*, **89**, 1222–1235.

FODA M. S., YOUSSEF A. F., SHAFEEK M. A. & KUSSEM K. A. (1962) Hysterography in diagnosis of abnormalities of the uterus. I. Congenital abnormalities. *Brit. J. Radiol.*, **35**, 115–121.

HAY D. (1958) The diagnosis and significance of minor degrees of uterine abnormality in relation to pregnancy. *J. Obst. Gynaec. Br. Emp.*, **65**, 557–582.

HUNG W. & LOPRESTI J. M. (1967) The high frequency of abnormal excretory urograms in young patients with gonadal dysgenesis. *J. Urol.*, **98**, 697–700.

HUNT A. B. (1934) Fenestrae and pouches in the broad ligament as an actual and potential cause of strangulated intra-abdominal hernia. *Surg. Gynec. Obst.*, **58**, 906–913.

IGNA E. J. & DARLING M. A. (1949) Anomalies of the ovary. *Obst. Gynec. Survey*, **4**, 159–174.

JARCHO J. (1946) Malformations of the uterus. *Amer. J. Surg.*, **71**, 106–166.

JOHANSEN K. (1972) Uterus didelphys with unilateral haematocolpos. *J. Obst. Gynaec. Br. Cwth.*, **79**, 85–89.

KAFKA R. M. (1966) Ureteral deviation in haematocolpos. *Radiology*, **87**, 903.

KATZEN P. & TRACHTMAN B. (1954) Diagnosis of vaginal ectopic ureter by vaginogram. *J. Urol.*, **72**, 808–811.

KEATS T. E. & BURNS T. W. (1964) The radiographic manifestations of gonadal dysgenesis. *Radiol. Clin. N. Amer.*, **2**, 297–313.

KERLANDER G. J. (1967) Roentgenology of imperforate anus. *Amer. J. Radiol.*, **100**, 190–202.

KOSOWICZ J. (1960) The deformity of the medial tibial condyle in nineteen cases of gonadal dysgenesis. *J. Bone Jt Surg.*, **42A**, 600.

KOSOWICZ J. (1962) The carpal sign in gonadal dysgenesis. *J. Clin. Endocrinol*, **22**, 949–952.

KOSOWICZ J. (1965) The roentgen appearance of the hand and wrist in gonadal dysgenesis. *Amer. J. Roentgenol.*, **93**, 354–361.

LEVIN B., RAMBAR A. C. & SHAPIRO I. J. (1953) Female pseudohermaphrodism. *Amer. J. Roentgenol.*, **69**, 948–952.

MCDONOUGH P. G. & SIMMONS R. G. (1971) Pelvic pneumoperitoneum in intersex states. *Obst. Gynec.*, **37**, 368–371.

MCKUSICK V. A., BAUER R. L., KOOP C. E. & SCOTT R. B. (1964) Hydrometrocolpos as a simply inherited malformation. *J. Amer. Med. Assoc.*, **189**, 813–816.

MEAKER S. R. (1940) Female genital hypoplasia. *J. Obst. Gynaec. Br. Emp.*, **47**, 40–48.

MILLER N. F. & STOUT W. (1957) Congenital absence of the vagina. *Obst. Gynec.*, **9**, 48–54.

MULLER P. (1968) Malformations génitales et urinaires associée chez la femme. *Gynaecologia*, **165**, 285–294.

PERSKY L. & OWENS R. (1971) Genitourinary tract anomalies in Turner's syndrome (gonadal dysgenesis). *J. Urol.*, **105**, 309–313.

PHELAN J. T., COUNSELLER V. S. & GREENE L. F. (1953) Deformities of the urinary tract with congenital absence of the vagina. *Surg. Gynec. Obst.*, **97**, 1–3.

PONTIFEX G., TRICHOPOULOS D. & KARPATHIOS (1972). Hystero-salpingography in the diagnosis of infertility (statistical analysis of 3427 cases). *Fertil. Steril.* **23**, 829–833.

POZNANSKI A. K., STERN A. M. & GALL J. C. (1970) Radiographic findings in the hand-foot-uterus syndrome. *Radiology*, **95**, 129–134.

PREGER L., STEINBACK H. L., MOSKOWITZ P., SCULLY A. L. & GOLDBERG M. B. (1968) Roentgenographic abnormalities in phenotypic females with gonadal dysgenesis. *Amer. J. Roentgenol.*, **104**, 899–910.

REED M. H. & GRISCOM N. T. (1973) Hydrometrocolpos in infancy. *Amer. J. Roentgenol.*, **118**, 1–13.

REENKOLA M. (1949) The form and position of the hysterogram in women investigated for primary sterility. *Acta Obstet. Gynec. Scan.*, **29**, 311–328.

REVENO J. S. & PALUBINSKAS A. J. (1966) Congenital renal abnormalities and gonadal dysgenesis. *Radiology*, **86**, 49–51.

RHAMME R. C. & DERRICK F. C. (1973) Gartner's duct involving urinary tract. *J. Urol.*, **109**, 60–61.

ROLEN A. C., CHOQUETTE A. J. & SEMMENS J. P. (1966) Rudimentary uterine horn: obstetric and gynecologic implications. *Obst. Gynec.*, **27**, 806–813.

SCHUMACKER H. B. (1938) Congenital anomalies of the genitalia associated with unilateral renal agenesis. *Arch. Surg.* **37**, 586–606.

SHOPFNER C. E. (1967) Radiology in pediatric gynecology. *Radiol. Clin. N. Amer.* **5**, 151–167.

SPASOV S. A., DOKUMOV S. I., DIANKOV L. A., BALKOV I. M. & SARKANYATZ A. M. (1976) Efficiency of pneumogynecography in the diagnosis of Meyer-Rokitansky-Küster-Hauser syndrome. *Amer. J. Roentgenol.*, **126**, 413–415.

STERN A. M., GALL J. C., PERRY B. L., STIMSON C. W., WEITKAMP L. R. & POZNANSKI A. K. (1970). The hand-foot-uterus syndrome. *J. Pediat.*, **77**, 109–116.

SWAHN G., LUNDERQUIST A. & RAFSTED S. (1966) Gynaecography in diagnosis and treatment evaluation in Turner's syndrome. *Acta Radiol. (Diag.)*, **4**, 529–535.

THOMPSON J. D., WHARTON L. R. & TE LINDE R. W. (1957) Congenital absence of the vagina. *Amer. J. Obst. Gynec.*, **74**, 397–404.

TRISTAN T. A., EHERLEIN W. R. & HOPE J. W. (1956). Roentgenologic investigation of patients with heterosexual development. *Amer. J. Roentgenol.*, **76**, 562–568.

TURENEN A. & UNNERUS C. E. (1967) Spinal changes in patients with congenital aplasia of the vagina. *Acta Obst. Gynec. Scandinav.*, **46**, 99–106.

VANHOUTTE J. J. (1970) Ureteral ectopia with a Wolffian duct remnant (Gartner's duct or cysts) presenting as a urethral diverticulum in girls. *Amer. J. Roentgenol.*, **110**, 540–545.

WEPFER J. F. & SINSKY J. E. (1958) Gartner's duct. *Amer. J. Roentgenol.* **80**, 686–689.

WESTERHAUT F. C., HODGMAN J. E., ANDERSON G. V. & SACK R. A. (1964) Congenital hydrocolpos. *Amer. J. Obst. Gynec.*, **89**, 957–961.

WESTON W. J. (1960) Radiographic demonstration of Gartner's duct. *Brit. J. Radiol.*, **33**, 370–373.

WILLOWS R. L. & WALL M. B. (1959) Hematometra in a rudimentary uterine horn. *Obst. Gynec.*, **13**, 103–106.

WILLS S. A. (1957) Intestinal obstruction associated with a hiatus in the broad ligament. *Amer. J. Obst. Gynec.*, **74**, 1143–1145.

WOOLFE R. B. & ALLEN W. M. (1953) Concomitant malformations. *Obst. Gynec.*, **2**, 236–265.

CHAPTER 6

Inflammatory Disease of the Female Genital Tract

Pelvic inflammatory disease is due to a variety of organisms, including gonococci, staphylococci, coliforms and tubercle bacilli. Most non-tuberculous organisms enter via the vagina, but infection sometimes spreads to the pelvic organs from adjacent viscera. Acute salpingitis is often associated with uterine and peritoneal inflammation and there may be resultant damage to the tubal mucosa and reactive fibrosis. Adhesions may form following infection, especially at the fimbriated ends of the Fallopian tubes, and the eventual outcome may be a distended, thin walled tube which becomes chronically filled with clear fluid when the infection is quiescent (hydrosalpinx) or with pus (pyosalpinx). When pus becomes pocketed around the ovary, as well as within the Fallopian tube, a tubo-ovarian abscess is the result. An abscess limited to the ovary is another possible sequel of pelvic inflammation. In some cases, usually during investigation for infertility, a hydrosalpinx is found without any past history to suggest an infective origin and is then usually secondary to endometriosis or to low grade salpingitis in childhood.

PLAIN RADIOGRAPHIC FINDINGS IN ACUTE SALPINGITIS AND PELVIC PERITONITIS

Radiology is of limited value in cases of acute salpingitis. The normal pelvic fat lines may be obliterated by inflammatory exudate. Moderately dilated loops of small intestine with fluid levels are sometimes seen in the lower part of the abdomen and represent local ileus. A more generalized paralytic ileus and free peritoneal fluid may result from a widespread peritonitis in more severe cases. Peritoneal adhesions resulting from pelvic inflammatory disease will occasionally cause a mechanical intestinal obstruction. An intrauterine contraceptive device may be associated with acute pelvic inflammatory disease.

HYDROSALPINX

Magnusson (1954) considered that bilateral proximal tubal occlusion was usually associated with puerperal pelvic infection or with abortion, while salpingitis in other circumstances tended to cause distal tubal obstruction. When the more usual perifimbrial fibrosis is present hysterosalpingography shows tubal dilatation, especially of the ampulla, with absent or limited peritoneal spillage of contrast medium with loculation (Fig. 6.1). The dilated tubes may be fixed, or in an abnormal position, due to adhesions. If there is doubt concerning tubal patency at the time of screening or on the routine radiograph taken ten or fifteen minutes later, then a delayed radiograph should be taken at one hour, by which time the contrast medium is completely absorbed except in cases of tubal obstruction (Fig. 6.2). Turning the patient into a prone position may help to increase peritoneal spillage in cases of doubtful tubal patency.

A comparative study of laparoscopy and hysterosalpingography in sterility (Ladipo, 1976) found complete agreement between both diagnostic modalities in the assessment of tubal patency in 70% of cases, with laparoscopy giving a better appraisal of tubal structure

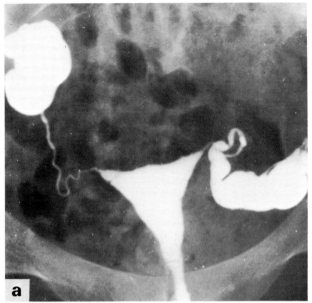

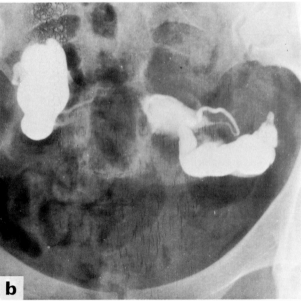

FIG. 6.1   (a) Hysterosalpingogram of a normal uterus. Gross bilateral hydrosalpinx due to perifimbrial adhesions.

(b) 15 minutes later a small residue of contrast medium remains in the uterus, and loculation persists in the Fallopian tubes with no free peritoneal spill.

and of the state of the pelvic peritoneum than hysterosalpingography.

PYOSALPINX, TUBO-OVARIAN AND OVARIAN ABSCESS

Hysterosalpingography is contraindicated in patients who have evidence of active pelvic inflammatory disease. Occasionally an apparently quiescent hydrosalpinx may flare up with acute inflammation, or even abscess formation, following hysterosalpingography.

An adnexal abscess is rarely due to a primary gonococcal infection, but is usually due to reinfection or secondary bacterial invasion by other organisms. Septic abortion, and intrauterine manipulation in general, may also provoke a pyogenic adnexal abscess. Ovarian and sometimes tubo-ovarian abscesses may occur after pelvic operations, especially vaginal hysterectomy (Ledger *et al.*, 1969).

A tubo-ovarian abscess shows as a radiographic soft tissue mass in most cases. Small radiolucent bubbles of gas may be visible within tubo-ovarian and ovarian abscesses.

Perforation of the abscess, especially when it is the relatively unprotected ovarian type, may result in a generalized peritonitis if the infection is not enveloped by pelvic adhesions (Pedowitz & Bloomfield, 1964). A 'silent' pyosalpinx has been reported by Brantley *et al.* (1960) as rupturing into the peritoneal cavity following hysterosalpingography. Adnexal abscesses may also rupture into the intestine (Fig. 6.3), urinary bladder and vagina, and these fistulae have been demonstrated by hysterosalpingography (Rozin, 1954). However, many adnexal abscesses with fistulae are tuberculous in nature.

Pelvic pneumography, although now mainly replaced by laparoscopy, shows peritubal and general pelvic adhesions as well as inflammatory masses (Fig. 6.4). These appearances may be impossible to differentiate from endometriosis.

Ureteral dilatation is found on intravenous urography in over 40% of cases of pelvic inflammatory disease (Klempner, 1952), and in 80% of tubo-ovarian abscesses (Phillips, 1974). The ureter is obstructed at or just below the pelvic brim (Fig. 6.5). Phillips also found that the ureter may be deviated in either a lateral or medial direction, the latter being unusual in other types of pelvic mass lesion. Regression of the ureteral obstruction occurs

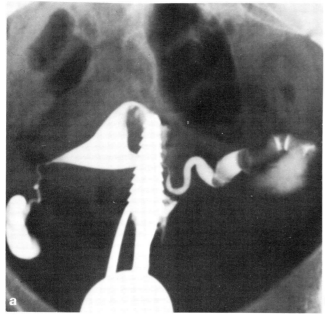

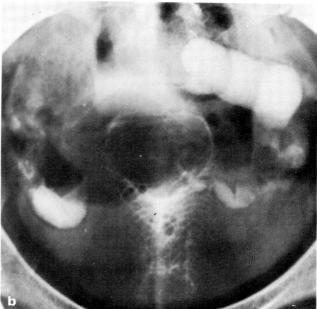

FIG. 6.2 (a) Hysterosalpingogram of a retroverted uterus showing delineation of dila⁺ed Fallopian tubes.

(b) 15 minutes later, contrast medium persists in dilated tubes, although there is some limited peritoneal spill.

(c) At 1 hour, contrast medium persists in dilated left tube. The bladder is opacified by excreted contrast medium which has been absorbed from the peritoneum.

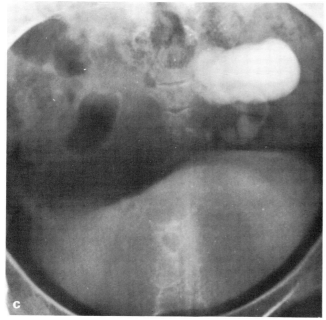

the presence of pelvic inflammatory masses, especially when there is loin pain.

Pelvic inflammatory disease may cause a 4–8 cm long narrowing in the rectosigmoid region of the large bowel, due to adhesions between the adnexa and the bowel (Marshak, 1947).

PELVIC INFLAMMATORY DISEASE OF EXTRAGENITAL ORIGIN

Diverticulitis

The symptoms of acute diverticulitis may mimic various forms of pelvic inflammatory disease, especially pyosalpinx and tubo-ovarian abscess. Chronic diverticulitis may cause a symptomless pelvic mass, sometimes with no relevant history to suggest intestinal disease. A barium enema may be inconclusive, as an adnexal inflammatory

in only 40% of cases following treatment, which is less frequent as well as occurring slower than with other benign pelvic lesions (Klempner, 1952) because of peri-ureteral scarring. Intravenous urography is indicated in

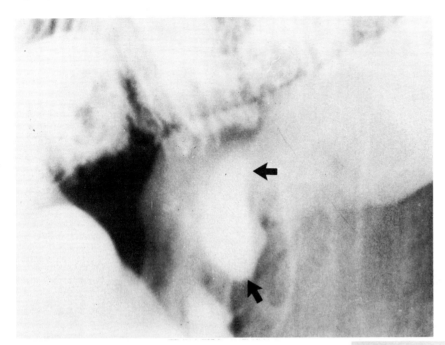

FIG. 6.3 Barium enema showing fistula between sigmoid colon and pyosalpinx (arrows); confirmed at operation.

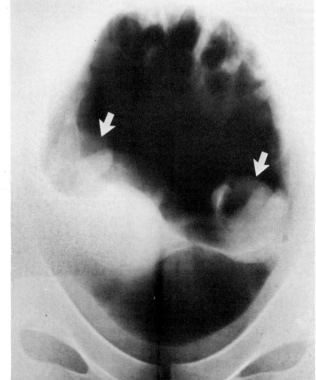

FIG. 6.4 Pelvic pneumography showing bilateral hydrosalpinx (arrows) in a woman aged 21 years.

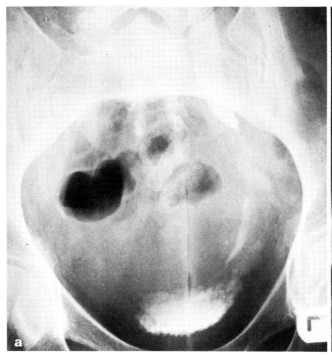 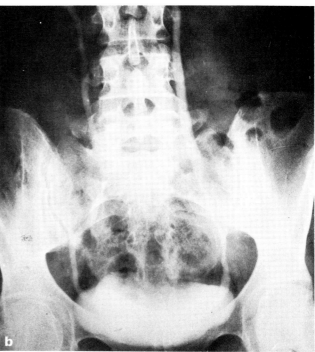

FIG. 6.5   (a) Tubo-ovarian abscess causing soft tissue pelvic mass, and narrowing of pelvic portion of left ureter with obstruction on intravenous urography.

(b) Left ureter almost normal on repeat urography 2 months after surgical drainage of abscess.

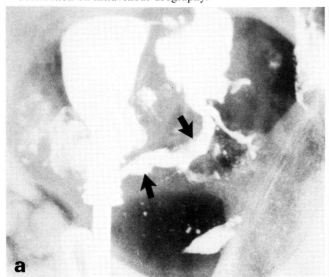 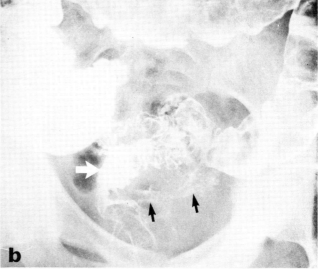

FIG. 6.6   Uterocolic fistula. (a) Hysterogram shows delineation of fistulous tract (black arrows) leading from cervix to sigmoid colon.

(b) Delineation of uterus (white arrow) and vagina via fistula from diverticular disease of sigmoid segments. Paget's disease of pelvis.

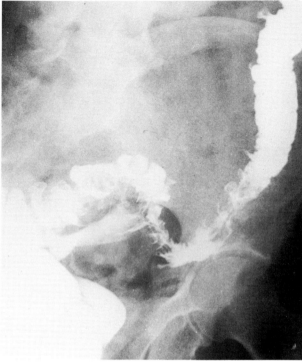

mass may coexist with diverticular disease (Balz, 1968). A diverticular abscess may rupture into the female genital tract, causing a uterocolic (Fig. 6.6) or vaginocolic fistula (Fig. 6.7). The fistula may not be revealed on the filling phase of a barium enema, but only after evacuation (Fig. 6.8). Left sided salpingitis may result from diverticulitis.

Appendicitis

Right sided salpingitis may be caused by spread from adjacent appendicitis. Hysterosalpingography may subsequently show ampullary dilation of the right Fallopian tube with restricted spillage of contrast medium due to perifimbrial adhesions.

Crohn's disease

Salpingitis, usually unilateral, and tubo-ovarian abscess may be due to direct involvement of adnexa from the adjacent rectosigmoid or terminal ileum (Fig. 6.9) affected by Crohn's disease (Hudson, 1963). Unilateral acute salpingitis may occasionally be the presenting feature of

FIG. 6.7 Vaginocolic fistula demonstrated by barium enema in diverticular disease.

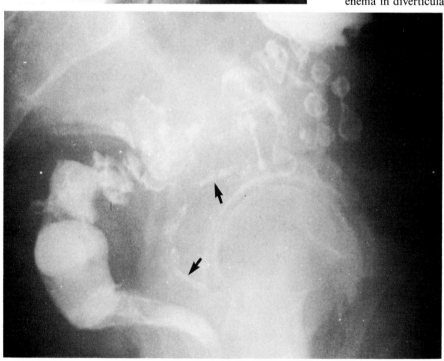

FIG. 6.8 Lateral view of rectosigmoid postevacuation shows diverticular disease and barium in vagina (arrows) from vaginocolic fistula.

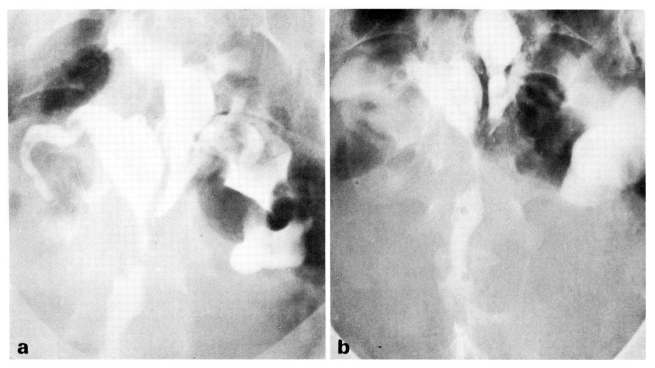

FIG. 6.9 Hysterosalpingogram showing loculation of contrast medium in the pelvic peritoneal cavity and tubal obstruction due to adhesions in a patient with Crohn's disease of the terminal ileum and colon. There was a five year history of primary infertility. (a) During tubal filling. (b) Delayed film.

Crohn's disease (Measday & Buckle, 1963). Rectovaginal fistula is another manifestation of Crohn's disease.

DIVERTICULOSIS OF THE FALLOPIAN TUBES (SALPINGITIS ISTHMICA NODOSA)

Minute loculations of contrast medium are seen adjacent to the tubal lumen on hysterosalpingography in diverticulosis of the Fallopian tubes. These diverticula are up to 2 mm in diameter, usually clustered together over a length of 1 to 2 cm but occasionally over a longer segment, and often involve both Fallopian tubes (Fig. 6.10). Freakley *et al.* (1974) found the diverticula to be confined to the proximal portion of the Fallopian tube in two-thirds of cases, and infrequently involving the distal parts alone. There is a definite association between diverticulosis of the Fallopian tubes and ectopic pregnancy (Persaud, 1970), and also tubal obstruction (Freakley

et al., 1974). These authors also found the condition to be more frequent in West Indians than in Europeans. Inflammatory changes are often found in association with tubal diverticulosis, but Benjamin & Beaver (1951) considered that infection is not likely to be the sole cause and may sometimes be a secondary event. Histologically, the diverticula have an epithelial lining and penetrate into the muscle coat, often associated with hypertrophy of adjacent muscle, and associated fibrosis and leucocytic infiltration is the rule. The hysterosalpingographic appearances have to be differentiated from tuberculous salpingitis, but the consistently nodular appearance of the diverticula is the main discriminating feature.

UTERINE INFECTIONS

Gas gangrene

Gas gangrene of the uterus usually follows septic abortion and is due to *Clostridium welchii* or occasionally infection

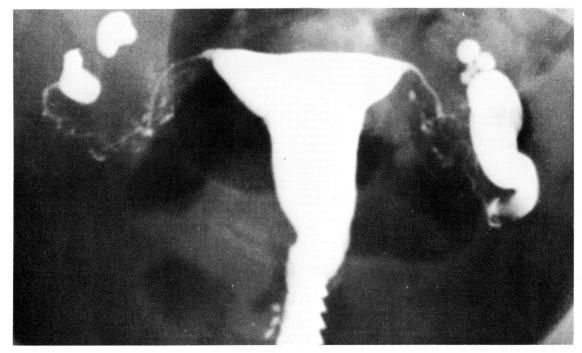

FIG. 6.10   Hysterosalpingogram of bilateral diverticulosis of the Fallopian tubes.

by other Clostridial organisms. The first case to be described with accompanying radiographs was by Poppel & Silverman (1941), demonstrating globules of gas within an enlarged uterus. The gas bubbles may be seen in layers within the uterine wall, with an onion peel configuration (Doehler *et al.*, 1960). The gas may extend into the retroperitoneal space and into the parametrium (Holly *et al.*, 1960).

Physopyometra

A large, rounded pelvic mass containing gas and a fluid level may be a pyometra (Walker & Pearson, 1955). A pyometra occurs secondary to cervical stenosis, particularly when due to a carcinoma of the cervix or following radium treatment.

Weintraub & Tilos (1964) described the radiological appearances of a large pelviabdominal mass with a gas/fluid level, lying outside the colon in a pyrexial woman. The cause was shown to be an abscess within a uterine leiomyoma, with *E. coli* being the responsible organism.

Cervicitis

Gross dilatation of cervical (Nabothian) glands and ulceration of the endocervix are found in endocervicitis (Fig. 6.11). Prominence of the normally delineated plicae palmatae is not by itself indicative of cervical inflammation (Fullenlove, 1953). Cystically dilated glandular elements in the cervical canal are regarded by Slezak & Tillinger (1976) as often being a normal appearance. Adenomyosis does not generally cause cavities in the lower half of the uterus, and does not account for cystic spaces greater than 5 mm in diameter.

Asplund (1952) considered that the diagnosis of cervicitis cannot be made from hysterographic appearances alone. Nonspecific inflammatory changes may be found in curettings where cervical contours are either smooth or only slightly irregular on hysterography, and a normal microscopic structure may be associated with a very irregular and protuberant cervical contour. Dufresne *et al.* (1959) found that a hysterographic diagnosis of endocervicitis was substantiated by pathological ex-

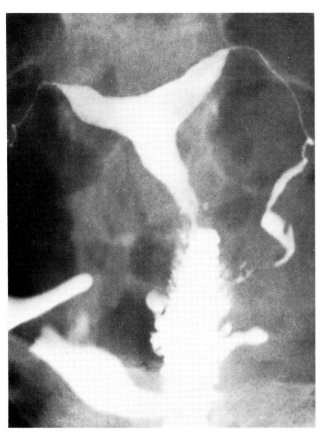

FIG. 6.11 Hysterogram showing irregularity of endocervix with Nabothian cysts.

amination in only 10% of cases. A longitudinal fold pattern to the cervical mucosa may indicate healing of a previous endocervicitis. Postpartum infection or cervicitis following surgical dilatation may, according to Asplund, cause a permanent stenosis of the internal os.

SOME DISTANT EFFECTS OF PELVIC INFLAMMATORY DISEASE

Sherman & Schneider (1955) have described three cases of vertebral osteomyelitis complicating postabortal and postpartum infection. Septic arthritis of the hip may be a consequence of perforation of a variety of abdominal and pelvic organs, including the uterus after radiotherapy (Smith & Ward, 1966).

Severe pelvic adhesions have caused fixation of the superior mesenteric artery and subsequent vascular compression of the third part of the duodenum (Haddad & Decker, 1959).

VAGINITIS

Vaginitis is the commonest gynaecological condition in the paediatric age group. Some of these cases are due to a vaginal foreign body. Anteroposterior and lateral radiographs will localize radio-opaque foreign bodies within the vagina. Non-opaque foreign bodies may be demonstrated by positive contrast vaginography.

Emphysematous vaginitis is a benign, self limiting condition in which gas filled cysts are present in the lamina propria of the vaginal wall and cervix. Many of the patients are pregnant, but this is not an invariable association. There is evidence that emphysematous vaginitis is due to *Trichomonas* infection (Wilbanks & Carter, 1963). The radiolucent cystic areas are of varying size and are situated behind and above the symphysis, and a lateral view shows them to have a rectangular disposition in the midsaggital plane (Wepfer & Sinsky, 1968). The radiological differential diagnosis includes emphysematous cystitis, gangrene of the uterus, pelvic abscess and bowel gas.

TUBERCULOSIS OF THE GENITAL TRACT

Tuberculous involvement of the female genital tract tends to be a latent disease, with little in the way of symptoms and often no palpable abnormality of the pelvic viscera. However, genital tuberculosis is found in 3–5% of cases investigated for infertility (Sherman, 1952; Francis, 1964). Amenorrhoea is the next commonest presenting feature (Francis, 1964). The muscular layer of the Fallopian tubes is generally the primary site of the infection in the genital tract from bloodborne infection, with subsequent spread to the serosa and mucosa. Occasionally, the adnexa may be involved directly by spread from peritoneal tuberculosis. The uterus is secondarily affected in about half the cases of tuberculous salpingitis, so that failure to culture tubercle bacilli from endometrial curettings does not exclude the possibility of genital tuberculosis.

Evidence of pulmonary tuberculosis is found in

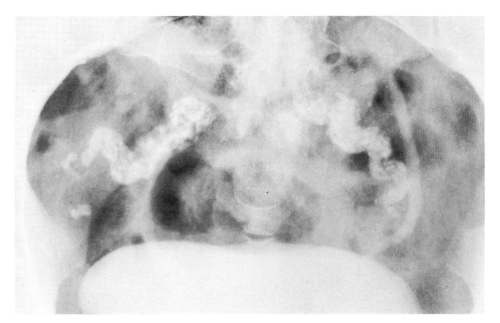

FIG. 6.12 Intravenous urography showing tubal calcification due to tuberculous salpingitis.

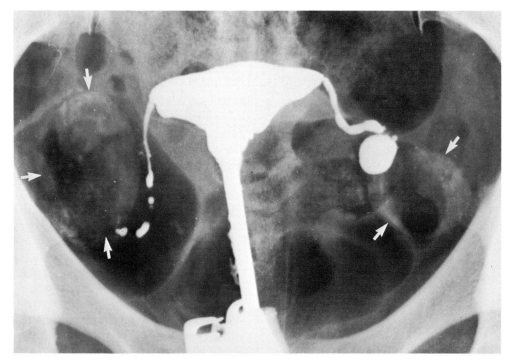

FIG. 6.13 Hysterosalpingography showing tuberculous salpingitis with total bilateral tubal occlusion but only moderate dilatation. Calcification in the region of both ovaries (arrows).

30–37% of females with genital tuberculosis (Zummo *et al.*, 1955; Schaefer, 1970), and an 8% incidence of genital tuberculosis has been found at autopsy among women dying from pulmonary involvement (Schaefer, 1970). Overbeck (1966) found genital tuberculosis in almost 10% of women with renal tuberculosis, and vice versa.

Radiology of tuberculous salpingitis

Calcification related to totally or partially occluded Fallopian tubes and calcified pelvic lymph nodes were originally noted to be a feature of tuberculous salpingitis by Robins & Shapira (1931) (Fig. 6.12). Stones may form within the tubal lumen (Rozin, 1952) and true ossification may also occur with caseous material inside the Fallopian tube (Adoni & Polliack, 1969). Calcification may also occur in the ovaries (Fig. 6.13).

Tubal occlusion is very common and is usually bilateral (Pontifex *et al.*, 1972), although the tubes may remain patent in proven disease (Ekengren & Ryden, 1951). Very dilated hydrosalpinges are not typical of tuberculous salpingitis, dilatation usually being moderate or only slight with club-like appearances even in the presence of total tubal occlusion (Madsen, 1947) (Figs. 6.13 and 6.14). The site of tubal occlusion may be the isthmus or the ampulla. The longitudinal mucosal folds of the Fallopian tubes may be thickened in either tuberculous or pyogenic chronic salpingitis, but gross thickening is very suggestive of tuberculosis (Fig. 6.15).

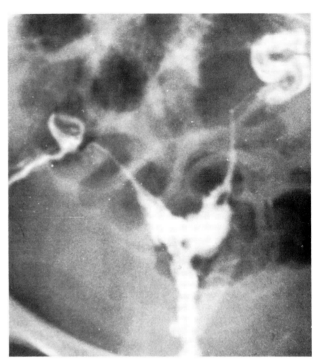

FIG. 6.15 Hysterosalpingogram in tuberculosis. Contracted, irregular uterus with strictures. Both tubes are occluded, with coarse mucosal folds.

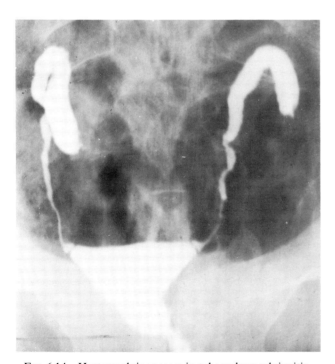

FIG. 6.14 Hysterosalpingogram in tuberculous salpingitis. Elevation and fixation of both Fallopian tubes which are club shaped and show total occlusion.

The tubal contours are often smooth, but an irregular or rugged outline, the presence of cavities or multiple tubal strictures giving a beaded or 'rosary' appearance are strong diagnostic pointers to tuberculous salpingitis. Small fistulae, sometimes at the point of tubal occlusion (Fig. 6.16), or irregular tubal recesses are also characteristic features. The Fallopian tubes may be rigid and straightened to give a 'pipestem' appearance (Magnusson, 1947) or may be in an abnormal situation (Fig. 6.14). On the whole, tuberculosis causes its greatest damage in

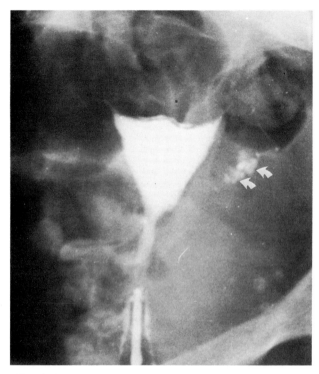

FIG. 6.16   Hysterosalpingogram in tuberculous salpingitis. The 'double' uterine fundal contour is a normal variant. Both Fallopian tubes are occluded, but there is irregular cavitation at the point of tubal obliteration on the left (arrows).

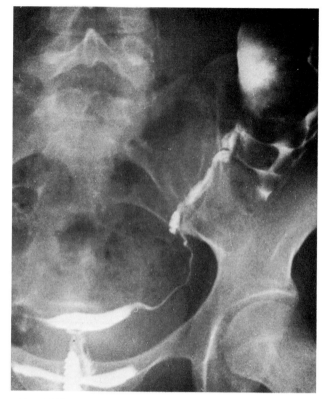

FIG. 6.17   Hysterosalpingography in tuberculous salpingitis. Fistula between left Fallopian tube and proximal part of sigmoid colon.

the ampullary portion of the tube. Patients on anti-tuberculous therapy tend to have a reversion towards normal of otherwise progressive changes (Ekengren, 1955). Primary carcinoma of the Fallopian tube is occasionally associated with tuberculous salpingitis, but this is regarded as being a coincidental combination of lesions (Dickson *et al.*, 1952).

Adhesions of a tuberculous pyosalpinx to an adjacent hollow viscus and subsequent breaking down of the separating wall leads to tubointestinal and tubovesical fistulae. The lumen of an involved tube in these cases is usually dilated, and the fistula may be demonstrated on hysterosalpingography (Rozin, 1954) (Fig. 6.17). Adnexal tuberculosis is regarded as the most frequent cause of these spontaneous tubal fistulae.

Pneumopelvigraphy has demonstrated tubal thicken-ing, adhesions, and the closely related calcific densities in pelvic tuberculosis (Stein, 1934).

Radiology of uterine tuberculosis

Tubal changes are anticipated in all cases of tuberculous uterine involvement. Hysterography may reveal poly-poid lesions, hyperplastic endometrium and a ragged saw-toothed uterine contour, although these findings are not specific for tuberculous endometritis (Ekengren & Ryden, 1951). Recesses and fistulae may extend into the myometrium and are a characteristic feature when combined with strictures in advanced cases. In time, the uterus may become shivelled and deformed (Fig. 6.15). Venous intravasation of contrast medium may occur secondary to uterine involvement by tuberculosis (Fig. 6.18) or when the Fallopian tubes are occluded (Kika,

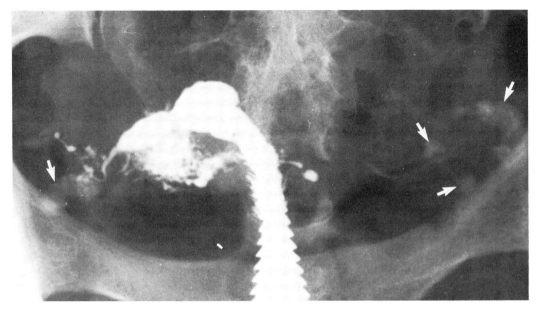

FIG. 6.18 Hysterosalpingogram in tuberculosis. Deformed uterus with stricture formation and gross intravasation. Bilateral tubal occlusion with fistulous tracts from right Fallopian tube, and calcification in the region of both ovaries (arrows).

1954). Uterolymphatic intravasation from a shrunken and deformed uterus with obstructed Fallopian tubes is invariably associated with tuberculosis (Drukman & Rozin, 1951; Kika, 1954) and gives a cloudy, persistent opacification of the whole uterine wall on hysterography.

REFERENCES

ADONI A. & POLLIACK A. (1969) Heterotopic bone formation in tuberculous salpingitis. *Amer. J. Obst. Gynec.*, **104**, 918–919.

ASPLUND J. (1952) The uterine cervix and isthmus under normal and pathological conditions. *Acta Radiol. Suppl.*, **91**.

BALZ F. F. (1968) Diverticulitis as a diagnostic problem in gynecology. *Amer. J. Roentgenol.*, **101**, 372–376.

BENJAMIN C. L. & BEAVER D. C. (1951) Pathogenesis of salpingitis isthmica nodosa. *Amer. J. Clin. Path.*, **21**, 212–222.

BRANTLEY W. M., DELVALLE R. A., AABY G. V. & SCHOEN-BUCHER A. K. (1960) Rupture of a silent pyosalpinx following a hysterosalpingogram. *Obst. Gynec.*, **16**, 483–485.

DICKSON W. P. G., LODGE K. V. & WOODCOCK A. S. (1952) A case of primary carcinoma of the Fallopian tube associated with tuberculosis salpingitis. *J. Obst. Gynaec. Br. Emp.*, **59**, 834–837.

DOEHLER G. A., KLINGES K. G. & PISANI B. J. (1960) The X-ray diagnosis of gas gangrene of the uterus. *Amer. J. Obst. Gynec.*, **79**, 542–544.

DRUKMAN A. & ROZIN S. (1951) Uterovenous and uterolymphatic intravasation in hysterosalpingography. *J. Obst. Gynaec. Br. Emp.*, **58**, 73–78.

DUFRESNE M. R., GERIN-LAJOIE L. & MALTAIS R. (1959) Problems in hysterosalpingography. *J. Amer. Med. Ass.*, **170**, 1169–1171.

EKENGREN K. (1955) Roentgenographic diagnosis of genital tuberculosis in the female and roentgenographic effects of antibiotic treatment. *Acta Radiol. Supp.*, **123**.

EKENGREN K. & RYDEN A. B. V. (1951) Roentgen diagnosis of tuberculous endometritis. *Acta Radiol.*, **36**, 485–494.

FRANCIS W. J. A. (1964) Female genital tuberculosis. *J. Obst. Gynaec. Br. Emp.*, **71**, 418–428.

FREAKLEY G., NORMAN W. J., ENNIS J. T. & DAVIES E. R. (1974) Diverticulosis of the Fallopian tubes. *Clin. Radiol.*, **25**, 535–542.

FULLENLOVE T. M. (1953) Uterosalpingography. With special reference to the cervical canal. *Amer. J. Roentgenol.*, **69**, 74–77.

HADDAD G. H. & DECKER W. H. (1959) Superior mesenteric syndrome following pelvic inflammatory disease. *Amer. J. Obst. Gynec.*, **78**, 1301–1303.

HOLLY L. E., HARTWELL S. W., McNAIR J. N. & LOWRY R. A. (1960) Mural emphysema of the uterus. *Amer. J. Roentgenol.*, **84**, 913–922.

HUDSON C. N. (1963) Gynaecological manifestations of Crohn's disease. *J. Obst. Gynaec. Br. Emp.*, **70**, 437–442.

KIKA K. (1954) A clinical analysis of the 'angiograms' found in the course of hysterosalpingography with special reference to tuberculosis of the female genitals. *Amer. J. Obst. Gynec.*, **67**, 56–63.

KLEMPNER E. (1952) Gynecological lesions and ureterohydronephrosis. *Amer. J. Obst. Gynec.*, **64**, 1232–1241.

LADIPO O. A. (1976) Tests of tubal patency. Comparison of laparoscopy and hysterosalpingography. *Brit. Med. J.*, **2**, 1297–1298.

LEDGER W. J., CAMPBELL C., TAYLOR D. & WILLSON J. R. (1969) Adnexal abscess as a late complication of pelvic operations. *Surg. Gynec. Obst.*, **129**, 973–978.

MADSEN V. (1947) Hysterograms in genital tuberculosis in women. *Acta Radiol.*, **28**, 812–823.

MAGNUSSON W. (1947) Further experiences in the roentgen diagnosis of tuberculous salpingitis. *Acta Radiol.*, **28**, 824–832.

MAGNUSSON W. (1954) On the localization of tubal obstruction in cases of sterility from different causes. *Acta. Radiol.*, **141**, 513–516.

MARSHAK R. H. (1947) Extrinsic lesions affecting the rectosigmoid. *Amer. J. Roentgenol.*, **58**, 439–450.

MEASDAY B. & BUCKLE R. M. (1963) Unilateral salpingitis as the presenting feature of Crohn's disease. *J. Obst. Gynaec. Br. Emp.*, **70**, 307–310.

OVERBECK L. (1966) Is tuberculosis of the female genital tract an entity? *J. Obst. Gynaec. Br. Emp.*, **73**, 624–628.

PEDOWITZ P. & BLOOMFIELD R. D. (1964) Ruptured adnexal abscess (tubo-ovarian) with generalized peritonitis. *Amer. J. Obst. Gynec.*, **88**, 721–729.

PERSAUD V. (1970) Etiology of tubal ectopic pregnancy. *Obst. Gynec.*, **36**, 257–263.

PHILLIPS J. C. (1974) A spectrum of radiologic abnormalities due to tubo-ovarian abscess. *Radiology*, **110**, 307–311.

PONTIFEX G., TRICHOPOULOS D. & KARPATHIOS S. (1972) Hysterosalpingography in the diagnosis of infertility (statistical analysis of 3437 cases). *Fertil. Steril.*, **23**, 829–833.

POPPEL M. H. & SILVERMAN M. (1941) Gas gangrene of the uterus. *Radiology*, **37**, 491–492.

ROBINS S. A. & SHAPIRA A. A. (1931) The value of hysterosalpingography. A study of 1000 cases. *New Engl. J. Med.*, **205**, 380–395.

ROZIN S. (1952) The X-ray diagnosis of genital tuberculosis. *J. Obst. Gynaec. Br. Emp.*, **59**, 59–63.

ROZIN S. (1954) The diagnosis of tubointestinal and tubovesical fistulae by hysterosalpingography. *Amer. J. Obst. Gynec.*, **68**, 1525–1534.

SCHAEFER G. (1970) Tuberculosis of the female genital tract. *Clin. Obst. Gynec.* **13**, 965–998.

SHERMAN A. (1952) Genital T.B. in the female. *J. Obst. Gynaec. Br. Emp.*, **59**, 721–728.

SHERMAN M. & SCHNEIDER G. T. (1955) Vertebral osteomyelitis complicating postabortal and postpartum infection. *South Med. J.*, **48**, 333–338.

SLEZAK P. & TILLINGER K. G. (1976) The incidence and clinical importance of hysterographic evidence of cavities in the uterine wall. *Radiology*, **118**, 581–586.

SMITH W. S. & WARD R. M. (1966) Septic arthritis of the hip complicating perforation of abdominal organs. *J. Amer. Med. Assoc.*, **195**, 1148–1150.

STEIN I. F. (1934) Oxygen pneumoperitoneum in the diagnosis and treatment of tuberculosis of the genitalia, intestine and peritoneum. *Surg. Gynec. Obst.*, **58**, 567–577.

WALKER A. H. C. & PEARSON D. (1955) A case of physometra. *J. Obst. Gynaec. Br. Emp.*, **62**, 540–541.

WEINTRAUB R. A. & TILOS F. (1964) Gas abscess within a leiomyoma of the uterus. *Amer. J. Roentgenol.*, **92**, 400–403.

WEPFER J. F. & SINSKY J. E. (1968) Roentgen manifestations of vaginitis emphysematosa. *Amer. J. Roentgenol.*, **102**, 946–950.

WILBANKS G. D. & CARTER B. (1963) Vaginitis emphysematosa. *Obst. Gynec.*, **22**, 301–309.

ZUMMO B. P., SERED H. & FALLS F. H. (1955) The diagnosis and prognosis of female genital tuberculosis. *Amer. J. Obst. Gynec.*, **70**, 34–43.

CHAPTER 7

Uterine Tumours

FIBROIDS (FIBROMYOMAS)

A fibroid is a benign tumour consisting mainly of smooth muscle, but with some fibrous tissue, and with a thin layer of connective tissue separating it from the surrounding myometrium. Fibroids may be multiple or occur singly and are found in 20% of women over the age of thirty years. Most fibroids are either intramural or subserosal, but 5% are submucosal in situation.

Plain radiographic findings

Multiple and large fibroids may show as a soft tissue pelvic mass. The outline of the mass is characteristically lobulated in the presence of multiple fibroids (Fig. 7.1).

Calcification occurs in fibroids following necrosis in pregnancy or is secondary to postmenopausal degeneration. Finkle *et al.* (1954) found only five instances of calcified fibroids on radiographs of over four thousand adult females, all except one being in women over the age of fifty years. Initially, punctate or small irregular scattered calcifications are seen and these increase in number and size, coalescing to form coarse aggregates (Figs. 7.1 and 7.2). A less common finding is a peripheral rim of calcification (Fig. 7.3). Rarely, metaplasia within fibroids may lead to ossification.

Hysterosalpingography

Dufresne *et al.* (1959) found hysterosalpingography to have an overall accuracy of only 58% in the diagnosis of uterine fibroids, mainly because subserosal and small intramural fibroids often gave a normal picture. This contrasts with the experience of Pietilä (1969) who, in over eight hundred patients with fibroids, found a preoperative hysterographic diagnosis to be correct in 88% of all cases. In Pietilä's series there was agreement of radiological and operative findings in all cases of submucosal fibroids, and a correct radiological diagnosis in 73% of intramural and 62% of subserosal fibroids.

Fibroids which are clinically palpable may cause no hysterographic abnormality, and there is probably a greater tendency for fibroids to grow outwards and become subserosal, rather than submucosal in situation. However, curettage may fail to demonstrate very large submucosal fibroids which form a false smooth wall misinterpreted as a normal uterine cavity (Marshak *et al.*, 1950), whereas hysterography will establish the diagnosis in such cases (Fig. 7.4). In general, however, submucosal fibroids may be expected to cause distortion of the hysterographic contour. A single fibroid will cause a smooth, round filling defect (Fig. 7.5), while multiple submucosal fibroids are associated with separate filling defects and sometimes gross distortion of the uterine cavity (Figs. 7.6 and 7.7). Large fibroids may also cause a crescentic or spindle shape and perhaps elongation of the cavity (Fig. 7.8). The uterine cavity is enlarged in the presence of submucosal intramural fibroids (Fig. 7.9) in just over half the cases (Pietilä, 1969), secondary to the actual increase in uterine size and because of hypotonicity of the uterine musculature. A globular uterine configuration is also associated with the presence of fibroids. Small submucosal fibroids may be missed on hysterography unless there is fractioned injection of contrast medium (Fig. 7.10). Pietilä found uterine deformity

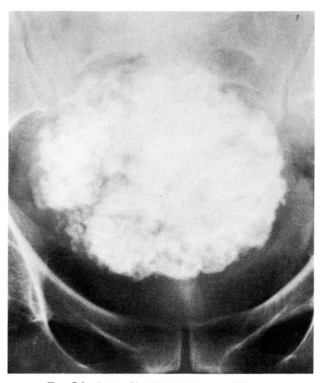

FIG. 7.1 Several calcified fibroids with typical flocculent pattern. The uterus is enlarged with a lobulated margin.

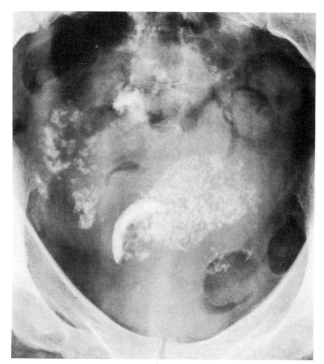

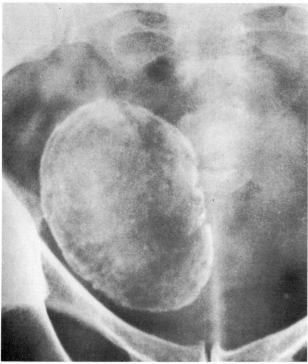

FIG. 7.2 Large fibroid with dense calcification.

due to fibroids to be visible only on the lateral view in a significant number of cases.

Small sessile, polypoidal submucosal fibroids may be difficult to differentiate from endometrial polyps, but they tend to be more regular in outline (Fig. 7.11). Pedunculated fibroids cast a lacunar image and may occupy nearly all of the uterine cavity (Fig. 7.12). Occasionally, a pedunculated fibroid descends into a dilated and elongated cervical canal, but its smooth and rounded contour distinguishes it from a cervical polyp (Rozin, 1956). Fibroids arising from the cervix itself may also elongate and distort the cervical outline. Asymmetry and blunting of the cornua is an important and sometimes subtle sign caused by the presence of fibroids (Fig. 7.9), and there may be obstruction to tubal filling.

FIG. 7.3 Rim calcification in a fibroid.

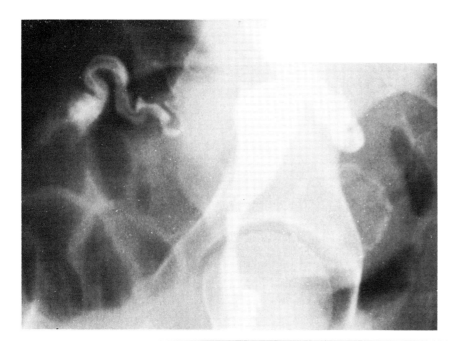

FIG. 7.4   A large right-sided myometrial fibroid with submucosal element was missed in curettage, but caused smooth indentation of the right uterine wall on hysterography with slight displacement of the uterine cavity and elevation of the right uterine tube. Calcified subserosal fibroid on the left.

FIG. 7.5 Large submucosal fibroid with smooth, lobulated margins on hysterography.

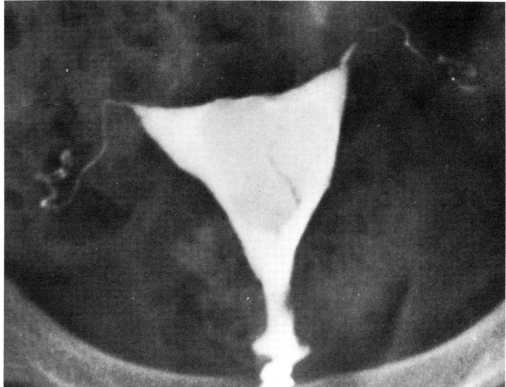

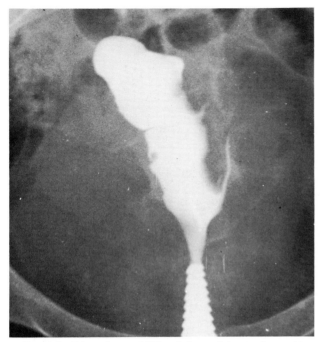

FIG. 7.6 Distortion and filling defects of the uterine cavity by fibroids.

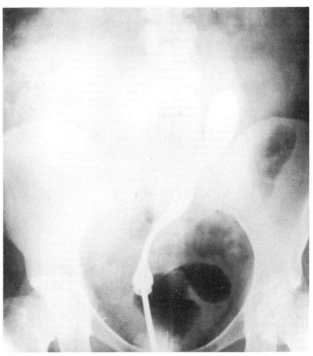

FIG. 7.8 Elongation of the cavity of a large fibroid uterus.

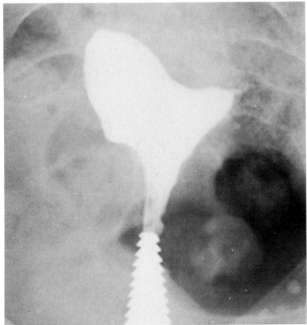

FIG. 7.7 Distortion of the uterine outline by myometrial fibroids with submucosal extensions.

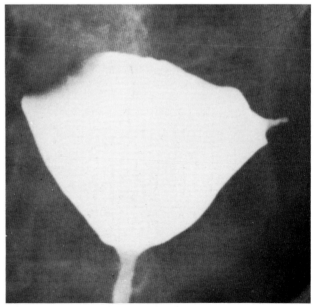

FIG. 7.9 Large, globular fibroid uterus with rounded filling defect obliterating right cornu and distorting left cornu. No tubal filling.

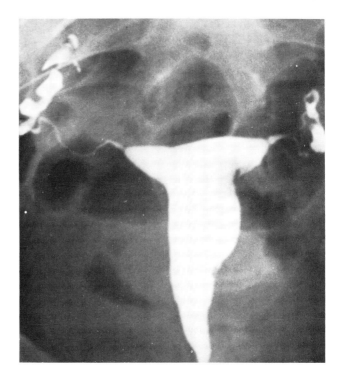

FIG. 7.10 Small submucosal fibroid partly obscured by contrast medium on hysterography.

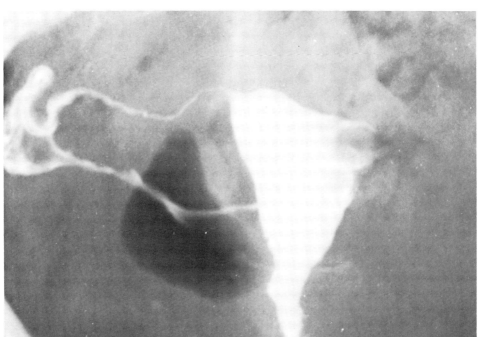

FIG. 7.11 Two rounded, well circumscribed fibroids in the left cornual region. Non-filling of left Fallopian tube.

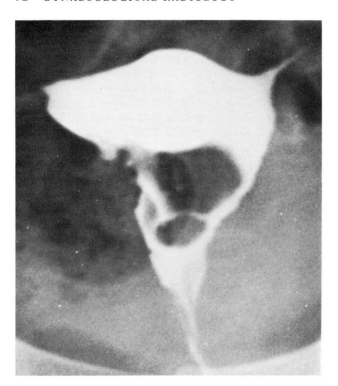

FIG. 7.12 Large, pedunculated fibroid.

Subserous fibroids usually give no definite signs on hysterosalpingography, but may sometimes be so large as to cause deformity of the uterine cavity with compression and deviation of a Fallopian tube. Peritoneal spillage of contrast medium may delineate subserous fibroids. A sinus tract between the uterine cavity and the inside of a calcified and presumably necrotic fibroid has been demonstrated by hysterography (Alpert & Lecher, 1954).

Hysterography should be performed in order to show the extent of uterine deformity after myomectomy, before allowing the patient to become pregnant (Fig. 7.13).

Intravenous urography and cystography

Under optimal conditions, it is possible to demonstrate uterine fibroids in 85% of cases during the 'vascular' phase of the intravenous urogram (Imray, 1975). It is preferable to use an infusion of contrast medium, 300 ml of 30% methylglucamine diatrizoate over a period of ten

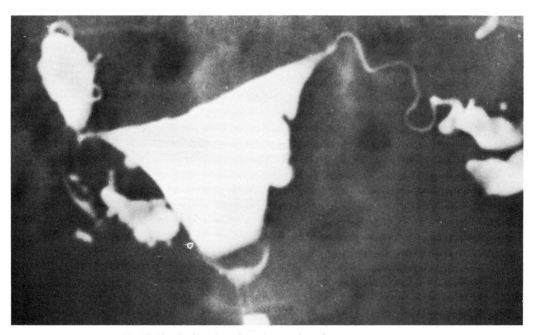

FIG. 7.13 Deformity of uterine cavity after myomectomy.

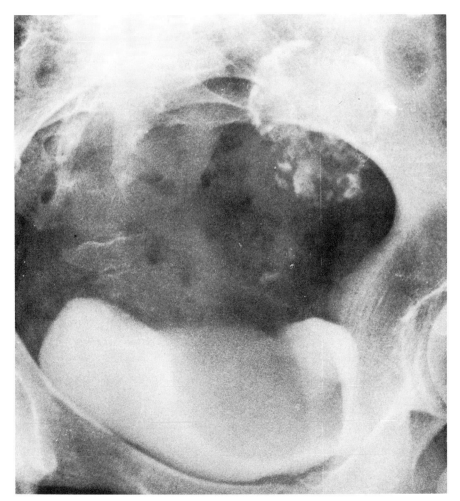

FIG. 7.14   Intravenous urogram showing lobulated bladder dome, secondary to impingement from fibroid uterus. Calcified fibroid present.

minutes being suitable. Infusion allows prolongation of the passive accumulation of contrast medium within fibroids compared to bolus injection. Preliminary AP tomography is performed prior to the infusion, and further tomograms of the pelvic region are taken after five minutes of the start of the infusion. Peck *et al.* (1975) recommend that tomography should initially be performed at 6 cm from the table top, with the patient supine, if the pelvic mass is 8 cm or less in diameter, and at 12 cm if the mass is more than 10 cm in size. The opacification of fibroids is usually diffuse (Love *et al.*, 1974; Imray, 1975).

The pelvic portions of the ureters may be poorly delineated due to compression by the enlarged uterus. Fibroid masses cause ureteral obstruction and hydronephrosis in 44 to 48% of cases (Long & Montgomery, 1952; Klempner, 1952). A very severe degree of ureteral obstruction may be present without urinary tract symptoms. As in all cases of large pelvic masses, a preoperative assessment of the urinary tract is important when there is a large fibroid uterus. Because of the benign nature of the condition, reversion of the ureters to the normal state is anticipated after hysterectomy. Ureteral obstruction is usually bilateral, but the right

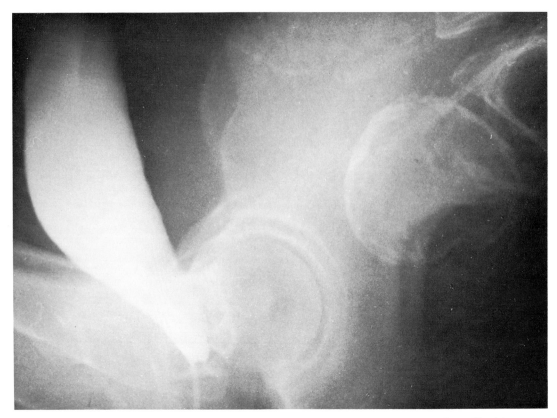

FIG. 7.15   Cystogram showing marked anterior compression and displacement of the bladder by a fibroid uterus. Calcified fibroid present.

ureter was found by Bryk (1966) and by Long & Montgomery to be more frequently and severely dilated than the left ureter.

Large fibroid masses may cause vesical compression with flattening or concavity of the dome of the bladder. Multiple pressure defects on the bladder contour occur secondary to the lobulation of the fibroid uterus (Fig. 7.14). Occasionally, extrapelvic extension of a large uterine mass may pull the uterus upwards so that the bladder has a smooth convex dome (Bryk, 1966) (Fig. 7.15). The indentation into the bladder by a subserosal fibroid may be so pronounced as to simulate a primary vesical tumour (Peterson, 1962). Cervical fibroids, or a retroverted fibroid uterus, may cause deformity and obstruction of the bladder neck on cystography (Donaldson & Ratliff, 1944). Rarely, a fistula may develop

between a fibroid and the bladder, presumably due to necrosis of the fibroid and fixity by adhesions (Nagyfy *et al.*, 1955).

Barium enema

Bryk (1967) has described barium enema findings with large fibroid masses. The sigmoid segment may be compressed at pelvic inlet level and may be deviated downwards, especially with larger masses, or upwards and to the left. The compression is smooth and the mucosal pattern remains intact (Marshak, 1947).

Fibroids may become adherent to bowel. Little & Barnhard (1960) described an unusual case of a calcified fibroid which was not only adherent to terminal ileum

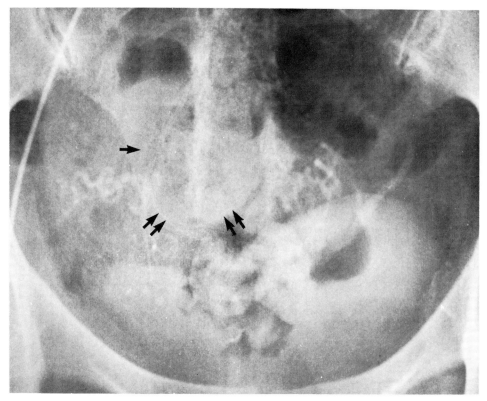

FIG. 7.16 Arteriography in presence of large fibroid. Lateral displacement and straightening of marginal part of uterine artery (single arrow). Displacement and straightening of intramural branches around fibroid (double arrow). Tumour blush is seen in late arterial phase.

but had eroded through the intestinal wall into the lumen and had caused obstruction.

Angiography

Arteriography is rarely performed in cases of suspected uterine fibroids, especially since the advent of ultrasonography, but may be helpful in the differentiation of pelvic masses in the occasional patient.

The arteriographic findings in cases of uterine fibroids have been extensively described by Lang (1967) using selective internal iliac angiography. The blood supply of fibroids is derived from the uterine artery. The marginal segment of the uterine artery shows loss of tortuosity and lateral displacement in the presence of large fibroids (Fig. 7.16). The intramural vessels also show straightening in the region of the fibroid with opacification of the splayed capsular vessels around the tumour, depending on its size and position.

Small fibroids usually have a paucity of supply arteries, but larger fibroids are often very vascular and contain numerous small intercommunicating irregular vessels (Borell *et al.*, 1952). A tumour blush is seen in larger fibroids, except when there is avascular necrosis (Radberg & Wickbom, 1967), although necrotic areas sometimes facilitate pooling of blood and thus show opacification (Smith, 1971). Pedunculated submucosal fibroids show tortuous dilated vessels entering the pedicle of the tumour.

Transmyometrial pelvic venography gives variable appearances in the presence of uterine fibroids. Bellina *et al.* (1969) have described circumscribed avascular areas within a distorted uterine outline.

CARCINOMA OF THE CERVIX

Carcinoma of the cervix is the second most common malignancy in women after breast cancer, and accounts for 11% of all cancers in females. Cervical carcinoma constitutes two-thirds of malignant tumours found in the female genital tract. Women may develop cervical carcinoma from the early twenties to long after the menopause, but most occur between the late thirties and the middle of the sixth decade.

The absence of a defining membrane around the cervix and the presence of a rich lymphatic drainage are contributing factors to the spread of cervical carcinoma. Direct spread from the cervix to the vagina and the parametrial tissues is common. Extension on to the anterior wall of the vagina may reach the bladder and result in a vesicovaginal fistula, but direct infiltration of the bladder may also occur from the supravaginal portion of the cervix. Infiltration of the parametrium is a frequent early occurrence, with ureteral obstruction being a complication. Later, the tumour may spread along ligamentous structures to the pelvic walls. The rectum is involved late and infrequently because of the separation of the rectum from the cervix by the pouch of Douglas. The tumour may spread upwards to involve the uterine body.

Lymphatic spread tends to occur frequently and early in the disease, and is notoriously difficult to assess by clinical means. The lymph nodes of the parametrium and the obturator, internal and external iliac nodes are primarily involved, with later spread to the common iliac and para-aortic lymph nodes.

Blood borne metastases reach many organs, but the lungs, bones and liver are the most frequently involved distant sites.

The International Staging of carcinoma of the cervix is as follows:

Stage 0   – Carcinoma *in situ*
Stage I   – Confined to the cervix
Stage II – Spread to the parametrium (but not extending to pelvic wall) and/or involvement of upper third of vagina
Stage III – Fixation to the pelvic wall and/or involvement of lower two-thirds of vagina
Stage IV – Extension to the bladder or rectum, or distant metastases

Carcinoma *in situ* is treated by conisation or total hysterectomy. Surgery or radiotherapy are used to treat Stage I disease. The Wertheim or radical hysterectomy (total hysterectomy, bilateral salpingo-oophrectomy, partial vaginectomy and pelvic lymph node dissection) may be employed in Stage I and sometimes in Stage II cases. Intracavitary and external irradiation, sometimes in combination, may be used in all stages of cervical carcinoma. The choice between surgery and radiotherapy, as well as between different modes of applying the latter, varies from centre to centre, depending on personal preferences and expertise.

Radiological investigation

The soft tissues of the pelvic cavity may show little appreciable change, even in the presence of extensive neoplastic involvement. Tumour masses may occasionally cause deviation of pelvic phleboliths on serial radiographs (Steinback, 1960). Obstruction of the cervical canal by advanced disease may cause dilation of the uterus which may be radiographically visible as a round mass.

LYMPHOGRAPHY

Bipedal lymphography is a very useful means of assessing the extent of metastasis to pelvic and para-aortic lymph nodes in carcinoma of the cervix, leading to a rational treatment programme. The unreliability of clinical staging has been revealed by lymphography, para-aortic lymph node metastases being demonstrated in 6% of patients with clinical Stage I and II, and in 10% with Stage III carcinoma of the cervix (Douglas *et al.*, 1972). The overall accuracy of lymph node metastasis detection by lymphography is on average 80–85% (Fuchs & Böök-Hederström 1964; Averette *et al.*, 1969). Averette *et al.* (1969) found false positives (22%) to be commoner than false negatives (13%), while metastases were found in 71% of cases when the lymphographic appearances were suspicious of metastatic involvement without being classified as definitively positive. Palpation of para-aortic lymph nodes at operation is also less reliable than lymphography in the detection of metastases. Although the internal iliac and obturator lymph nodes are not delineated by pedal lymphography, these nodes are included in standard radiotherapy fields.

The signs of lymph node metastases are filling defects within nodes or failure of nodes to opacify, enlargement

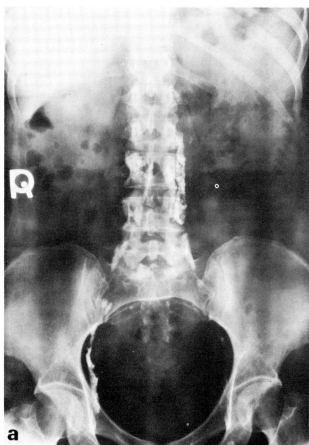

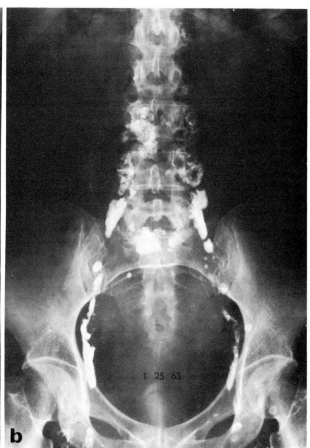

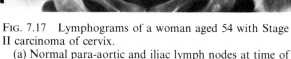

FIG. 7.17 Lymphograms of a woman aged 54 with Stage II carcinoma of cervix.

(a) Normal para-aortic and iliac lymph nodes at time of presentation.

(b) Repeat lymphogram 6 months later, following intra-cavitary radium and external radiotherapy, shows metastases in para-aortic lymph nodes. These nodes are enlarged and have rounded filling defects.

of nodes, displacement or matting of nodes (Fig. 7.17), distorted lymphatic anatomy, stasis in lymph vessels and opacification of collateral lymph nodes. Metastases are initially detected as filling defects at the periphery of the node. Further replacement of normal tissue gives the nodes a fragmented or amputated appearance. Finally, the lymph nodes will be totally replaced by tumour, and this failure of opacification will usually be associated with collateral lymphatic flow and stasis in lymph vessels.

The feasibility of surgery depends on confinement of the neoplasm to the pelvic cavity. The addition of chlorophyll to the Lipiodol has been used to facilitate identifica-tion of lymph nodes by their resulting green colour at operation (Averette et al., 1963). However, the chlorophyll distorts the lymphographic appearances and its use is not recommended for this reason. Radiographs in theatre at the time of the operation are useful to assess the completeness of lymphadenectomy. The postoperative development of lymphocysts and lymphoedema of the leg is assessed by lymphography (Chapter 11).

Treatment planning for external beam therapy is aided by lymphography, involved lymph nodes being included in the treatment field. Follow up radiographs allow assessment of response to radiotherapy. With a good response, metastases are seen to gradually reduce in size and may disappear. After complete regression the lymph nodes appear normal except for a slightly irregular outline and smaller size (Jing *et al.*, 1964). In some cases, radiotherapy may cause obstruction with extravasation of contrast medium and a reduction in opacified lymph nodes in the pelvis, signs which could also be attributed to persistence or recurrence of the carcinoma (Averette *et al.*, 1969). Apart from this, tumour recurrence in lymph nodes can be diagnosed from follow up radiographs (Fig. 7.17). Sequential radiographs confirm the presence of reactive hyperplasia, fibrosis or fatty foci and infective changes which are the differential diagnosis of metastases.

Intravenous urography is often performed routinely at the time of the 24-hour lymphographic series. Pelvic and para-aortic lymph node metastases may cause ureteral displacement and obstruction, lymphography being useful in confirming the cause and demonstrating the extent of the lymphatic spread.

The presence of lymphographically demonstrated metastases gives an important determination of prognosis. Tawil & Belanger (1973) found that only 12% of patients with positive lymphograms were alive at five years. The number of involved lymph nodes also correlates with survival time (Hsu *et al.*, 1972).

PELVIC VENOGRAPHY

Before the advent of lymphography in the early 1960s pelvic venography was the main method of determining the presence and recurrence of lymph node metastases and the response to treatment. Naturally, this was a coarse and inaccurate method and positive findings were the indentation, displacement or non-filling of pelvic veins (Carlsson *et al.*, 1961). Only 60% of patients with positive lymphograms had abnormalities on pelvic venography and inferior vena cavography, and even large lymph node masses may not cause impression on the inferior vena cava or iliac veins (Baum *et al.*, 1963). Despite these limitations, interosseous (trochanteric) venography may show pronounced venous alterations and extensive tumour invasion in the absence of clinical evidence of venous obstruction (Noriega *et al.*, 1964). Venography still has a limited role in the investigation of leg oedema in carcinoma of the cervix, a situation which is most likely to be due to tumour recurrence invading the vein and tending to cause thrombosis, or to post-irradiation pelvic fibrosis with venous compression. Envelopment

and obstruction of the pelvic portions of the ureters by cervical carcinoma will often cause similar effects on the adjacent iliac vein. Smith & Bosniak (1974) have used iliac venography to differentiate benign and malignant causes for the ureteral obstruction in these cases, finding that a normal pelvic venogram in the presence of an obstructed ureter favoured a benign aetiology for the latter.

UROGRAPHY

The pelvic portion of the ureter is vulnerable to spread of cervical carcinoma to the parametrium. In the majority of cases of ureteral obstruction, the cause is neoplastic compression or direct invasion of the ureter, perhaps by initial spread to periureteral lymphatics, although oedema and inflammation adjacent to the tumour may also contribute to the obstruction. Uraemia due to ureteral obstruction is the commonest cause of death in carcinoma of the cervix. Intravenous urography is mandatory in the pretreatment assessment of all cases of carcinoma of the cervix, and is an important investigation after treatment especially in cases with demonstrated prior ureteral involvement.

The incidence of ureteral obstruction (Fig. 7.18), as would be expected, increases with each clinical Stage (Table 7.1). Other authors have found incidences of ureteral involvement of 42% (Klempner, 1952), 53.4% (Long & Montgomery, 1952) and 23% (Dearing, 1953) prior to treatment. Ureteral involvement has a grave prognostic significance, only 41.7% surviving one year, while 77.8% with normal urograms survived one year after irradiation (Stander *et al.*, 1961). Waggoner & Spratt (1969) showed a recurrence rate of 93.5% after radiotherapy when pretreatment ureteral obstruction was present, independent of the clinical Stage of the dis-

TABLE 7.1 Percentage incidence of ureteral obstruction found on urography in carcinoma of the cervix, prior to treatment.

| | *Stage* | | | | |
	I	*II*	*III*	*IV*	*Total*
Howes & Strauss (1939)	2.0	25.0	31.0	52.0	52.0
Pomeroy (1947)	0	1.8	14.6	42.5	15.2
Aldridge & Mason (1950)	0	9.0	16.0	29.0	34.0
Kerr (1961)	6.0	12.0	24.0	48.0	17.0
Stander *et al.* (1961)	2.5	5.6	17.5	45.0	12.7
Rhamy & Stander (1962)	4.1	6.6	16.7	59.5	14.1

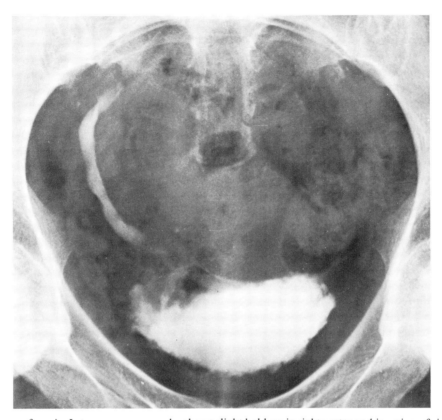

FIG. 7.18   Carcinoma of cervix. Intravenous urography shows slight hold-up in right ureter and invasion of right side of bladder by tumour.

ease. The persistence or development of obstructive ureteropathy after irradiation is associated with tumour recurrence in the great majority of cases. It is rare for ureteral obstruction to be caused by irradiation. While oedema from irradiation may precipitate complete occlusion where partial occlusion previously existed, ureteral obstruction which is progressive after the immediate effects of irradiation have subsided is indicative of active neoplastic disease (Kickham, 1961). Miller & Spear (1973) described cases in which urography demonstrated tapered narrowing of the abdominal portion of the ureter, secondary to metastatic involvement of lymph nodes and connective tissue surrounding the ureter.

Isotope renography, using I^{131} hippuran, has been found to be a more sensitive indicator of ureteral obstruction than intravenous urography in carcinoma of the cervix (Dische *et al.*, 1963; Mogensen *et al.*, 1973). When an abnormality is found on a routine pretreatment isotope renogram, subsequent urography may be used for confirmation and for anatomical localization of the obstruction (Evez *et al.*, 1968). The isotope technique is also useful for repeated follow up investigation (Gerlie *et al.*, 1961) and offers a practical alternative to intravenous urography in cases of iodine sensitivity and severe renal failure.

Mallik (1962) described irregular deformity of one side of the bladder fundus with lateral displacement of the corresponding ureter following spread of the tumour to the parametrium. Invasion of the bladder by cervical carcinoma occurs in only 1.7% of cases (Millim *et al.*, 1972). Early bladder invasion may not be apparent on radiological investigation, although associated oedema causes an ill defined filling defect in the bladder. The presence of tumour in the bladder wall is associated with

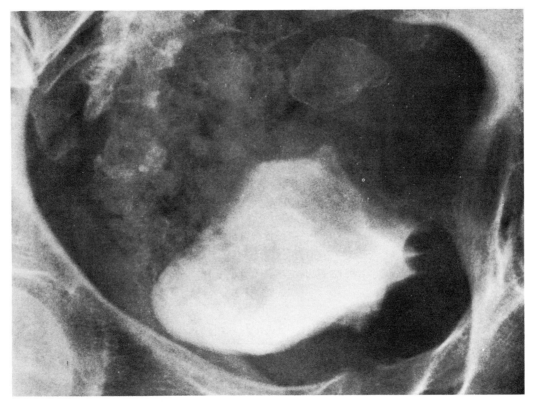

FIG. 7.19   Intravenous urography showing irregularity and filling defect on left side of bladder from direct spread by carcinoma of cervix.

an irregular localized filling defect and, when advanced, in reduction of bladder capacity (Figs 7.18 and 7.19). Vesicovaginal fistula in carcinoma of the cervix is usually a complication of hysterectomy or irradiation. The presence of tumour may itself be a direct cause of vesico-vaginal fistula, two-thirds of such cases being found at presentation, one-quarter occurring within a year of treatment and the rest developing later, with all patients dying within two years in the series of Kerr (1961), although Millim *et al.* had a 30% five year survival rate. There is often ureteral involvement by tumour when a malignant vesicovaginal fistula is present. One third of all vesico-vaginal fistulae are associated with carcinoma of the cervix and pelvic irradiation, while two thirds are due to gynaecological and obstetric procedures (Everett & Mattingly, 1956).

Pelvic pneumography has been used for the assessment of parametrial extension and in radiotherapy planning.

Although adnexal involvement and occasionally lymph node masses may be shown (Herbeau *et al.*, 1958), pelvic pneumographic changes are inconsistent and similar appearances may be found with pelvic inflammatory disease (Sala *et al.*, 1962).

PELVIC ARTERIOGRAPHY

Lang & Greer (1969) found that the accuracy of clinical staging was increased from 36% to 86% by the use of arteriography. Most cervical carcinomas show a characteristic tumour blush in the late capillary phase of the angiographic series (Fig. 7.20b). Briet (1967) claims that these vascular tumours are likely to be radiosensitive and are associated with a 50% two year survival rate, compared to a 20% two year survival for angiographically avascular tumours. Abnormal corkscrew-like vessels often supply the neoplasm (Fig. 7.20a and c). Multiple arteriovenous shunts are a common finding in histio-

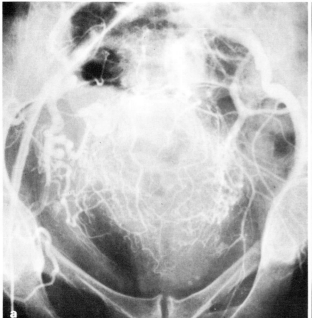

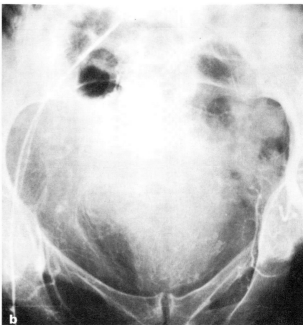

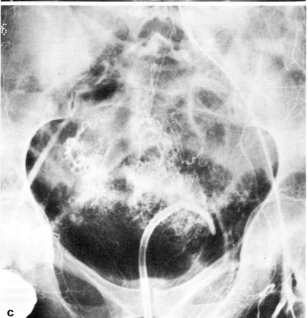

FIG. 7.20 Angiography in carcinoma of the cervix which has spread to the pelvic wall.

(a) Arterial phase shows many corkscrew-like arteries in cervix and in parametria.

(b) Tumour blush seen in pelvic cavity in capillary phase.

(c) Following ligation of both internal iliac arteries there is extensive tumour circulation supplied by collateral pelvic arteries.

four seconds suggests the presence of tumour and co-incidental inflammatory disease. Displacement and splaying of the cervical branch of the uterine artery is regarded as proof of tumour extension into the parametrium. Arteriography may also demonstrate tumour circulation in spread to the iliac lymph nodes and to the vesicovaginal septum. The internal iliac artery may be displaced by large lymph nodes. Successful radiotherapy should result in disappearance of the angiographic signs of cervical carcinoma, although it may be difficult to exclude a neoplastic recurrence of avascular tumours after high doses of irradiation which itself may cause some abnormality of small arteries (Briet, 1967).

The arteriographic investigation of cervical carcinoma has not been a common practice, partly because of difficulties in interpreting the findings. Lang & Greer

logically undifferentiated tumours which do not show a tumour blush (Lang & Greer, 1969). The same authors found that persistence of a vascular blush for longer than

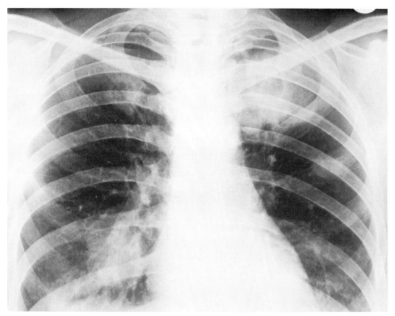

FIG. 7.21 Carcinoma of cervix. Multiple pulmonary metastases, some of which show cavitation.

FIG. 7.22 Mediastinal lymphadenopathy due to metastases from carcinoma of the cervix.

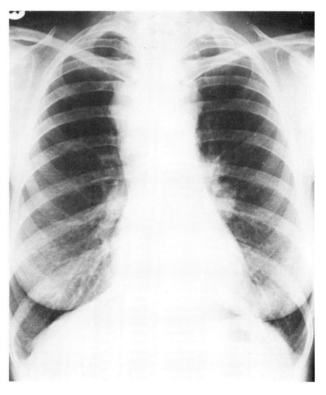

(1969) use concurrent pelvic pneumography to give improved visualization of these subtle angiographic changes.

Zeit *et al.* (1960) have used catheters inserted into the internal iliac arteries for continuous cytotoxic infusion of cervical carcinoma, although this method is not generally considered successful.

Barium enema

Spread of cervical carcinoma to the recto-sigmoid may cause a smooth, long segment of persistent narrowing, but with an intact mucous membrane (Marshak, 1947). These changes are not pathognomonic and may also be seen in retroperitoneal sarcomas, or when a fibroid uterus is associated with endometriosis or pelvic inflammatory disease. Parker & Friedman (1966) found that 7% of patients with cervical carcinoma had bowel involvement on barium enema, which is of grave prognostic significance. Colon involved by tumour does not return to normal after treatment.

Distant spread of cervical carcinoma

The usual spread of cervical carcinoma is by local extension to the parametrium and to regional lymph

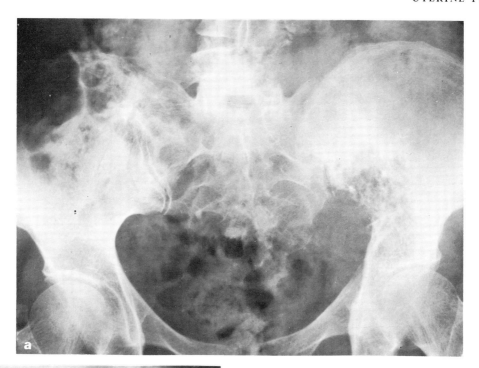

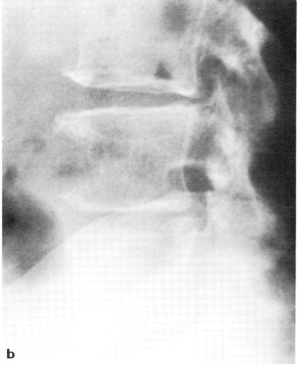

FIG. 7.23a and b   Osteolytic metastases to pelvis, sacrum and lumbar spine, consistent with invasion from involved overlying iliac and para-aortic lymph nodes.

nodes. The liver, lungs and bone are the most common sites of distant metastases, in that order. Golding (1950) found bone metastases in 2.29% and lung metastases in 3.34% of a large series of cervical carcinoma.

Parker & Friedman (1966) found lung or pleural metastases in 2.2% of cases not previously treated, and subsequently in 6% of those who had normal pretreatment chest radiographs. The lung metastases are often multiple and may show cavitation (Fig. 7.21). Solitary pulmonary metastases, sometimes with cavitation, may be indistinguishable from bronchial carcinoma (Seaman & Arneson, 1953). Mediastinal lymphadenopathy (Fig. 7.22), occasionally with lymphangitis carcinomatosa, may be seen (Buchsbaum, 1970) and is presumably due to collateral drainage to mediastinal lymph nodes via lymphatic channels in the abdominal wall when there is high pelvic neoplastic obstruction (Hreshchyshyn & Sheehan, 1965).

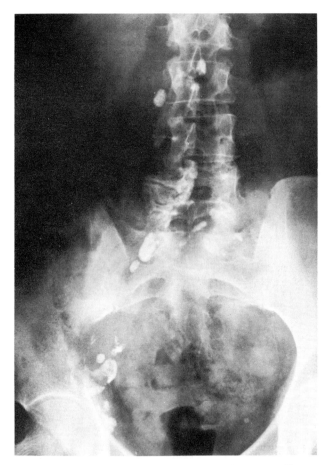

FIG. 7.24 Lymphogram in carcinoma of cervix. Filling defects and non-opacification in iliac lymph nodes with invasion of underlying right ileum.

Bone metastases often occur in the presence of widespread involvement of other organs, usually when the patient has undergone treatment and when the disease is of long standing. The metastases are osteolytic in type. The lumbar spine and pelvis, including the sacrum, are the most frequent sites of bone involvement (Fig. 7.23), in many cases due to direct invasion of underlying bone from iliac and para-aortic lymph node metastases (Fig. 7.24). However, metastatic spread to the lumbar vertebrae may be facilitated by the vertebral venous plexus. Direct lateral extension of the tumour to the pelvic wall may cause protrusio acetabulae (Elder & Maltheau, 1942).

CARCINOMA OF THE ENDOMETRIUM

Cervical carcinoma is three times more common than endometrial cancer. The peak incidence of endometrial carcinoma is between fifty-five and sixty years of age. The commonest symptoms are postmenopausal haemorrhage, irregular intermenstrual bleeding and offensive discharge. The uterus is often moderately enlarged, but may be normal in size. Pyometra, with a tender enlarged uterus, is sometimes an outcome. Endometrial carcinoma will gradually infiltrate the myometrium and tends to permeate along lymphatic channels.

Hysterosalpingography

Norman (1950) and Dufresne *et al.* (1959) have found hysterography to be a very accurate method of diagnosing the presence and extent of endometrial carcinoma, and have described two types of radiological appearance. The tumour may be circumscribed and focal, with a predilection for the upper part of the uterus. The mass is often irregular and ulcerated in these cases, but is generally well demarcated (Fig. 7.25).

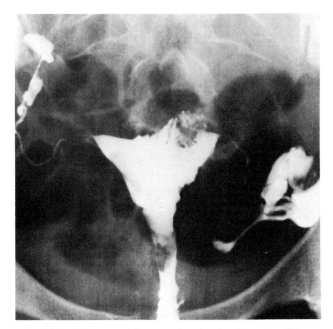

FIG. 7.25 Hysterosalpingography showing irregular filling defect with some intravasation of contrast medium in uterine fundus, due to carcinoma of endometrium.

In the diffuse variety the tumour usually involves a large area of the uterine cavity and bulges only slightly, although it is very irregular and has a shaggy outline. Large, relatively smooth, expansive tumours tend to have poorly differentiated cells; those with a markedly irregular contour will probably have better differentiation. Venous intravasation of contrast medium is found on hysterography in 10–15% of cases of endometrial carcinoma (Fig. 7.25) (Norman, 1955). Johnsson (1973) considers that intravasation may be more frequent when the tumour is poorly differentiated, and that tubal opacification is less common in the presence of poorly differentiated carcinomas. Metastases are much more frequent when there is spread to involve the cervix.

Hysterography yields more detailed information than curettage on the extent of the tumour and the presence of cervical involvement, and may be positive when curettage fails to reveal tumour tissue. Norman (1950) considers hysterography to be indicated in cases where curettage is normal despite clinical symptoms of a carcinoma. The hysterographic demonstration of tumour topography provides useful information for treatment planning.

The differential diagnosis on hysterography includes fibroids, but these have a smooth and rounded configuration. Mucosal polyps are irregular, sharply defined and are usually small. Retained placental fragments show as well defined filling defects. Localized endometrial hyperplasia has a more regular and consistent appearance than carcinoma. The early changes of tuberculous endometritis may give difficulty in differentiation, especially in Oriental patients (Fullenlove, 1969), although advanced uterine tuberculosis will show marked distortion, contraction and sinuses. Uterine sarcoma is indistinguishable from endometrial carcinoma.

Norman (1952) has noted that well defined, smooth, bulging masses may occur after irradiation and he attributes this to radionecrosis of the tumour. Follow up hysterograms show gradual diminution and eventual disappearance of this change.

Lymphography

As in carcinoma of the cervix, lymphography has been found to be valuable in the assessment and rational treatment planning of endometrial cancer. Douglas *et al.* (1972) found positive lymphograms in 19% of patients with endometrial carcinoma, with demonstrable para-aortic metastases in 9% of cases. Tumours low in the uterine body behave like carcinoma of the cervix and spread initially to hypogastric lymph nodes. Cervical involvement by the tumour increases the chance of lymphatic metastasis. Spread from the uterine body occurs directly to para-aortic lymph nodes.

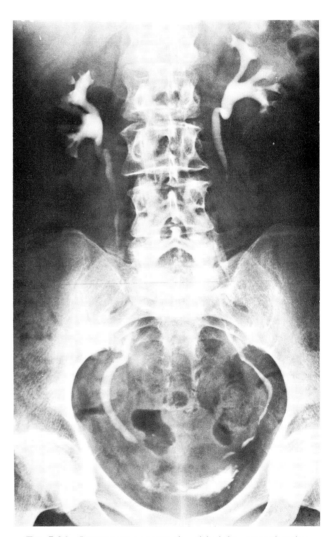

FIG. 7.26 Intravenous urography with right ureter showing some dilatation with hold-up due to endometrial carcinoma. The bladder, although underfilled, is extensively invaded by the tumour.

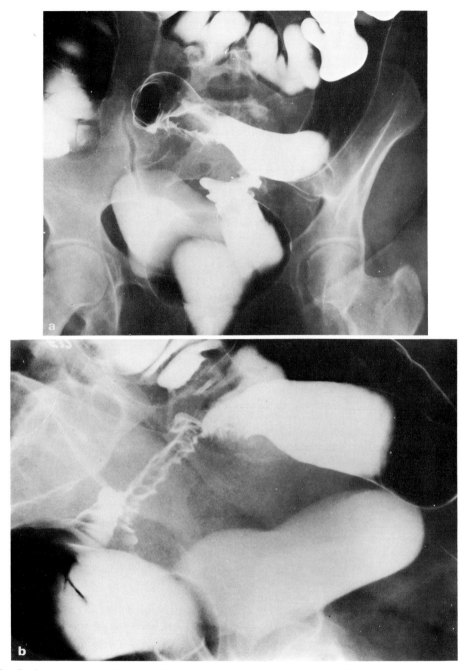

FIG. 7.27a and b   Barium enema showing serosal spread of endometrial carcinoma which has caused irregular narrowing and distortion of the sigmoid colon.

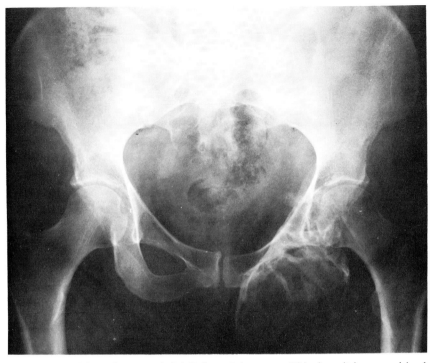

FIG. 7.28   Metastasis of endometrial carcinoma to left inferior pelvic ramus. This deposit is unusual in showing marked bony expansion. This feature is also occasionally seen in metastases from cervical carcinoma.

Urography

Endometrial neoplasms show no opacification during infusion urography (Imray, 1975). Klempner (1952) found ureteral obstruction in 40% and Long & Montgomery (1952) in 31% of cases of endometrial carcinoma (Fig. 7.26). Pre-treatment urography is therefore a part of case management.

Angiography

In the experience of Lang (1967) even considerable over-all enlargement of the uterus in endometrial carcinoma, unlike fibroids, did not cause loss of tortuosity of the marginal segment of the uterine arteries. In fact, there was often increased tortuosity of these arterial segments because of increased blood flow through the tumour. A constant feature in Lang's series was marked hyper-vascularity, with 'striate' tumour vessels and arterio-venous shunts. Vascular lakes were occasionally seen and often indicated frank necrosis in larger tumours. The presence of arteriovenous shunts resulted in very early venous opacification.

Distant metastases

Metastases outside the pelvic cavity are frequent when the carcinoma has extended outside the body of the uterus (Bunker, 1959) and usually spread to the peritoneum (Fig. 7.27) and liver.

BONE

The incidence of bone involvement is low, being found in 4.5% (Golding, 1950) to 5.6% (Geschickter & Copeland, 1949) of cases. As in carcinoma of the cervix, there is a tendency for invasion of the pelvic bones and lumbar vertebrae in endometrial carcinoma by direct spread from involved iliac and para-aortic lymph nodes. Bone metastases are osteolytic in type (Fig. 7.28).

LUNG

Lung metastases are found in 4.5% of cases (Golding, 1950).

SARCOMA OF THE UTERUS

Uterine sarcomas are a heterogenous group of tumours, comprising only 0.56% of all cases of uterine malignancy (Reich, 1949). A history of previous pelvic irradiation is found in 12% of patients with uterine sarcoma, most tumours being of the mixed mesodermal type (Norris & Taylor, 1965). The following subgroups of uterine sarcoma are identified:

1. Leiomyosarcoma and its variants arise in less than 0.25% of uterine fibroids (Gudgeon, 1968) and are the commonest sarcomatous tumours of the female genital tract.
2. Malignant mixed mesodermal tumour is the second commonest uterine sarcoma. A form of this tumour arising from the cervix is known as sarcoma botryoides.
3. Endometrial stromal sarcoma is a relatively rare tumour.

The peak incidence of sarcoma of the uterus is 40 to 60 years, but sarcoma botryoides arising from the cervix or vagina occurs typically in infancy.

Radiological features

LEIOMYOSARCOMA

Pulmonary metastases may occur secondary to leiomyosarcoma. In some well differentiated tumours, it may be difficult to assess malignancy on histological grounds and survival may be prolonged in these cases even in the presence of slow growing pulmonary or lymph node metastases (Bachman & Wolff, 1976).

As well as lung and para-aortic lymph node metastases, bone secondaries are sometimes seen in leiomyosarcoma. These are often osteolytic in nature, but osteoblastic metastases have also been found (Robbins, 1943).

Leiomyosarcoma is characterized by tumour vessels on pelvic angiography. Eroded vessels result in the formation of vascular lakes within necrotic tissue (Lang, 1967).

MIXED MESENCHYMAL TUMOURS

An osteosarcomatous element in this group of tumours may show calcification (Scheffey et al., 1956).

Very undifferentiated uterine sarcomas are distinguished by marked hypervascularity and 'anarchism' of the angiographic vascular pattern, with dissimilarity of the vascular pattern within various areas of the tumour (Lang, 1967).

SARCOMA BOTRYOIDES

Sarcoma botryoides in infancy, arising from upper vagina and cervix, may produce polypoidal masses which may fill the vagina. Vaginography, cystography and barium enema may be helpful in evaluating the extent of the tumour.

HYDATIDIFORM MOLE AND CHORIOCARCINOMA

A variety of abnormalities occurring in the chorion include hydatidiform mole, non-invasive and invasive (chorioadenoma destruens) in type, and choriocarcinoma. The incidence of these lesions varies in different parts of the world, but they affect one in every two thousand pregnancies in the United Kingdom and in the United States of America.

A hydatidiform mole is an irregular mass of grape-like vesicles of varying sizes, often mixed with fibrin, clotted blood and necrotic tissue. Microscopically, there is cystic dilatation of the placental villi, which are filled with a myxomatous hydropic stroma. There is an absence of blood vessels within the abnormal villi. It seems that the primary abnormality probably lies in the trophoblast, with excessive fluid within the villi, the destruction of blood vessels and death of the embryo being secondary to this abnormality. A rapid increase in uterine size results, with abortion occurring in most cases within a few weeks of conception. Hydatidiform mole is associated with elevated levels of chorionic gonadotrophin.

In some cases molar tissue penetrates deeply into the uterine wall, resulting in destruction of the myometrium. This is known as the invasive type of hydatidiform mole, although the histological appearances are indistinguishable from the noninvasive type, the difference being purely due to location and behaviour. Perforation of the uterine wall, secondary to invasion by the mole, results in haemorrhage into the peritoneal cavity or broad ligaments. Occasionally, parts of the invasive mole spread to the lungs via the circulation and 'metastases' result.

Choriocarcinoma is a highly malignant tumour of the

embryonic chorion, but is fortunately much less frequent than hydatidiform mole. However, choriocarcinoma is preceded by a hydatidiform mole in 50% of cases, and by normal pregnancy and abortion in about equal proportion in the rest. The twenty-one to thirty year age group is especially affected, and the risk of developing choriocarcinoma is greatest in first pregnancies. The tumour is usually diagnosed within a few weeks of pregnancy, and occasionally late in the course of a normal pregnancy or soon after delivery. Rarely, the tumour may become manifest years after a pregnancy. Haemorrhagic tumour masses arise from the lining of the uterine body. Irregular extensions of the tumour invade uterine muscle, erosion of blood vessels resulting in intrauterine bleeding. Necrosis frequently occurs within the tumour. Haematogenous spread of metastases may occur to almost any part of the body, the lungs and vagina being the most frequent sites. A history of recent abortion or pregnancy followed by persistent bleeding should always raise the suspicion of choriocarcinoma, especially in the presence of a poorly involuted uterus. Characteristically, there is a high and rising titre of urinary chorionic gonadotrophin. The treatment of choice is aggressive chemotherapy.

Radiology of hydatidiform mole

Prior to the widespread use of ultrasonography, the direct transabdominal injection of contrast medium into a hydatidiform mole (Fig. 7.29) had been employed to demonstrate hydatidiform moles (Senties *et al.*, 1969). An average of 20 to 30 ml of water-soluble contrast medium was injected along a No. 18 spinal needle, or via a thin trochar and cannula, which had been inserted into the uterine cavity under local anaesthesia. Typically, round or radiolucent filling defects, 5–15 mm in diameter, were surrounded by the contrast medium. Ultrasound is now regarded as an accurate method of detecting and assessing hydatidiform mole and has replaced the direct contrast study.

ANGIOGRAPHY

The role of arteriography is to distinguish the type of trophoblastic lesion and to evaluate the possibility of an invasive trophoblastic tumour following a molar pregnancy. The uterine arteries, and in most cases the ovarian arteries, are enlarged in length and calibre. Enlargement of the uterus causes increased separation of the marginal segments of the uterine arteries, with stretching of the fundal branches over the upper pole of the uterus. The intramural branches are not clearly seen and are less conspicuous than in a normal pregnant patient with a uterus of corresponding size (Cockshott *et al.*, 1964). After the arterial phase, the opacified intervillous spaces are widely dispersed and show poor opacification. A consistent feature is the disparity in size between the hypertrophied vascular supply to the uterus and the relatively avascular uterine contents. Borell & Fernström (1961) described smooth rounded filling defects, due to hydropic vesicles, at the edge of the opacified intervillous spaces, although this is not always a conspicuous feature as there may be small and widely scattered intervillous spaces without recognizable filling defects (Hirsch & Ben-Aderet, 1967). Normally, the intervillous spaces have frayed, irregular contours. Borell & Fernström (1961) also noticed that the intervillous spaces are fewer in number and more widely separated than in normal cases. The uterine arteries may remain hypertrophied for at least a week after evacuation of the mole, but no vascular pooling is then seen within the uterus (Cockshott *et al.*, 1964). Dilution of the contrast medium within the bulky uterus necessitates an injection of the order of 60 ml into the aorta.

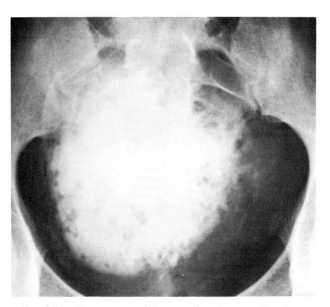

FIG. 7.29 Percutaneous injection of contrast medium into uterus. Multiple rounded filling defects within the contrast opacification are due to hydropic vesicles.

LUNG LESIONS

Pulmonary emboli from the invasive type of hydatidiform mole may show as rounded nodules on chest radiographs. Spontaneous regression, with histological evidence of necrosis, is the eventual outcome of these 'benign' pulmonary deposits (Jacobson & Enzer, 1959; Meyer, 1966).

Radiology of choriocarcinoma

ANGIOGRAPHY

Arteriography has been helpful in distinguishing between retained hydatidiform mole and choriocarcinoma in problem cases, and to provide a means of early detection of choriocarcinoma in those patients whose chorionic gonadotrophin levels remain elevated after molar pregnancy. The effectiveness of chemotherapy on the uterine tumour may be judged by arteriography, but this is done more accurately and simply by serial chorionic gonadotrophic assay. Unfortunately, the primary tumour may regress in the pelvis while distant metastases persist. Internal iliac perfusion has been used as a method of giving chemotherapy.

The uterine arteries are usually greatly increased in size (Fig. 7.30), more so than with a uterus of similar size containing either a normal pregnancy or a hydatidiform

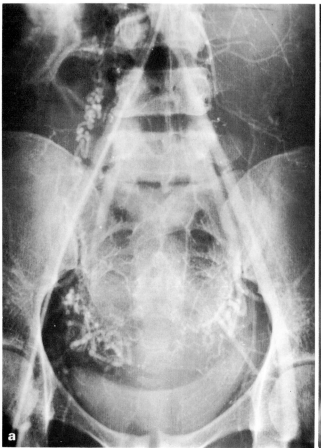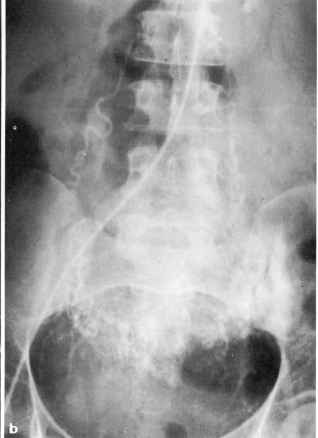

FIG. 7.30   Aortogram in choriocarcinoma.
(a) Arterial phase showing dilatation and tortuosity of uterine and ovarian arteries.

(b) Late arterial phase shows irregular tumour vessels, vascular spaces within the uterine cavity, and opacification of iliac veins due to arteriovenous shunting.

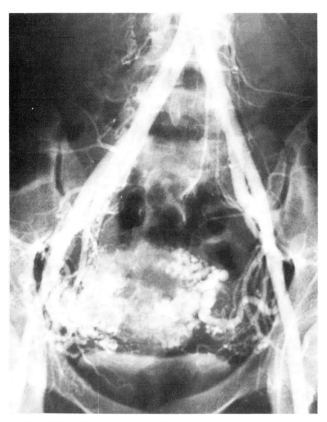

FIG. 7.31 Aortogram in choriocarcinoma showing enlarged uterine arteries and intramural branches and florid intrauterine tumour circulation.

mole (Cockshott *et al.*, 1964). The intramural arteries are also dilated (Fig. 7.31), especially those in the region of the tumour (Brewis & Bagshawe, 1968). Vascular spaces of irregular size and shape are a consistent feature, with florid shunting from these spaces into draining veins (Fig. 7.30). Sometimes there may be frank arteriovenous shunting (Borell *et al.*, 1955). Areas of abnormal vascularity often show central avascularity, due to blood clot or amorphous fibrinoid material (Brewis & Bagshawe, 1968). When there is spread into the uterine wall and beyond the uterus, similar vascular changes may be seen with dilatation of arteries to the region of involvement, vaginal and ovarian metastases having been demonstrated by Brewis & Bagshawe. Tumours as small as 1 cm in diameter have been shown on arteriography (Kolstad *et al.*, 1969).

Selective catheterization of the ovarian arteries shows enlargement of these vessels, and Lathrop & Frates (1970) have claimed that it is possible to identify these tumours more accurately than by aortic or internal iliac arteriography. Contrast medium injected into ovarian arteries passes directly to diseased areas, with improved delineation and a reduction in dilutional effects. Shimkin *et al.* (1971) have found selective internal iliac arteriography to be particularly good in the detection and localization of choriocarcinomas, especially when there is extrauterine spread, and in the demonstration of residual pelvic disease after chemotherapy.

It is usually possible to distinguish between noninvasive hydatidiform mole and choriocarcinoma by angiography, but the diagnostic differentiation of choriocarcinoma and invasive mole may be difficult and relies on subtle distinctions (Takahashi & Nagata, 1971). Kolstad *et al.* (1969) claimed a higher detection rate for angiography than curettage in the diagnosis of choriocarcinoma, although Brewis & Bagshawe (1968) failed to find some tumours on angiography which had been detected by other means.

Arteriovenous shunting in the uterus may persist after successful chemotherapy in choriocarcinoma (Cockshott & Hendrickse, 1967; Stern *et al.*, 1968).

Levin *et al.* (1975) found ultrasonography to be as sensitive as, and perhaps more specific than, angiography in the detection of choriocarcinoma, with the added advantages of being noninvasive and easily repeatable. However, they considered that arteriography had a role in cases in which ultrasonography was equivocal and where there was a suspicion of local invasion.

METASTASES

The vagina and other extrauterine pelvic structures are common sites of metastasis. Obstructive uropathy and bladder involvement may be demonstrated by intravenous urography.

The lungs are the most frequently recognized site of extrapelvic metastases from choriocarcinoma. Usually these metastases are nodular, multiple, and of varying size, but may occasionally be solitary. Less often they show as localized or diffuse patchy infiltrative changes often difficult to differentiate from pneumonia, varying in size from small areas to nearly complete consolidation of both lungs and from soft homogenous confluent shadowing to a more nodular configuration (Fig. 7.32)

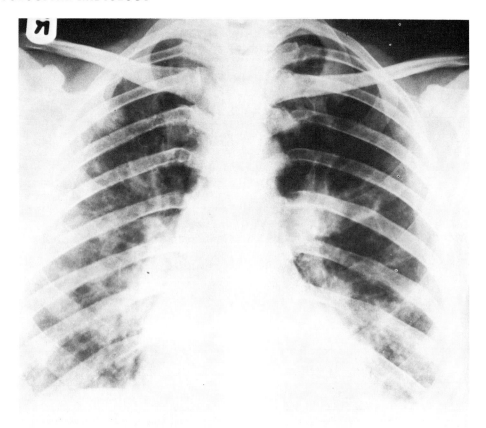

FIG. 7.32   Multiple ill-defined pulmonary metastases in choriocarcinoma.

(Hilbish & Schulz, 1960). Multiple tiny nodules, about 3 mm in diameter and giving a miliary pattern, may be seen (Lemahieu *et al.*, 1958). This pattern is associated with intra-arterial metastases which slowly progress until there is eventual occlusion of a pulmonary artery. Occasionally, pulmonary metastases may be the presenting feature of choriocarcinoma (Louisson & Foote, 1957). Large arteriovenous shunts may be demonstrated by angiography in pulmonary metastases and persist after successful treatment (Green *et al.*, 1973). It has been claimed that pulmonary metastases may rarely regress spontaneously after hysterectomy (Chun & Hou, 1957; Garber & Morrison, 1958). Calcification rarely occurs at the site of pulmonary metastases which have been successfully treated with chemotherapy (Cockshott & Hendrickse, 1969). Malignant pleural effusion, either alone or in combination with pulmonary metastases, may be

the first sign of metastatic disease. Occasionally, pleural haemorrhage of sudden onset may also be seen.

Isotope brain and liver scans are useful in showing metastases to these organs. Metastases to the small intestine and epidural lumbar invasion have been demonstrated radiologically by Hilbish & Schulz (1960). Skeletal and lymph node involvement is very rare.

REFERENCES

Fibroids

ALPERT M. & LECHER B. D. (1954) Opacification of a calcified leiomyoma during hysterosalpingography. *J. Canad. Ass. Radiol.*, **5**, 38–41.
BELLINA J. H., DOUGHERTY C. M. & MICKAL A. (1969) Transmyometrial pelvic venography. *Obst. Gynec.*, **34**, 194–199.

BORELL U., FERNSTRÖM I., LINDBLOM K. & WESTMAN A. (1952) The diagnostic value of arteriography of the iliac artery in gynaecology and obstetrics. *Acta Radiol.*, **38**, 247–263.

BRYK D. (1966) Roentgen evaluation of large uterine and ovarian masses. *Obst. Gynec.*, **28**, 630–636.

BRYK D. (1967) Barium enema examination in the evaluation of large pelvic masses. *Amer. J. Roentgenol.*, **101**, 970–977.

DONALDSON S. W. & RATLIFF R. K. (1944) Extravesical lesions causing bladder neck obstruction. *Radiology*, **43**, 319–324.

DUFRESNE M. R., GERIN-LATJOIE L. & MALTAIS R. (1959) Problems in hysterosalpingography. *J. Amer. Med. Assoc.*, **170**, 1169–1171.

FINKLE A. L., PRINCE C. L. & SCARDINO P. L. (1954) On the incidence of calcified uterine fibroids. *Amer. J. Obst. Gynec.*, **67**, 79–84.

IMRAY T. J. (1975) Evaluation of pelvic masses during infusion excretory urography. *Amer. J. Roentgenol.*, **125**, 60–65.

KLEMPNER E. (1952) Gynecological lesions and ureterohydronephrosis. *Amer. J. Obst. Gynec.*, **64**, 1232–1241.

LANG E. K. (1967) Arteriography in gynecology. *Radiol. Clin. N. Amer.*, **5**, 133–139.

LITTLE E. E. & BARNHARD J. H. (1960) Uterine leiomyoma as a cause of small bowel obstruction. *Amer. J. Roentgenol.*, **84**, 281–284.

LONG J. P. & MONTGOMERY J. B. (1952) The incidence of ureteral obstruction in benign and malignant gynecological lesions. *Amer. J. Obst. Gynec.*, **59**, 552–562.

LOVE L., MELAMED M., COOPER R. A., MONCADA R. & SCHWARTZ H. (1974) Infusion tomography of the female pelvis. *Amer. J. Roentgenol.*, **122**, 299–307.

MARSHAK R. H. (1947) Extrinsic lesions affecting the rectosigmoid. *Amer. J. Roentgenol.*, **58**, 439–450.

MARSHAK R. H., GOLDBERGER M. A. & EPSTEIN W. A. (1950) Value of hysterography in the diagnosis of large submucous uterine fibroids. *Radiology*, **55**, 725–727.

NAGYFY S. F., HOCK E. & COURTRAGE W. H. (1955) Vesicouterine fistula associated with a calcified leiomyoma. *Amer. J. Obst. Gynec.*, **69**, 861–864.

PECK A. G., YODER I. C. & PFISTER R. C. (1975) Tomography of pelvic abdominal masses during intravenous urography. *Amer. J. Roentgenol.*, **125**, 322–330.

PETERSON C. G. (1962) Uterine fibromyoma simulating bladder tumour. *J. Urol.*, **87**, 363–364.

PIETILÄ K. (1969) Hysterography in the diagnosis of uterine myoma. *Acta Obstet. Gynecol. Scandinav.*, **48**, Suppl. 5.

RADBERG C. & WICKBOM I. (1967) Pelvic angiography and pneumoperitoneum in the diagnosis of gynaecologic lesions. *Acta Radiol. (Diag.)*, **6**, 133–144.

ROZIN S. (1956) The diagnosis of submucous fibroids by hysterography. *J. Obst. Gynaec. Br. Emp.*, **63**, 917–919.

SMITH R. S. (1971) Pelvic arteriography in the differential diagnosis of pelvic mass. *Amer. J. Obst. Gynec.*, **111**, 952–958.

Carcinoma of the cervix

ALDRIDGE C. W. & MASON J. T. (1950) Ureteral obstruction in carcinoma of the cervix. *Amer. J. Obst. Gynec.*, **60**, 1272–1280.

AVERETTE H. E., VIAMONTE M. I. & FERGUSON J. H. (1963) Lymphangioadenography as a guide to lymphadenectomy. *Obst. Gynec.*, **21**, 682–686.

AVERETTE H. E., LE MAINE W. J. & LE PAGE J. R. (1969) Lymphography, arteriography and venography in gynecologic cancer. *Clin. Obst. Gynec.*, **12**, 372–397.

BAUM S., BRON K. M., WEXLER L. & ABRAMS H. L. (1963) Lymphangiography, cavography and urography. Comparative accuracy in the diagnosis of pelvic and abdominal metastases. *Radiology*, **81**, 207–218.

BRIET A. (1967) *Angiography of Uterine Tumours and their Recurrences*. George Thieme, Stuttgart, Germany.

BUCHSBAUM H. J. (1970) Lympangitis carcinomatosis secondary to carcinoma of cervix. *Obst. Gynec.*, **36**, 850–860.

CARLSSON E., HOLTZ S. & SHERMAN A. I. (1961) Demonstration of lymph node metastases by pelvic venography. *Amer. J. Roentgenol.* **85**, 21–28.

DEARING R. (1953) A study of the renal tract in carcinoma of the cervix. *J. Obst. Gynaec. Br. Emp.*, **5**, 165–174.

DISCHE S., CAPLAN L. & KRAMER S. (1963) The isotope renogram in carcinoma of the cervix. *Amer. J. Roentgenol.*, **90**, 149–156.

DOUGLAS B., MACDONALD J. S. & BAKER J. W. (1972) Lymphography in carcinoma of the uterus. *Clin. Radiol.*, **23**, 286–294.

ELDER J. R. & MALTHEAU N. M. (1942) Invasion of the bony pelvis by carcinoma of the cervix uteri as a cause of pathologic central dislocation of the hip. *Ann. Surg.*, **116**, 1–5.

EVERTEE H. S. & MATTINGLY R. F. (1956) Vesicovaginal fistula. *Amer. J. Obst. Gynec.*, **72**, 712–724.

EVEZ S., JORDAN W. M., KAPLAN A. L. & BURDINE J. A. (1968) Use of radioisotope renography and intravenous pyelography in carcinoma of the cervix. *Amer. J. Obst. Gynec.*, **101**, 947–953.

FUCHS W. A. & BÖÖK-HEDERSTRÖM G. (1964) Lymphography in the diagnosis of metastases with special reference to the carcinoma of the uterine cervix. *Acta Radiol. (Diag.)*, **2**, 161–171.

GERLIE A. B., FLANAGAN C. L. & WOODBURY L. P. (1961) The radioisotope renogram. A method of evaluation of urinary tract dysfunction associated with gynecological operations; preliminary report. *Obst. Gynec.*, **18**, 44–51.

GOLDING F. C. (1960) Metastatic tumours of bone – diagnostic aspects. *J. Fac. Radiol.*, **1**, 246–252.

HERBEAU J., VERHAEGHE M. & LEQUINT A. (1958) Gaseous pelvigraphy. Its use in the evaluation of endopelvic extension of cervical cancer. *J. Radiol. Électrol.*, **39**, 1–12.

HOWES W. E. & STRAUSS H. (1939) The significance of urological surveys in cervical carcinoma. *Amer. J. Roentgenol.*, **41**, 63–68.

HSU C-T., CHENG Y-S. and SU S-C. (1972) Prognosis of uterine cervical cancer with lymph node metastases. *Amer. J. Obst. Gynec.*, **114**, 954–962.

HRESHCHYSHYN M. M. & SHEEHAN F. R. (1965) Collateral lymphatics in patients with gynecologic cancer. *Amer. J. Obst. Gynec.*, **91**, 118–121.

JING B-S, MCGRAW J. P. & RUTLEDGE F. N. (1964) Gynecologic applications of lymphangiography. *Surg. Gynec. Obst.*, **119**, 763–772.

KERR W. K. (1961) The significance of urinary tract complications in carcinoma of the cervix uteri. *Surg. Gynec. Obst.*, **113**, 219–226.

KICKHAM C. J. E. (1961) Urologic problems in carcinoma of the cervix. *Surg. Gynec. Obst.*, **112**, 27–32.

KLEMPNER E. (1952) Gynecological lesions and ureterohydronephrosis. *Amer. J. Obst. Gynec.*, **64**, 1232–1241.

LANG E. K. & GREER J. L. (1969) The value of pelvic arteriography for the staging of carcinoma of the cervix. *Radiology*, **92**, 1027–1034.

LONG J. P. & MONTGOMERY J. B. (1952) The incidence of ureteral obstruction in benign and malignant gynecologic lesions. *Amer. J. Obst. Gynec.*, **59**, 552–562.

MALLIK M. K. B. (1962) Radiological appearances of the urinary bladder in carcinoma of the cervix, before and after treatment. *J. Obst. Gynaec. Br. Cwth.*, **69**, 66–70.

MARSHAK R. H. (1947) Extrinsic lesions affecting the rectosigmoid. *Amer. J. Roentgenol.*, **58**, 439–450.

MILLER W. A. & SPEAR J. L. (1973) Periureteral and ureteral metastases from carcinoma of the cervix. *Radiology*, **107**, 533.

MILLIM R. R., RUTLEDGE F. & FLETCHER G. H. (1972) Stage IV carcinoma of the cervix with bladder invasion. *Amer. J. Obst. Gynec.*, **113**, 239–246.

MOGENSEN P., RØDHO P. & LEFEVRE H. (1973) Radioisotope renography in the surgical management of carcinoma of the cervix. *Acta Obst. Gynec. Scand.*, **52**, 109–112.

NORIEGA J., SAN MARTIN G. R. & FALCO J. (1964) Intraosseous phlebography and lymphadenography in carcinoma of the cervix and other pelvic neoplasia. *Radiology*, **83**, 219–227.

PARKER R. G. & FRIEDMAN R. F. (1966) A critical evaluation of the roentgenographic examination of patients with carcinoma of the cervix. *Amer. J. Roentgenol.*, **96**, 100–107.

POMEROY L. A. (1947) Examination of the urinary and lower intestinal tracts before treatment of carcinoma of the cervix uteri. *Amer. J. Roentgenol.*, **57**, 453–454.

RHAMY R. K. & STANDER (1962) Pyelographic analysis of radiation therapy in carcinoma of the cervix. *Amer. J. Roentgenol.*, **87**, 41–43.

SALA J. M., KEATS T. E. & DOLAN K. D. (1962) The pelvic pneumogram in carcinoma of the cervix. *Radiology*, **78**, 274–276.

SEAMAN W. B. & ARNESON A. N. (1953) Solitary pulmonary metastases in carcinoma of the cervix. *Obst. Gynec.*, **1**, 165–176.

SMITH T. R. & BOSNIAK M. (1974) Evaluation of ureteral obstruction in the bony pelvis with iliac vein venography. *Amer. J. Roentgenol.*, **120**, 124–129.

STANDER R. W., RHAMY R. K., HENDERSON W. R., LANSFORD K. G. & PEARCY M. (1961) The intravenous pyelogram and carcinoma of the cervix. *Obst. Gynec.*, **17**, 26–29.

STEINBACK H. L. (1960) Identification of pelvic masses by phlebolith displacement. *Amer. J. Roentgenol.*, **83**, 1063–1066.

TAWIL E. & BELANGER R. (1973) Prognostic value of the lymphangiogram in carcinoma of the uterine cervix. *Radiology*, **109**, 597–599.

WAGGONER C. M. & SPRATT J. S. (1969) Prognostic significance of radiographic ureteropathy before and after irradiation therapy for carcinoma of the cervix uteri. *Amer. J. Obst. Gynec.*, **105**, 1197–1200.

ZEIT P. R., HUGHES C. R., CAHILL J. J. & HAMILTON J. G. (1960) Hypogastric ureterography prior to continuous infusion of malignant tumours of uterine cervix and vagina. Preliminary report. *Cleveland Clin. Quart.*, **27**, 119–124.

Carcinoma of the endometrium

BUNKER M. L. (1959) The terminal findings in endometrial carcinoma. *Amer. J. Obst. Gynec.*, **77**, 530–538.

DOUGLAS B., MACDONALD J. S. & BAKER J. W. (1972) Lymphography in carcinoma of the uterus. *Clin. Radiol.*, **23**, 286–294.

DUFRESNE M. R., GERIN-LAJOIE L. & MALTAIS R. (1959) Problems in hysterosalpingography. *J. Amer. Med. Assoc.*, **170**, 1169–1171.

FULLENLOVE T. M. (1969) Experience with over 2,000 uterosalpingographies. *Amer. J. Radiol.*, **106**, 463–471.

GESCHICKTER C. F. & COPELAND M. M. (1949) *Tumors of Bone.* Lippincott, Philidelphia.

GOLDING F. C. (1950) Metastatic tumours of bone–diagnostic aspects. *J. Fac. Radiol.*, **1**, 246–252.

IMRAY T. J. (1975) Evaluation of pelvic masses during infusion excretory urography. *Amer. J. Radiol.*, **125**, 60–65.

JOHNSSON J. G. (1973) Hysterography and diagnostic curettage in carcinoma of the uterine body. *Acta Radiol. Suppl.*, 326.

KLEMPNER E. (1952) Gynecological lesions and ureterohydronephrosis. *Amer. J. Obst. Gynec.*, **64**, 1232–1241.

LANG E. K. (1967) Arteriography in gynecology. *Radiol. Clin. N. Amer.*, **5**, 133–149.

LONG J. P. & MONTGOMERY J. B. (1952) The incidence of ureteral obstruction in benign and malignant gynecologic lesions. *Amer. J. Obst. Gynec.*, **59**, 552–562.

NORMAN O. (1950) Hysterography in cancer of the corpus of the uterus. *Acta Radiol. Suppl.*, 79.

NORMAN O. (1952) Hysterographically visualized radionecrosis following intrauterine radiation of cancer of the corpus of the uterus. *Acta Radiol.*, **37**, 96–102.

NORMAN O. (1955) Recent advances in hysterosalpingography and angiography in gynaecological diagnosis. *J. Obst. Gynaec. Br. Emp.*, **62**, 816–825.

Sarcoma of the uterus

BACHMAN D. & WOLFF M. (1976) Pulmonary metastases from benign-appearing smooth muscle tumors of the uterus. *Amer. J. Radiol.*, **127**, 441–446.

GUDGEON D. H. (1968) Leiomyosarcoma of the uterus. *Obst. Gynec.*, **32**, 96–100.

LANG E. K. (1967) Arteriography in gynecology. *Radiol. Clin. N. Amer.*, **5**, 133–149.

NORRIS M. J. & TAYLOR H. B. (1965) Post-irradiation sarcomas of the uterus. *Obst. Gynec.*, **26**, 689–694.

REICH S. B. (1949) Sarcoma of the uterus. *Amer. J. Roentgenol.*, **61**, 830–838.

ROBBINS L. L. (1943) Roentgenologic demonstration of spinal metastases from leiomyosarcoma of the uterus. *Arch. Surg.*, **47**, 462–467.

SCHEFFEY L. C., LEVINSON J., HERBUT P. A., HEPLER T. K. & GILMORE G. H. (1956) Osteosarcoma of the uterus. *Obst. Gynec.*, **8**, 444–450.

Hydatidiform mole and choriocarcinoma

BORELL U., FERNSTRÖM I. & WESTMAN A. (1955) The value of pelvic arteriography in the diagnosis of mole and chorionepithelioma. *Acta Radiol.*, **44**, 378–384.

BORELL U. & FERNSTRÖM I. (1961) Hydatidiform mole diagnosis by pelvic angiography. *Acta Radiol.*, **56**, 113–118.

BREWIS R. A. L. & BAGSHAWE K. D. (1968) Pelvic arteriography in invasive trophoblastic neoplasia. *Brit. J. Radiol.*, **41**, 481–495.

CHUN D. & HOU P. C. (1957) Spontaneous regression of pulmonary metastases in a case of chorionepithelioma. *J. Obst. Gynaec. Br. Emp.*, **64**, 222–226.

COCKSHOTT W. P., EVANS K. T. & HENDRICKSE J. P. DE V. (1964) Arteriography of trophoblastic tumours. *Clin. Radiol.*, **15**, 1–8.

COCKSHOTT W. P. & HENDRICKSE J. P. DE V. (1967) Persistent arteriovenous fistulae following chemotherapy of malignant trophoblastic disease. *Radiology*, **88**, 329–334.

COCKSHOTT W. P. & HENDRICKSE J. P. DE V. (1969) Pulmonary calcification at the site of trophoblastic metastases. *Brit. J. Radiol.*, **42**, 17–20.

GARBER E. C. & MORRISON R. H. (1958) Spontaneous regression of pulmonary metastases following hysterectomy for choriocarcinoma. *Amer. J. Obst. Gynec.*, **76**, 812–816.

GREEN J. D., CARDEN T. S., HAMMOND C. B. & JOHNSTRUDE I. S. (1973) Angiographic demonstration of arteriovenous shunting in pulmonary metastatic choriocarcinoma. *Radiology*, **108**, 67–70.

HILBISH T. F. & SCHULZ E. (1960) Roentgenologic manifestations of trophoblastic tumours. *Amer. J. Roentgenol.*, **83**, 66–77.

HIRSCH M. & BEN-ADERET N. (1967) Angiography in diagnosis of benign hydatidiform mole. *Obst. Gynec.*, **30**, 498–506.

JACOBSON F. J. & ENZER N. (1959) Hydatidiform mole with 'benign' metastasis to lung. *Amer. J. Obst. Gynec.*, **78**, 868–875.

KOLSTAD P. & LIVERUD K. (1969) Pelvic arteriography in malignant trophoblastic neoplasia. *Amer. J. Obst. Gynec.*, **105**, 175–182.

LATHROP J. C. & FRATES R. E. (1970) Selective ovarian angiography in trophoblastic disease. *Obst. Gynec.*, **35**, 844–851.

LEMAHIEU S. F., LAMIROY H. & PANNIER R. (1958) Pulmonary manifestations of choriocarcinoma. *J. belge de radiol.*, **41**, 195–217.

LEVIN D. C., STAIANO S., SCHNEIDER M. & BECKER J. A. (1975) Sonography and arteriography in the management of uterine choriocarcinoma. *Amer. J. Roentgenol.*, **125**, 462–468.

LOUISSON G. I. & FOOTE A. (1957) A case of chorionepithelioma. *J. Obst. Gynaec. Br. Emp.*, **64**, 442–447.

MEYER J. S. (1966) Benign pulmonary metastasis from hydatidiform mole. *Obst. Gynec.*, **28**, 826–829.

SENTIES L., PERDOMO A. & LUNA R. (1969) Diagnosis of hydatidiform mole by hysterography through transabdominal injection. *Obst. Gynec.*, **33**, 352–357.

SHIMKIN P. M., VAN THIEL D. H. & ROSS G. T. (1971) Selective hypogastric arteriography in uterine choriocarcinoma. *Amer. J. Roentgenol.*, **111**, 535–546.

STERN W. Z., LOPEZ F. & HERZIG N. (1968) Persistent angiographic abnormalities after cure of malignant trophoblastic disease. *Radiology*, **91**, 1019–1021.

TAKAHASHI M. & NAGATA Y. (1971) Angiography of trophoblastic tumours. *Amer. J. Roentgenol.*, **112**, 779–787.

CHAPTER 8

Cysts and Tumours of the Ovaries

NON-NEOPLASTIC CYSTS OF THE OVARIES

Follicular cysts

Ovarian follicles normally enlarge up to 1.5 cm in diameter, but usually involute with the death of the ovum. Follicular cysts result when an atretic follicle becomes distended with fluid and are usually 3 to 10 cm in diameter. They may be associated with endometrial hyperplasia and metropathia haemorrhagica. Most follicular cysts are symptomless, although larger cysts may be associated with heaviness and discomfort in the pelvis. Torsion and rupture may occur and cause abdominal pain. Follicular cysts often undergo spontaneous regression.

Lutein cysts

GRANULOSA LUTEIN CYSTS

These are due to haemorrhage into a corpus luteum at the time of vascularization. Resorption of the blood may initiate a subsequent accumulation of fluid. The resultant cyst is usually 1 to 4 cm in diameter. Intracapsular haemorrhage may cause pelvic pain, and rupture of the cyst results in intraperitoneal haemorrhage (Chapter 1). Spontaneous regression or persistence of the cyst will otherwise result.

THECA LUTEIN CYSTS

The luteinization of theca cells of atretic follicles is responsible for this type of cyst, a process associated with excessive chorionic gonadotrophin in cases of hydatidiform mole and choriocarcinoma. The ovaries are polycystic and vary in size from slight enlargement to filling of the pelvic cavity and lower abdomen.

Radiology

Non-neoplastic cysts are shown on plain radiographs as well defined, rounded soft-tissue masses within the pelvic cavity and sometimes extending into the abdomen (Fig. 8.1). They are seen to be distinct from the urinary bladder, and from the uterus when it is visible, although a distended bladder may give diagnostic difficulties. Large ovarian cysts tend to appear as essentially midline masses. Calcification is absent from these simple cysts. Ovarian cysts elevate the small intestine (Fig. 8.1) and, when very large, also cause lateral displacement of bowel shadows. This is an important differential point between those cysts which are so large that their borders cannot be readily defined and which cause bulging of the flanks, and ascites which extends as homogenous soft tissue opacification beyond the centrally situated bowel (Fig. 8.2).

UROGRAPHY

Tomography of an ovarian cyst during infusion of urographic contrast medium shows the mass lesion to be avascular because of a failure of opacification. However, a thin curvilinear zone of opacification is seen at the margin of at least half of ovarian cysts (Fig. 8.3), the so-called 'rim sign' (Phillips *et al.*, 1974; Imray, 1975). This effect is particularly well seen in the rare ovarian cysts of the newborn (Carlson & Griscom, 1972). Large ovarian cysts may cause hydronephrosis with dilatation

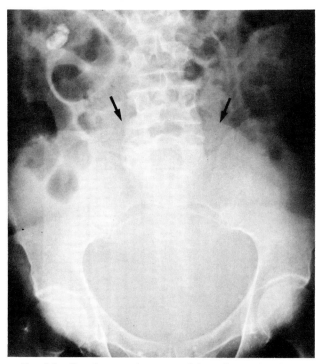

FIG. 8.1 Ovarian cyst shown on plain radiograph as large, well defined and rounded mass rising out of the pelvic cavity into the abdomen (arrows). Elevation of small intestine is also present.

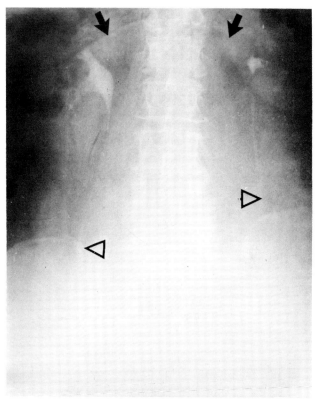

FIG. 8.2 Huge ovarian cyst, the upper border of which is well defined (closed arrows). Lateral and upward displacement of bowel. Lateral displacement of ureters (open arrows) shown on intravenous urography.

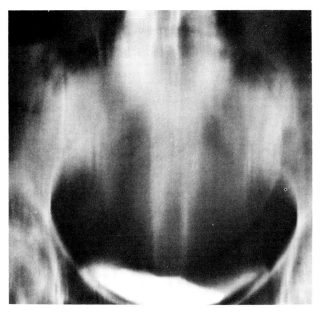

and lateral deviation of the ureters (Fig. 8.4). Long & Montgomery (1952) found the incidence of ureteral obstruction by benign ovarian masses to be 58%, while Klempner (1952) quotes the incidence as 32% in these cases. The right ureter, as in Fig. 8.4, tends to be more severely affected than the left ureter. The stretched ureters are often underfilled by contrast medium. The bladder is compressed from above by ovarian masses, so that its dome is flattened and concave (Fig. 8.5). Sometimes the compression is bipartite, with a localized concavity due to the normal uterine impression and a

FIG. 8.3 'Rim sign' of opacified thin wall of ovarian cyst during infusion urography (tomogram).

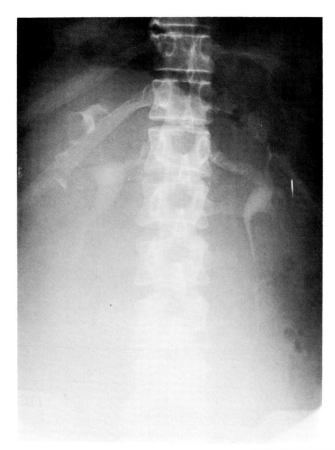

generalized flattening due to the ovarian mass (Bryk, 1966).

HYSTEROSALPINGOGRAPHY

Large ovarian cysts cause displacement of the uterus and the ipsilateral Fallopian tube is stretched around the mass (Fig. 8.6).

BARIUM ENEMA

Relatively mobile benign ovarian masses which are completely intra-abdominal have no effect on the sigmoid colon and rectum, although large masses may cause lateral deviation of the descending colon and elevation of the caecum and transverse colon. Flattening of the anterior aspect of the sigmoid segment may be present at pelvic brim level, especially on the post-evacuation radiograph, when the ovarian mass lesion is in the pelvic colon (Bryk, 1967) (Fig. 8.7).

ANGIOGRAPHY

Ovarian cysts cannot be demonstrated with certainty using arteriography, but may be differentiated by pelvic pneumography from other poorly vascularized pelvic masses (Radberg & Wickbom, 1967). Ovarian cysts will

FIG. 8.4 Intravenous urography showing very large ovarian cyst causing lateral displacement of both ureters and right-sided hydronephrosis.

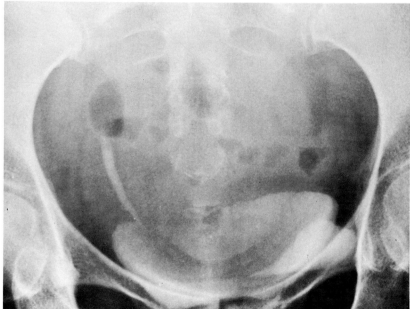

FIG. 8.5 Flattening and concavity of bladder by large ovarian cyst. The localized concavity on the right side of the dome may be due to the uterine impression.

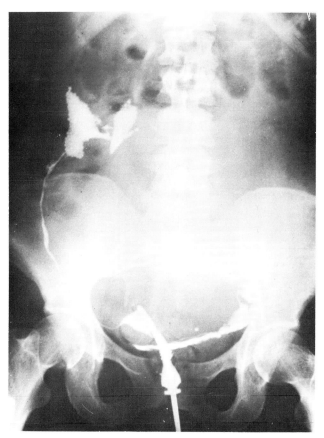

FIG. 8.6 Hysterosalpingogram showing the uterus deviated to the right and the right Fallopian tube stretched around a large ovarian cyst.

cause displacement of tubo-ovarian branches of the uterine artery (Altemus, 1969).

STEIN-LEVENTHAL SYNDROME

The Stein-Leventhal syndrome typically consists of amenorrhoea and sterility in the second and third decades, with a variable degree of hirsutism in 50% of patients and obesity in 10% of cases (Stein, 1945). The breasts may be fully developed or show hypoplasia. The ovaries contain multiple follicular cysts, full of clear fluid which contains oestrogen, and thickening of the ovarian capsule. The hormone profile shows low or normal oestrogen levels, normal urinary 17-ketosteroids, and

normal or elevated FSH levels. As Jeffcoate (1964) states, the variation in the features described in the Stein-Leventhal syndrome causes its diagnosis to rest on an insecure basis, and probably reflects a widespread endocrine dysfunction. The treatment originally consisted of wedge resection of the ovaries, but more recently clomiphene has been given with success.

Pelvic pneumography

Pelvic pneumography was originally used by Stein & Leventhal (1935) to diagnose the presence of the bilateral polycystic ovaries (Fig. 8.8). Bimanual palpation, even under general anaesthesia, is an inaccurate method of assessing ovarian size in the Stein-Leventhal syndrome. However, determination of the size and shape of the ovaries by pelvic pneumography shows much inconsistency. While the ovaries tend to be enlarged (Stein & Leventhal, 1935; Edwards & Evans, 1963), they may often be of normal size (Daves et al., 1964; Weigen & Stevens,

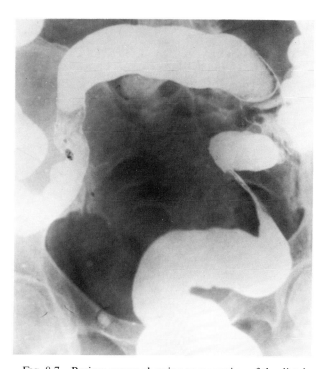

FIG. 8.7 Barium enema showing compression of the distal part of the sigmoid segment and elevation of its redundant proximal portion by an ovarian cyst.

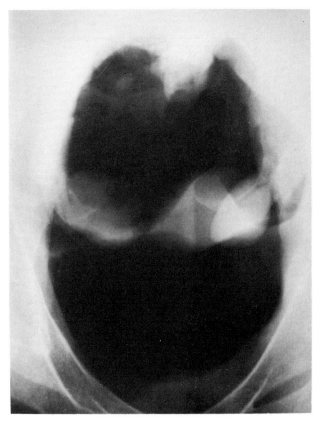

FIG. 8.8 Pelvic pneumogram showing enlarged lobulated ovaries in Stein-Leventhal syndrome.

1967). Ovarian size is often arbitrarily measured by the ovarian index, which is the maximum length multiplied by the maximum width on pelvic pneumography. Weigen & Stevens showed considerable overlap between the ovarian index in normal women (3.7–14.6 cm², average 9 cm²) and that found in Stein-Leventhal syndrome (6.0–38.0 cm³, average 16.8 cm²). Lobulations due to cysts may be seen in the syndrome, even when the ovaries are not enlarged (Kreel, 1972). At times, the ovarian enlargement is greater on one side than on the other (Stevens, 1967), but usually enlargement is fairly symmetrical with a rounded or elongated configuration (Weigen & Stevens, 1967).

Variation in the ovary–film distance and angulation of the ovaries will cause errors in the quantitative assessment of ovarian size. Abrahams et al. (1971) confirmed the large errors in estimating ovarian size from pelvic pneumography when compared with measurements obtained directly at laparotomy. Laparoscopy is probably the most appropriate investigation nowadays, especially with the advent of drug treatment for the condition.

Uterine hypoplasia is present in the Stein-Leventhal syndrome when the ovarian changes occur early in life, or when secondary amenorrhoea has persisted for some years (Stein, 1945). Relating the pneumographic size of the ovaries and uterus is invalid, not only because of the variation in uterine size but also because of the compounding of large errors which are inherent in the two individual measurements (Abrahams et al., 1971).

Mammography

Balcar et al. (1972) have found a decreased amount of glandular breast tissue for the patient's age on mammography in 87% of cases of Stein-Leventhal syndrome. This change persists even after wedge resection of the ovaries and subsequent pregnancy.

EPITHELIAL TUMOURS

Epithelial tumours account for more than half of all ovarian neoplasms, and occur as either mucinous or serous types which in turn may be either benign or malignant in form. Ovarian carcinomas may also be solid in nature. Cancer of the ovary causes more deaths than any other gynaecological malignancy, about four thousand per year in Britain.

Serous cystadenoma and cystadenocarcinoma

Benign tumours in this group tend to be mainly cystic in nature while malignant forms, comprising a quarter of serous tumours, have a larger solid component. The size may range from a few centimetres in diameter to enormous dimensions. The external and internal surfaces of both the benign or malignant form may be either smooth or studded with papillary masses. The papillarity of these tumours is a distinguishing feature when present, and is certainly related to a malignant potential. Serous tumours may be unilocular but often contain multiple loculations. Psammoma bodies are often present, in the stroma of both benign and malignant lesions. Both ovaries are involved in up to 50% of cases.

Serous carcinomas spread directly to the peritoneum, to the endometrium by lymphatic permeation or by direct implantation through the tubal lumen, and may also spread to the para-aortic lymph nodes.

Mucinous cystadenoma and cystadenocarcinoma

These tumours usually occur during the third to fifth decades, and vary in size from 5 cm to huge masses. Malignancy is present in only 5% of this group, and only 5% of mucinous tumours affect both ovaries. The tumour is generally multilocular with a smooth external surface. Papillary growth is far less frequent than in serous tumours. Mucinous tumours, whether benign or malignant, may rupture to give pseudomyxoma peritonei in 3.5% of cases. A similar condition may be associated with a mucocoele of the appendix. Malignant mucinous tumours may spread directly to the peritoneum and adjacent viscera, and may also metastasize to the uterus. Unlike serous cystadenocarcinoma, they do not often cause a 'frozen pelvis' and uncommonly metastasize to lymph nodes.

Solid carcinoma

The majority of solid ovarian carcinomas can be traced to pre-existent lesions such as cystadenomas and granulosa-cell tumours, but some are totally undifferentiated with no clue as to their origin.

While over a third of all primary ovarian carcinomas are papillary serous cystadenocarcinomas, most of the others are solid tumours. The treatment of malignant ovarian tumours is hysterectomy and bilateral salpingo-oophrectomy followed by radiotherapy. Peritoneal implants are treated by radioactive gold in the peritoneal cavity.

Radiology of epithelial tumours

PLAIN RADIOGRAPHS

Soft tissue pelvic mass lesions, often extending into the abdomen, are a visible feature. Psammoma body calcification is often visible in serous cystadenomas (Fig. 8.9) and in 12% of serous cystadenocarcinomas (Fig. 8.10) (Castro & Klein, 1962). Individually, psammoma bodies have a punctate calcific density and aggregations of them gives a granular, hazy opacification, less dense than any of the other common calcific lesions of the abdomen and often only slightly denser than normal soft tissues. Metastases of serous cystadenocarcinoma sometimes show calcification and these may be radiographically visible within the peritoneum, liver (Fig. 8.11),

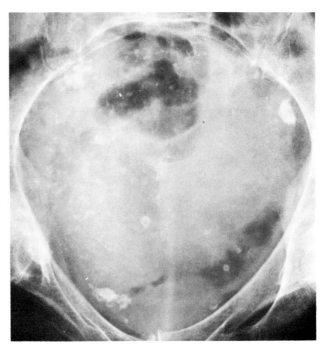

FIG. 8.9 Psammoma body calcification in serous cystadenoma of ovary.

abdominal lymph nodes, lung (Nathanson, 1950) and breast (Royen & Ziter, 1974). Metastases involving the intestine and causing ureteral obstruction may also be identified (Teplick *et al.*, 1976). Serosal metastases are often distributed along the course of the colon and may be initially mistaken for previously ingested barium (Fig. 8.12). Deposits along the lateral abdominal wall and adjacent to the properitoneal fat line are commonly visible, but the whole abdomen and pelvis may contain multiple masses of psammomatous calcification. A high uptake of technetium diphosphonate isotope has been seen in the calcified abdominal metastases (Teplick *et al.*, 1976). Bizarre dense calcifications with sharply defined margins may also be visible within serous cystadenocarcinomas (Fig. 8.12) (Lingley, 1942).

Ascites is common in ovarian carcinoma (Fig. 8.10) and, as would be expected, is usually associated with peritoneal spread. Studies using I^{131} tagged to human serum albumen unexpectedly showed that uninvolved peritoneum, not the cancer, produced most of the ascitic fluid (Hirabayashi & Graham, 1970). Occasionally, the

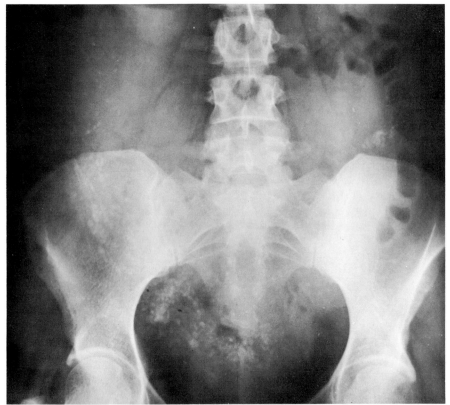

FIG. 8.10 Psammoma body calcification in cystadenocarcinoma of ovary in woman aged 34 years. The tumour was in the left ovary which was matted to the omentum and bowel. Eight litres of ascites were present.

ascites of ovarian carcinoma, and sometimes also pleural effusions, are not due to metastatic spread because they have not the characteristic features of malignant exudates and resolve spontaneously on removal of the tumour (Mueller-Heuback & Reisfield, 1970). These can be regarded as examples of pseudo-Meigs' syndrome (see p. 129) which has also been described with mucinous cystadenoma (Smith & Boronow, 1967) and other non-fibrous tumours. In general, however, pleural effusions in ovarian cancer have an ominous connotation, being related to pleural metastases with patients having an average life expectancy of 4.5 months (Graham et al., 1970).

Calcification in mucinous cystic ovarian tumours is uncommon on microscopy and its probably quite rare on radiography (Stevens, 1971), but curvilinear calcifications may develop in pseudomyxoma peritonei from mucinous cystadenocarcinoma (Moncada et al., 1974).

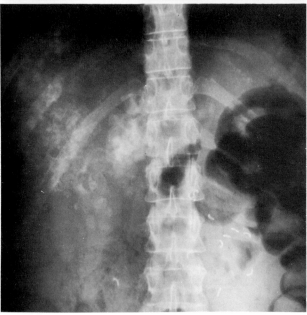

FIG. 8.11   Calcified liver metastases from serous cystadenocarcinoma.

Destruction of overlying bone by direct invasion from ovarian carcinoma is extremely rare (Fig. 8.13).

UROGRAPHY

The total body opacification effect will delineate some solid ovarian tumours (Imray, 1975). As with ovarian cysts, large tumours of the ovary compress and deviate the ureters (Fig. 8.14). Long & Montgomery (1952) found ureteral obstruction in 69% of malignant ovarian tumours and a 58% incidence with benign ovarian mass lesions. Klempner (1952) found lower incidences than these, 32% and 58% respectively for benign and malignant ovarian masses. While the ureters are usually deviated laterally by large pelvic masses, ovarian tumours sometimes cause medial deviation (Bryk, 1966).

BARIUM STUDIES

Khilnani *et al.* (1966) have described stretching, indentation and infiltration with narrowing of the rectosigmoid by extracolonic malignant pelvic masses (Fig. 8.15). The

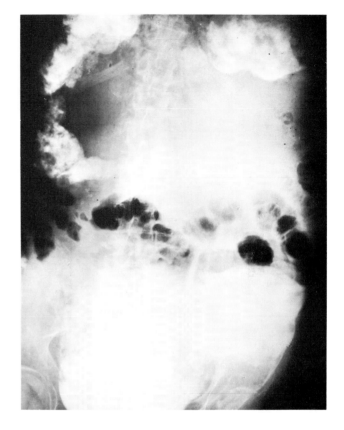

FIG. 8.12 Peritoneal metastases from serous cystadenocarcinoma along course of colon mimics residual barium with large bowel. Particularly dense calcification and curvilinear densities are also present.

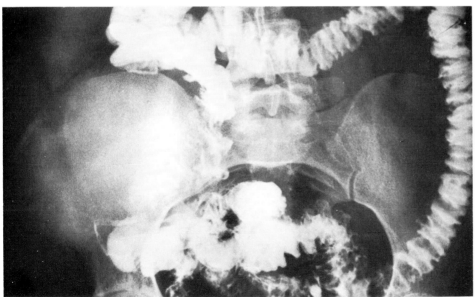

FIG. 8.13 Papillary cystadenocarcinoma of the ovary. The tumour has a high position, displaces the ascending colon medially, and has invaded the underlying right iliac crest.

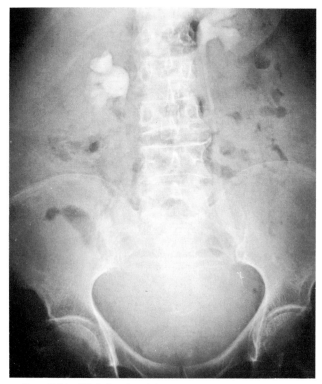

FIG. 8.14 Ill-defined pelvic mass, ascites and bilateral ureteral compression in carcinoma of the ovary.

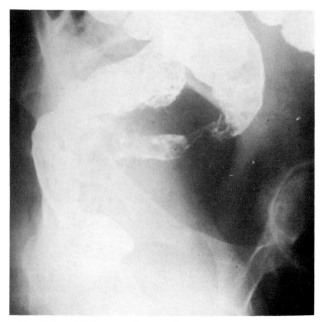

FIG. 8.15 Rigidity and narrowing of rectum and sigmoid segment by infiltration from ovarian carcinoma.

anterior aspect of the narrowed rectum will become irregular with numerous nodular defects. If the posterior wall remains distensible, it arches over the fixed area of involvement. A pattern of fixed transverse folds develops, but will be replaced by the nodular defects and mucosal ulceration. Complete obstruction may be the outcome.

Strictures and fixation of bowel, with alteration of mucosal pattern, will occur when peritoneal metastases invade underlying intestine (Fig. 8.16).

LYMPHOGRAPHY

Ovarian neoplasms metastasize to lymph nodes in 46% of cases (Athey et al., 1975). Tumours confined to the ovary metastasize to the para-aortic lymph nodes, but spread to adjacent pelvic viscera and to the peritoneum

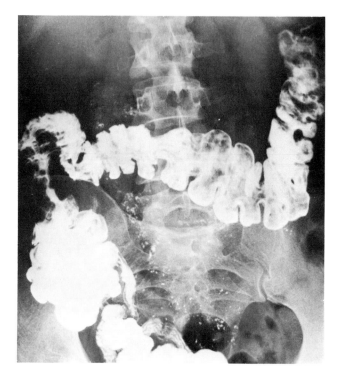

FIG. 8.16 Irregular stricture of ascending colon mimicking primary colonic carcinoma but due to invasion from ovarian carcinoma.

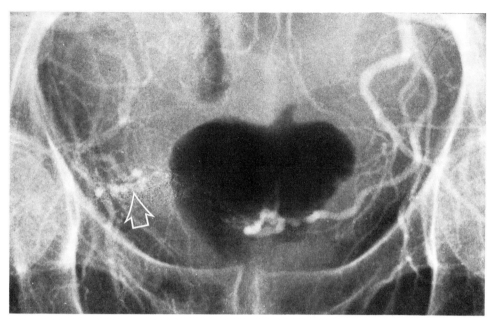

FIG. 8.17   Pelvic arteriogram. Small, irregular vessels derived from the displaced adrexal branch of the right uterine artery supply a carcinoma of the right ovary (arrow).

allows metastasis to the inguinal and iliac lymph nodes.

ANGIOGRAPHY

Ovarian tumours derive their blood supply from the adnexal branch of the uterine artery, the major sign of an ovarian tumour being stretching and straightening of this vessel although similar changes may be seen in chronic pelvic inflammatory disease (Altemus, 1969).

Ovarian carcinoma may appear relatively avascular, or very vascular overall or in part (Fig. 8.17). Pneumography has been used to differentiate between adnexal and uterine masses where angiography has shown the mass to have poor vascularity (Radberg & Wickbom, 1967).

TERATOID TUMOURS

Teratomas contain elements of all three germ layers and comprise 10% of all ovarian tumours (Novak, 1952). The vast majority of these (96.7%) are benign cystic teratomas, while only 2.95% are either malignant solid tumours or cystic teratomas with malignant degeneration (Caruso et al., 1971).

Benign cystic teratomas

The term 'dermoid cyst' would strictly be applicable for tumours whose elements are derived entirely from ectoderm. Many pathologists believe this to be a rare occurrence and, if sufficient histological sections are taken, elements from all three germ layers will be identified. 'Benign cystic teratoma' is therefore a preferable name for this tumour. Over 90% of cases present between the ages of fifteen and fifty years, with the majority in the third and fourth decades, and 10.5–11% affect both ovaries (Peterson et al., 1955; Caruso et al., 1971). Peterson et al. found 23.2% of their series of over a thousand cases of benign cystic teratomas to be asymptomatic, while pain and less often an abdominal mass or abnormal uterine bleeding were other presenting features. Benign cystic teratomas range from 2 to 45 cm in diameter, with an average size of 7.7 cm, 80% being 10 cm or less.

RADIOLOGY

The classic plain radiographic appearances are of a rounded soft tissue translucent mass in the pelvic cavity or lower abdomen, with a sharply defined capsule and

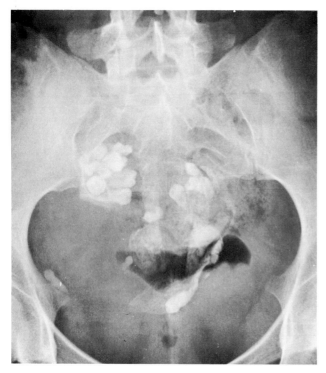

FIG. 8.18 Large benign cystic teratoma. Multiple well-formed teeth and bone are present.

signs in 64.5% of cystic teratomas. An analysis of the diagnostic criteria related to tumour sign was made by Sloan (1963). It was unusual to make a preoperative radiological diagnosis when cystic teratomas were less than 5 cm in diameter, less than a quarter of all cases being this size, while most of those between 6 and 15 cm in diameter tended to show the classic radiological appearances of intracystic calcifications, radiolucency and capsular density. Very large tumours, 16 cm or more in diameter, were difficult to diagnose because their overall density was often the same or more than that of the surrounding soft tissues, and any teeth or bone within these teratomas tended to lie well up in the abdominal cavity. Overall, Sloan found that 40% of all cystic teratomas had radiological signs which permitted a specific diagnosis.

Wollin & Ozonoff (1961) have described the case of a woman where the sequential appearance of three teeth occurred over a thirteen year period within a cystic

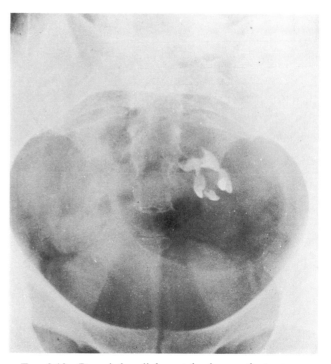

FIG. 8.19 Rounded radiolucent benign cystic teratoma with well-defined soft tissue capsule, and containing several dental elements.

containing identifiable dental or bony structures (Fig. 8.18 and 8.19). The radiolucency is due to fat-containing sebaceous material, but may have a mottled rather than homogenous appearance due to admixture with hair. The 'cystic' portion, therefore, contains mainly ectodermal derivatives such as hair and sebum, while the more solid structures tend to be aggregated in a 'plug' attached to the inner wall of the cyst (Fig. 8.20). Calcification within the cyst is often absent (Robins & White, 1940) (Fig. 8.21), but a rim of peripheral calcification may occasionally be seen (Burfield & Kemp, 1955). In a series of 225 cases, Blackwell et al. (1946) found teeth in 31% and bone in 41% of cystic teratomas. Peterson et al. (1955) and Georgakopoulos (1965) found cystic teratomas where calcification of the fatty contents, secondary to necrosis following torsion, gave the tumours a radiological appearance of a sharply defined mass of homogenous calcific density.

Peterson et al. (1955) found diagnostic radiological

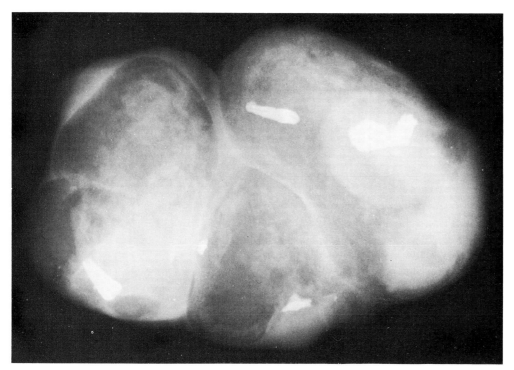

FIG. 8.20 Radiograph of excised benign cystic teratoma. Mottled appearance due to hair intermingled with radiolucent sebum. Solid 'plug' on left side. Several teeth are present.

teratoma, densely radio-opaque enamel being followed by the adjacent formation of calcified dentine. Levi (1951) and Engel *et al.* (1965) have described three cases where recurrence of cystic teratoma had followed local resection of such a tumour some years previously with conservation of the affected ovary. Bilateral ovarian cystic teratomas have been documented in triplets (Feld *et al.*, 1966).

Struma ovarii is the name given to cystic teratomas in which thyroid tissue composes more than 50% of tissue or when functioning thyroid tissue is present. In 15–25% of cases there is enlargement of the thyroid gland (Adcock, 1972). An isotope scan of the pelvic mass may show increased uptake of radioactive iodine, although this finding may also occur in haemorrhagic ovarian cysts which do not contain thyroid tissue (Nodine & Maldia, 1961). Thyroid adenocarcinoma occasionally develops in struma ovarii, tends to be slow growing and occasionally metastasizes to brain and bone.

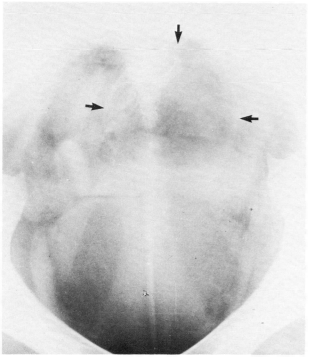

FIG. 8.21 Radiolucent benign cystic teratoma with well defined capsule, but not containing any calcification (arrows).

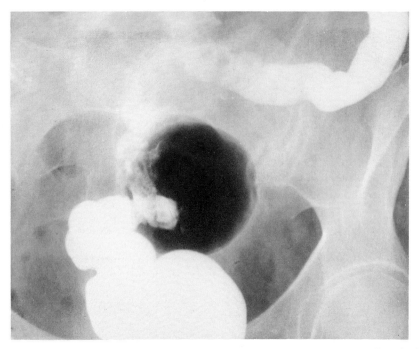

FIG. 8.22 Gas-containing infected benign cystic teratoma. The infection spread from adjacent diverticular disease, shown on barium enema.

Other complications of cystic teratoma

TORSION

Torsion has been variously reported in 7.5% (Blackwell *et al.*, 1946), 13% (Sloan, 1963) and 16% (Peterson *et al.*, 1955) of cystic teratomas, but only in 3.6% of those with malignant degeneration (Peterson, 1957). Torsion is especially prone to occur during pregnancy (Campbell, 1973) and childhood (Thatcher, 1963), circumstances where the tumours tend to lie in the abdomen and therefore have increasing mobility. If torsion is acute, gangrene is common and occasionally leads to rupture of the cyst. Chronic torsion may lead to the development of a collateral circulation via adhesions or parasitism, and occasionally to hyalinization with calcification.

RUPTURE

The intraperitoneal rupture of a benign cystic teratoma may be followed after a period of time by calcification of peritoneal implants, sometimes confused with tuberculous peritonitis or peritoneal carcinomatosis (Kistner,

1952). Acute symptoms with paralytic ileus may occur at the time of rupture (Abitbol *et al.*, 1959).

INFLAMMATION

This complication has been reported in 1.2% of cases (Peterson *et al.*, 1955) while predispositions to inflammation include pregnancy, torsion, tapping of the cyst and inflammatory disease of adjacent pelvic organs. Gas (Fig. 8.22) and a fluid level may be seen in an infected cyst (Sloan, 1963).

FISTULA FORMATION

Following infection of a benign cystic teratoma, there may be spontaneous rupture into the urinary bladder (Tancer *et al.*, 1955). Sebaceous material and hair are passed into the urine and there are accompanying symptoms of cystitis. Cystography will show contrast medium entering the cyst from the bladder. Bladder calculus is sometimes an occurrence in these cases (Detar, 1954). Occasionally, a cyst will perforate into the rectum

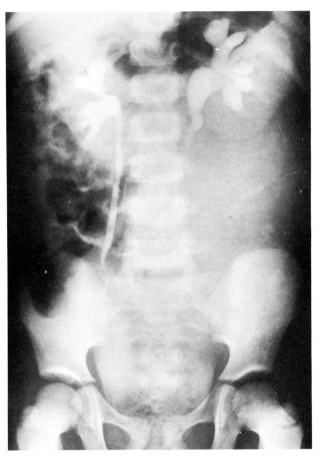

FIG. 8.23 Large malignant solid teratoma of the ovary in child aged 3 years. Linear and amorphous calcification in the large abdominal mass. Associated left-sided hydronephrosis seen on intravenous urography.

(Bacon & Eisenberg, 1951) or may rarely communicate with both bladder and rectum (Dandia, 1967).

MALIGNANT TERATOMA

The average age of presentation of malignant teratomas is 61 years (Caruso et al., 1971). Malignant transformation occurs in 2% of benign cystic teratomas (Malkasian et al., 1965), with direct invasion of surrounding tissues as well as pelvic and abdominal metastases. The malignant tissue is usually a squamous cell carcinoma, although other tumours such as sarcoma, carcinoid tumour, adenocarcinoma and melanoma sometimes occur. Ascites and

hydrothorax without pleural metastases have been described in association with malignant teratomas (Peterson, 1957).

The majority of solid teratomas are highly malignant and usually occur in childhood and adolescence. They may contain calcification in the form of linear and branching spicules (Fig. 8.23), recognizable teeth and bone being rare (Berger & Pochaczevsky).

MEIGS' SYNDROME

Meigs & Cass in 1937 described seven cases of ovarian fibroma associated with hydrothorax and ascites. Meigs (1954a) has defined the criteria necessary for the diagnosis of his syndrome: (1) The ovarian tumour must be benign and solid, with the gross appearance of a fibroma. Thecomas, granulosa cell tumours and Brenner's tumour, which also have a large fibrous element, are included within the criteria. (2) Ascites, which may be very small or enormous in amount. (3) Pleural effusion, usually on the right side but occasionally on the left and rarely in both pleural cavities (Fig. 8.24). (4) Spontaneous disappearance of the ascites and pleural fluid occurs on removal of the ovarian tumour. The serous exudate is usually clear and yellow, but occasionally is blood stained or serosanguinous in nature. On review of the literature and his own cases, Meigs (1954b) found the syndrome to occur in association with 13.7% of ovarian fibromas. However, while some large series have found the incidence of ascites to range from 18% (Fino, 1948) to 30% (Rubin et al., 1944) and 43% (Rökaeus, 1949), the association with pleural effusion was 12%, 4.3% and 3.2% respectively in these same series.

Occasionally, other ovarian lesions, including epithelial cysts, teratomas, primary cystadenocarcinomas (Calmenson et al., 1947; Meigs, 1954a), Krukenberg tumours (Brenner & Scott, 1968) as well as uterine fibroids (Martinez-Esteve & Orrico, 1950) have been associated with ascites and pleural effusion which are spontaneously resolved with their excision. These are best described as pseudo-Meigs' syndrome.

Gross oedema of the tumour (Calmenson et al., 1947; Meigs, 1954a) has been consistently observed in the ovarian fibromas in Meigs' syndrome, and may be associated with leakage of fluid from the tumour into the peritoneal cavity. The oedema may follow partial venous

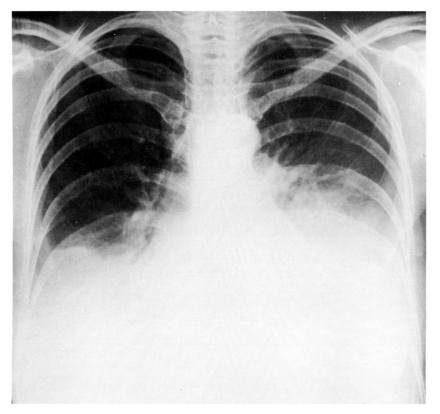

FIG. 8.24   Bilateral pleural effusions in Meigs' syndrome.

obstruction (Dockerty & Masson, 1944) and necrosis (Fino, 1948) within the tumour.

Hodari & Hodgkinson (1968) describe lymphography in one case of Meigs' syndrome. Contrast medium was recognized within pleural fluid, but not in the ascites, and the suggestion was made that the pleural fluid was derived via intrathoracic lymphatic connections from the thoracic duct. As described in Chapter 1, another explanation for the pleural fluid is that distention of the peritoneal sac may cause widened interstices between muscle bundles of the diaphragm, thus allowing the permeation of the fluid into the pleural cavity (Lieberman & Peters, 1970).

FIBROMA

Apart from Meigs' syndrome, other radiological manifestations of ovarian fibromas are calcification and ossification of the tumour. The calcification takes the form of diffuse stippled and mottled areas (Sotto *et al.*, 1956) and is the result of necrosis within the tumour (Dockerty & Masson, 1944). There is a rare association of ovarian fibromas with mesenteric cysts and Gorlin's syndrome (Clendenning *et al.*, 1963).

THECOMA

Rarely, a thecoma may contain fine granular calcifications which are sufficiently dense for radiographic demonstration (Mecca *et al.*, 1974).

GONADOBLASTOMA

Gonadoblastoma of the ovary may present with symptoms of precocious puberty, oestrogenic activity or with masculinization. Seymour *et al.* (1976) found circumscribed mottled or punctate calcification within the tumour in half the cases. Pelvic pneumography will confirm that the calcification is within the ovaries and will also demonstrate uterine hypoplasia in cases of masculinization. Gonadoblastomas may occasionally metastasize but are usually benign in nature.

DYSGERMINOMA

Dysgerminoma is an ovarian tumour consisting of cells which resemble primordial germ cells. This tumour has often been reported in hermaphrodites, pseudoherm-aphrodites and other patients with genital malformations. Brody (1961), however, considers the incidence in these conditions to be not as high as originally thought, and found the majority of dysgerminomas to occur in otherwise normal women.

It is a malignant neoplasm which tends to spread to other pelvic structures. Metastases occur in 20% of cases (Brody, 1961), usually to the peritoneal cavity. Ascites develops in 10% of cases. Sometimes metastases develop in iliac and para-aortic lymph nodes, and occasionally mediastinal lymphadenopathy is found. Haematogenous metastases spread to the liver, lungs and skeleton. The bone metastases are osteolytic in nature (Pendergrass & Selman, 1946) and may be associated with periosteal reaction (Feinberg, 1960).

KRUKENBERG TUMOURS

Characteristically these tumours consist of adenocarcinoma cells diffusely arranged through the stroma or, more often, arranged in clumps together with a cellular stroma of spindle-shaped cells. Many of the tumour cells have a signet ring appearance and contain mucin. The tumours affect both ovaries in the majority of cases. Hale (1968) found primary neoplasms in the stomach in 93%, in the colon in 4% and in the breast in 2.6% of cases. It is usual for the tumours to occur before the menopause and before the age of peak incidence of carcinoma of the alimentary tract and breast. The preservation of the ovarian form and the lack of local invasion suggest a lymphatic or haematogenous route of metastasis from the primary site. In rare instances, scrupulous and repeated search for a neoplasm in the gastrointestinal tract and breast fails to reveal a primary site, and in these

cases it must be presumed that the tumour arises *de novo* in the ovary.

Ascites may be radiologically visible and there may be evidence of generalized peritoneal metastases in some cases on barium follow through examination (Lowman & Kushlan, 1945).

REFERENCES

ABITBOL M. M., POMERANCE W. & MACKLES A. (1959) Spontaneous intraperitoneal rupture of benign cystic teratomas. *Obst. Gynec.*, **13**, 198–203.

ABRAHAMS O. L., HAWKINS D. F. & LAWRENCE D. M. (1971) Estimation of ovarian size with reference to Stein-Leventhal syndrome. *Obst. Gynec.*, **38**, 117–124.

ADCOCK L. L. (1972) Unusual manifestations of benign cystic teratomas. *Obst. Gynec. Survey.*, **27**, 471–474.

ALTEMUS R. (1969) Differentiating uterine and extrauterine masses by bilateral selective hypogastric arteriography. *Radiology*, **92**, 1020–1026.

ATHEY P. A., WALLACE S., JING B. S., GALLAGHER H. S. & SMITH J. P. (1975) Lymphangiography in ovarian cancer. *Amer. J. Roentgenol.*, **123**, 106–113.

BACON H. E. & EISENBERG S. W. (1951) Ovarian dermoid perforating the rectum in a child. *Ann. Surg.*, **133**, 408–410.

BALCAR V., SILINKOVA-MALKOVA E. & MATYS Z. (1972) Soft tissue radiography of the female breast and pelvic pneumoperitoneum in the Stein-Leventhal syndrome. *Acta Radiol.* (*Diag.*), **12**, 353–362.

BERGER N. and POCHACZEVSKY R. (1969) Astrocytoma-containing ovarian teratoma in childhood. *Amer. J. Roentgenol.*, **107**, 647–651.

BLACKWELL W. J., DOCKERTY M. B., MASSON J. C. & MASSEY R. D. (1946) Dermoid cysts of the ovary: their clinical and pathological significance. *Amer. J. Obst. Gynec.*, **5**, 151–172.

BRENNER W. E. & SCOTT R. B. (1968) Meigs-like syndrome secondary to Krukenberg's tumor. *Obst. Gynec.*, **31**, 40–44.

BRODY S. (1961) Clinical aspects of dysgerminoma of the ovary. *Acta Radiol.*, **56**, 209–230.

BRYK D. (1966) Roentgen evaluation of large uterine and ovarian masses. *Obst. Gynec.*, **28**, 630–632.

BRYK D. (1967) Barium enema examination in the evaluation of large pelvic masses. *Amer. J. Roentgenol.*, **101**, 970–977.

BURFIELD G. A. & KEMP F. H. (1955) The radiological evaluation of dermoid cysts of the ovary. *Brit. J. Radiol.*, **28**, 199–203.

CALMENSON M., DOCKERTY M. B. & BIANCO J. J. (1947) Certain pelvic tumors associated with ascites and hydrothorax. *Surg. Obst. Gynec.*, **84**, 181–191.

CAMPBELL J. B. (1973) Cystic teratomas of the ovary in pregnancy. *Amer. J. Roentgenol.*, **118**, 14–17.

CARLSON D. H. & GRISCOM N. T. (1972) Ovarian cysts in the newborn. *Amer. J. Roentgenol.*, **116**, 664–672.

CARUSO P. A., MARSH M. R., MINKOWITZ S. & KANTEN G. (1971) An intense clinico-pathologic study of 305 teratomas of the ovary. *Cancer*, **27**, 343–359.

CASTRO J. R. & KLEIN E. W. (1962) The incidence and appearance of roentgenologically visible psammomatous calcifications of papillary cystadenocarcinoma of the ovaries. *Amer. J. Roentgenol.*, **88**, 861–891.

CLENDENNING W. E., HERDT J. R. & BLOCK J. B. (1963) Ovarian fibromas and mesenteric cysts: their association with hereditary basal cell cancer of the skin. *Amer. J. Obst. Gynec.*, **87**, 1008–1012.

COOPERMAN L. R., HAMLIN J. & NG E. (1968) Gonadoblastoma. *Radiology*, **90**, 322–324.

DANDIA S. D. (1967) Rectovesical fistula following an ovarian dermoid with recurrent vesical calculus. *J. Urol.*, **97**, 85–87.

DAVES M. L., DINER W. C. & BRENNER G. H. (1964) Pelvic pneumography. *Amer. J. Roentgenol.*, **92**, 390–399.

DETAR J. H. (1954) Ovarian dermoid producing a hair growing bladder diverticulum. *J. Urol.*, **72**, 837–839.

DOCKERTY M. B. & MASSON J. C. (1944) Ovarian fibromas: a clinical and pathologic study of two hundred and eighty three cases. *Amer. J. Obst. Gynec.*, **47**, 741–752.

EDWARDS E. M. & EVANS K. T. (1963) Pelvic pneumography in the Stein-Leventhal syndrome. *Brit. J. Radiol.*, **36**, 46–48.

ENGEL T., GREELEY A. V. & SWEENEY W. J. (1965) Recurrent dermoid cysts of the ovary. *Obst. Gynec.*, **26**, 757–759.

FEINBERG S. R. (1960) Dysgerminoma of the ovary: unusual roentgen manifestations of metastases. *Minnesota Med.*, **43**, 179–181.

FELD D., LAHES J. & NATHANSON M. (1966) Bilateral ovarian dermoid cysts in triplets. *Obst. Gynec.*, **27**, 525–528.

FINO J. A. (1948) A report of eighty cases of benign solid tumors of the ovary with special reference to complications. *Amer. J. Obst. Gynec.*, **56**, 808–810.

GEORGAKOPOULOS P. A. (1965) An unusual case of benign cystic teratoma of the ovary. *Amer. J. Obst. Gynec.*; **92**, 573–574.

GRAHAM J., BURSTEIN P. & GRAHAM R. (1970) Prognostic significance of pleural effusion in ovarian cancer. *Amer. J. Obst. Gynec.*, **106**, 312–313.

HALE R. W. (1968) Krukenberg tumour of the ovaries. *Obst. Gynec.*, **32**, 221–225.

HIRABAYASHI K. & GRAHAM J. (1970) Genesis of ascites in ovarian cancer. *Amer. J. Obst. Gynec.*, **106**, 492–497.

HODARI A. A. & HODGKINSON C. P. (1968) Lymphangiography of Meigs' symdrome. *Obst. Gynec.*, **32**, 477–481.

IMRAY T. J. (1975) Evaluation of pelvic masses during infusion excretory urography. *Amer. J. Roentgenol.*, **125**, 60–65.

JEFFCOATE T. N. A. (1964) The androgenic ovary, with special reference to Stein-Leventhal syndrome. *Amer. J. Obst. Gynec.*, **88**, 143–156.

KHILNANI M. T., MARSHAK R. H., ELIASOPH J. & WOLF B. S. (1966) Roentgen features of metastases of the colon. *Amer. J. Roentgenol.* **96**, 302–310.

KISTNER R. W. (1952) Intraperitoneal rupture of benign cystic teratomas. *Obst. Gynec. Survey.*, **7**, 603–617.

KLEMPNER E. (1952) Gynaecological lesions and ureterohydronephrosis. *Amer. J. Obst. Gynec.*, **64**, 1232–1241.

KREEL L. (1972) Gynaecography. *Proc. Roy. Soc. Med.*, **65**, 295.

LEVI A. A. (1951) Reformation of an ovarian dermoid cyst. *New Engl. J. Med.*, **245**, 99.

LIEBERMAN F. L. & PETERS R. L. (1970) Cirrhotic hydrothorax: further evidence that an acquired diaphragmatic defect is at fault. *Arch. Int. Med.*, **125**, 114–121.

LINGLEY J. R. (1942) The significance of psammoma body calcification in the roentgen diagnosis of papillary tumours of the ovary. *Amer. J. Roentgenol.*, **47**, 563–570.

LONG J. P. & MONTGOMERY J. B. (1952) The incidence of ureteral obstruction in benign and malignant cynecologic lesions. *Amer. J. Obst. Gynec.*, **59**, 552–562.

LOWMAN R. M. & KUSHLAN S. D. (1945) 'The Krukenberg tumour'. The roentgen and gastroenterological aspects of secondary ovarian carcinoma. *Gastroenterology*, **4**, 305–322.

MALKASIAN G. D., SYMMONDS R. E. & DOCKERTY M. B. (1965) Malignant ovarian teratomas. *Obst. Gynec.*, **25**, 810–814.

MARTINEZ-ESTEVE P. & ORRICO J. R. (1950) Myoma of the uterus associated with ascites and hydrothorax. *West. J. Surg.*, **58**, 28–32.

MECCA J. T., ELGNEZABAL A. & BRYK D. (1974) Thecoma with extensive calcification. *Brit. J. Radiol.*, **47**, 492–493.

MEIGS J. V. (1954a) Fibroma of the ovary with ascites and hydrothorax – Meigs' syndrome. *Amer. J. Obst. Gynec.*, **67**, 962–987.

MEIGS J. V. (1954b) Pelvic tumors other than fibromas of the ovary with ascites and hydrothorax. *Obst. Gynec.*, **3**, 471–486.

MEIGS J. V. & CASS (1937) Fibroma of the ovary with ascites and hydrothorax. *Amer. J. Obst. Gynec.*, **33**, 249–251.

MONCADA R., COOPER R. A., CARCES M. & BADRINATH K. (1974) Calcified metastases from malignant ovarian tumours. *Radiology*, **113**, 31–35.

MUELLER-HEUBACH E. & REISFIELD D. R. (1970) Pseudo-Meigs' syndrome resulting from ovarian malignancy. *Obst. Gynec. Survey*, **25**, 815–824.

NATHANSON L. (1950) Calcified metastatic deposits in the peritoneal cavity, liver and right lung field from papillary cystadenocarcinoma of the ovary. *Amer. J. Roentgenol.*, **64**, 467–469.

NODINE J. H. & MALDIA G. (1961) Pseudostruma ovarii. *Obst. Gynec.*, **17**, 460–462.

NOVAK E. (1952) *Gynecologic and Obstetric Pathology*. W. B. Saunders, Philadelphia.

PENDERGRASS E. P. & SELMAN J. (1946) Dysgerminoma of the ovary with widespread metastases. *Radiology*, **46**, 377–379.

PETERSON W. F. (1957) Malignant degeneration of benign cystic teratomas of the ovary. *Obst. Gynec. Survey*, **12**, 793–830.

PETERSON W. F., PROVOST E. C., EDMUNDS F. T., HUNDLEY J. M. & MORRIS F. K. (1955) Benign cystic teratomas of the ovary. *Amer. J. Obst. Gynec.*, **70**, 368–382.

PHILLIPS J. C., EASTERLY J. E. & LANGSTON J. W. (1974) Contrast enhancement of pelvo-abdominal masses: the rim sign. *Radiology*, **112**, 17–21.

RADBERG C. & WICKBOM I. (1967) Pelvic angiography and pneumoperitoneum in the diagnosis of gynaecologic lesions. *Acta Radiol. (Diag.)*, **6**, 133–144.

ROBINS S. A. & WHITE G. (1940) Roentgen diagnosis of dermoid cysts of the ovary in the absence of calcification. *Amer. J. Roentgenol.*, **43**, 30–34.

RÖKAEUS S. (1949) Fibroma of the ovary and two cases of Meigs' syndrome. *Acta Obst. & Gynec. Scandinav.*, **28**, 403–411.

ROYEN P. M. & ZITER F. M. H. (1974) Ovarian carcinoma metastatic to the breast. *Brit. J. Radiol.*, **47**, 356–357.

RUBIN I. C., NOVAK J. & SQUIRE J. J. (1944) Ovarian fibromas and theca cell tumors: report of 78 cases with special reference to production of ascites and hydrothorax. (Meigs' syndrome). *Amer. J. Obst. Gynec.*, **48**, 601–616.

SEYMOUR E. Q., HOOD J. B., UNDERWOOD P. B. & WILLIAMSON H. O. (1976) Gonadoblastoma: an ovarian tumor with characteristic pelvic calcifications. *Amer. J. Roentgenol.*, **127**, 1001–1002.

SLOAN R. D. (1963) Cystic teratoma (dermoid) of the ovary. *Radiology*, **81**, 847–853.

SMITH J. P. & BORONOW R. C. (1967) Pseudo-Meigs' syndrome with mucinous cystadenoma. *Obst. Gynec.*, **30**, 121–126.

SOTTO L. S. J., POSTOLOFF A. V. & CARR F. (1956) A case of calcified ovarian fibroma with ossification. *Amer. J. Obst. Gynec.*, **71**, 1355–1358.

STEIN I. F. (1945) Bilateral polycystic ovaries. *Amer. J. Obst. Gynec.*, **50**, 385–398.

STEIN I. F. & LEVENTHAL M. L. (1935) Amenorrhoea associated with bilateral polycystic ovaries. *Amer. J. Obst. Gynec.*, **29**, 181–191.

STEVENS G. M. (1967) Pelvic pneumography with assessment of infertility. *Radiol. Clin. N. Amer.*, **5**, 87–103.

STEVENS G. M. (1971) *The Female Reproductive Tract*. Year Book Medical Publishers, Chicago.

TANCER M. L., ORSON A., BAKER J. D. & GREENBERGER M. E. (1955) Spontaneous rupture of ovarian teratoid tumour (dermoid cyst) into urinary bladder. *Obst. Gynec.*, **6**, 668–670.

TEPLICK J. G., HASKIN M. E. & ALAVI A. (1976) Calcified intraperitoneal metastases from ovarian carcinoma. *Amer. J. Roentgenol.*, **127**, 1003–1006.

THATCHER D. S. (1963) Ovarian cysts and tumors in children. *Surg. Gynec. Obst.*, **117**, 477–483.

WEIGEN J. F. & STEVENS G. M. (1967) Pelvic pneumography in the diagnosis of polycystic disease of the ovary, including Stein-Leventhal syndrome. *Amer. J. Roentgenol.*, **100**, 680–687.

WOLLIN E. & OZONOFF M. B. (1961) Serial development of teeth in an ovarian teratoma. A thirteen-year X-ray record. *New Engl. J. Med.*, **265**, 897–898.

CHAPTER 9

Miscellaneous Conditions of the Vulva, Vagina and Uterus

THE VULVA

Carcinoma

Squamous cell carcinoma of the vulva spreads directly to the vagina, urethra, groin and anus. Lymphatic spread is to the superficial inguinal lymph nodes, and subsequently to the deep inguinal and external iliac lymph nodes. Comas et al. (1969) claim an overall accuracy of 85% in detecting the presence or absence of lymphatic metastases by lymphography. Hagen & Bjørn-Hansen (1971) found lymphography of little or no value in carcinoma of the vulva because of a high number of false positive and false negative cases. The superior superficial inguinal lymph nodes are not often shown by pedal lymphography because they drain the buttock region, yet they may be involved by direct metastatic spread from the inferior inguinal group. Vulval carcinoma usually affects the elderly, at an age when lymph node fibrolipomatosis is especially common and gives a false impression of tumour involvement. Parry-Jones (1963) has shown a deep lymphatic pathway from the vulva to the internal iliac lymph nodes which are not opacified by lymphography. As with other lymph node metastases, those from the vulva cause nodal filling defects and blockage of afferent lymphatic vessels.

Haemangiopericytoma of the vulva is a rare tumour which may cause bone metastases many years later (Reymond et al., 1972).

Vulval varices

Varices of the vulva usually occur in multiparous women and are often associated with varicose veins of the legs. The symptoms include pruritus, discomfort and occasionally severe pain. Contrast medium may be injected directly into a vulvar varicose vein, although these are often friable, or opacified by interosseous pelvic phlebography (Lea Thomas et al., 1967). Three main venous drainage routes from vulvar varices may be demonstrated by these contrast studies prior to operative treatment (Lea Thomas et al., 1967; Dixon & Mitchell, 1970): (1) through the superficial and deep external pudental veins to the greater saphenous vein and thence to the femoral vein, (2) via the obturator vein to the internal iliac vein and (3) by the vein of the round ligament which runs through the inguinal canal to join the ovarian vein. There are numerous connections between these three systems and also with the veins draining the opposite side of the vulva. The best display of the venous pathways is obtained by positioning the patient 40° oblique towards the side under investigation by venography.

THE VAGINA

Congenital abnormalities of the vagina are described in Chapter 5 and vaginitis is discussed in Chapter 6.

Foreign bodies

A bloodstained or foul smelling vaginal discharge suggests the presence of a foreign body in the vagina. This occurrence is most frequent in the first decade of life. AP and lateral radiographs will accurately locate a radio-opaque foreign body within the vagina. Vaginography is occasionally useful for demonstrating a non-opaque foreign body. The local inflammatory response to a foreign body sometimes provokes fibrous stenosis of the vagina. Radio-opaque suppositories containing iodine may be confused with bladder calculi on AP radiographs.

Vaginal calculus

Vaginal calculi may be formed by the deposition of urinary salts when there is a continuous leakage of urine into the vagina from an ectopic ureter, through a urinary fistula, or as a result of urinary incontinence in patients with neurological disease. Occasionally, a calculus reaches the vagina by ulceration of a bladder stone through the vesicovaginal septum. Many cases of vaginal calculus result from the deposition of organic salts around foreign bodies inserted into the vagina. Congenital or acquired vaginal strictures probably predispose to the formation of vaginal calculi.

A vaginal calculus often contains sufficient calcium to become radio-opaque (Fig. 9.1) and sometimes shows lamination (Navani & Tessier, 1970).

Vaginal fistulae

URETEROVAGINAL FISTULA

This fistula most often results from ureteral severence or vascular compromise sustained during hysterectomy (see

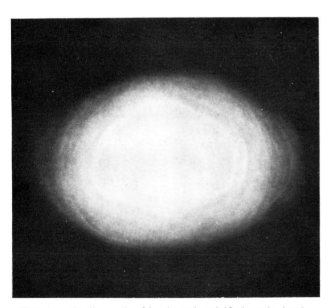

FIG. 9.1 Radiograph of laminated, calcified vaginal calculus (4 cm × 2.5 cm) removed from a bedridden patient with multiple sclerosis.

Fig. 11.5). Radiotherapy for uterine malignancy is another cause of ureterovaginal fistula.

VESICOVAGINAL FISTULA

In the extensive series of Chassar Moir (1973), 80% of vesicovaginal fistulae were due to gynaecological causes while the rest were obstetric in origin. Hysterectomy was the cause of 42% of fistulae in the gynaecological group (Chapter 11), while 24% were secondary to colporrhaphy. Obstetric vesicovaginal fistula results from necrosis of maternal soft tissues compressed between the pelvis and the fetal head during obstructed labour. Caesarean section is associated with vesicovaginal fistula when the bladder is not reflected far enough downwards before opening the lower uterine segment, when the bladder is torn during its reflection in the presence of dense adhesions between the uterus and bladder from previous Caesarean sections, or when a suture is inserted through the bladder wall during repair of the incision. Bladder calculi may complicate fistulae into the vagina, either in association with nonabsorbable sutures left in the bladder wall at previous repair operations or in stagnant urine below the level of the fistula (Lawson, 1972).

IV urography and cystography are standard methods for demonstrating vesicovaginal fistulae (see Figs. 11.9 and 11.15). A tampon may be left in the vagina during urography and is then radiographed after its removal, contrast medium in the tampon indicating a fistulous communication (Wesolowski & Meaney, 1977). Vaginography is sometimes useful in showing a fistula to the bladder.

URETHROVAGINAL FISTULA

This is most frequently due to ischaemic necrosis of the vaginal and urethral walls following anterior colporrhaphy, and infection after the excision of a urethral diverticulum (Gray, 1968). Occasionally an infected urethral diverticulum associated with stones or abscesses spontaneously ruptures into the vagina. Obstetric injury is nowadays an uncommon cause of urethrovaginal fistula.

RECTOVAGINAL AND SIGMOIDOVAGINAL FISTULAE

Most cases of sigmoidovaginal fistulae are due to diverticular disease (Fig. 9.2, and see Fig. 6.6). Other causes include irradiation for carcinoma of the cervix and granulomatous colitis. Rectovaginal fistulae may be

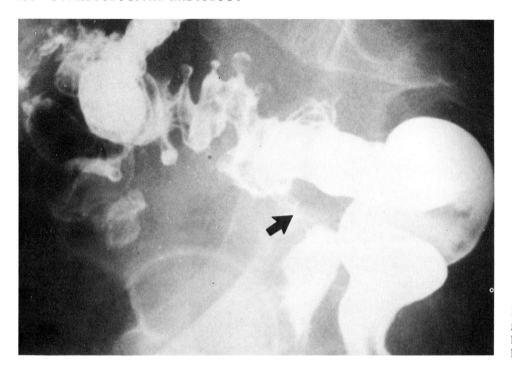

FIG. 9.2 Barium enema shows sigmoidovaginal fistula (arrow) secondary to diverticulitis.

FIG. 9.3 Hysterosalpingogram showing a smooth, pedunculated endometrial polyp.

secondary to carcinoma of the vagina, granulomatous proctitis and obstetric injury. Barium enema examination will demonstrate most cases of sigmoidovaginal fistula, although diluting the barium will increase the chance of delineation. The fistula may only become apparent after evacuation. It is difficult to demonstrate a rectovaginal fistula by barium enema. Vaginography is of particular use in such cases, and may also be helpful in the delineation of sigmoidovaginal fistulae.

Vaginal ectopic ureter

It is very difficult to directly catheterize an ectopic ureter which terminates in the vagina. Reflux of contrast medium may occur on vaginography (Katzen & Trachtman, 1954) although there is sometimes a stenosis of the ureteral orifice.

THE UTERUS

Endometrial polyps

Endometrial polyps are localized areas of endometrial hyperplasia. They are either sessile or pedunculated, have a smooth surface, are rarely larger than 1 cm, and may

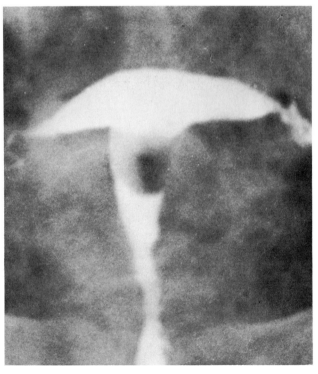

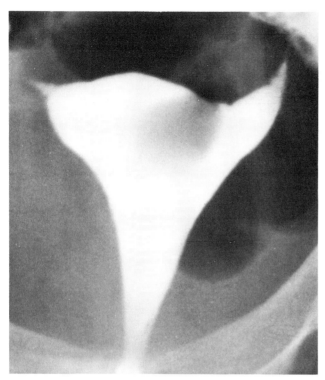

FIG. 9.4   Hysterosalpingogram showing a large smooth endometrial polyp arising from the fundal region.

be found anywhere in the uterine cavity (Figs. 9.3 and 9.4). Multiple polyps are sometimes present. These polypoid lesions occur at any time after the menarche and sometimes after the menopause. While endometrial polyps are often incidental findings on hysterography or curettage, it is widely held that they are associated with menorrhagia, intermenstrual and postmenopausal bleeding (Béclére, 1965). Slezak & Tillinger (1975) found polypoid filling defects in 2.5% of hysterograms, but endometrial polyps were present in only 8% of these and histological examination was normal in 78% of cases (see Fig. 2.24). There was no relationship to the secretory or proliferative phases in this respect, and no correlation was found by Slezak & Tillinger between the radiological evidence of polypoid filling defects and abnormal uterine bleeding. Armenia (1967) found that the risk of carcinoma developing in the body of the uterus was nine times greater in women with endometrial polyps. The incidence of the association of endometrial polyps and endometrial

carcinoma is 10%, according to Peterson & Novak (1956), although this applies primarily to postmenopausal women. In summary, Novak (1954) considered that while glandular hyperplasia of the endometrium was a common precursor of carcinoma, the latter occurred in only a small proportion of women with endometrial hyperplasia.

The typical hysterographic appearance is a sharply outlined, rounded and often pedunculated filling defect, usually 5 to 10 mm in diameter, which does not distort the uterine cavity. A pedunculated polyp is sometimes seen to move within the contract opacified uterine cavity, but may be differentiated from air bubbles because of the pronounced change in shape and position of the latter. Blood clots tend to be irregular and poorly circumscribed in outline. Sessile polyps are difficult to distinguish from submucosal polyps on hysterography (Fig. 9.5). Dufresne et al. (1959) found an accuracy rate of 75% in diagnosing endometrial polyps on hysterography.

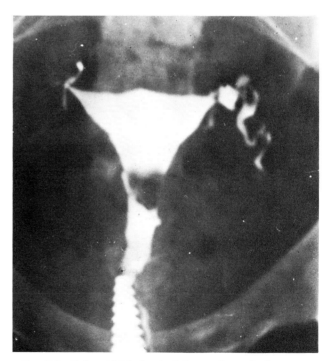

FIG. 9.5   Polypoidal lesion in isthmus shown by hysterography was later proven to be a fibroid.

Retained products of conception

The uterine cavity is invariably enlarged on hysterography in cases of missed abortion or retained products of conception. According to Foda *et al.* (1962) there are three possible hysterographic appearances. Multiple, very irregular filling defects may be present, resembling endometrial carcinoma. A more or less circumscribed filling defect occurs with retention of the majority or all of the ovum, with the delineated portion of the cavity flattened or displaced to one side as is seen in some cases of uterine fibroids. Occasionally, when the retained products of conception are of long standing, the uterine cavity is regular in shape with sharply circumscribed filling defects along the borders of the cavity (Fig. 9.6).

Adenomyosis

Uterine endometriosis, or adenomyosis, usually involves the body of the uterus, sometimes only in part, and

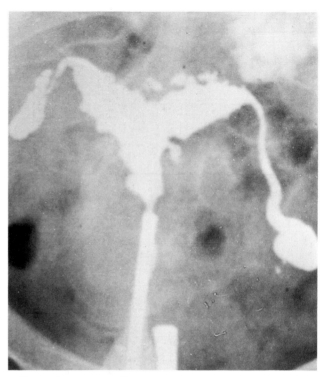

FIG. 9.7 Hysterosalpingogram in adenomyosis showing large uterine cavity and irregular contour with some spiculation. Courtesy of Dr Graham Russell.

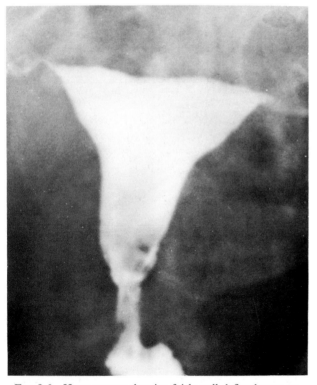

FIG. 9.6 Hysterogram showing fairly well-defined mass on left side of uterus and irregular filling defects on right side. These appearances were due to retained products of conception of several weeks' duration.

rarely involves the cervix. Glandular tissue with surrounding stroma grows diffusely into the uterine musculature, separating and destroying the muscle fibres and connective tissue. The glands of these ectopic endometrial foci often contain blood. Localized adenomyosis may grossly resemble a fibroid, although a distinctive feature of the former is the lack of a capsule. Fibroids are a fairly frequent associated finding in the presence of adenomyosis. The main symptom of adenomyosis is menorrhagia, although the patient may also complain of infertility and dysmenorrhoea.

On hysterography, the uterus is usually enlarged and, when present, the most striking feature consists of short spicules extending perpendicularly outwards from the uterine cavity for a depth of 1 to 4 mm (Fig. 9.7).

Occasionally, the spicules are considerably enlongated, reaching 1 to 2 cm in length with a circulatous or undulating course. This spiculation is only seen in 25%

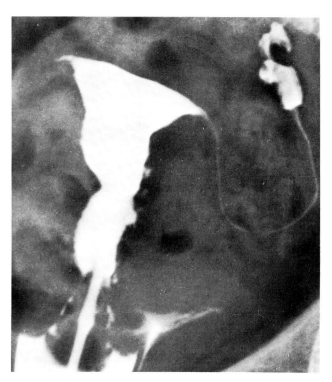

FIG. 9.8 Hysterosalpingogram shows glandular filling in lower half of uterine body and isthmus, regarded as being a normal variant.

of cases, because muscle overgrowth and the presence of secretions, clotted blood and desquamated epithelium may block the endometrial channels. The projections terminate in small rounded sacs, 2 to 4 mm in diameter in 30% of cases (Marshak & Eliasoph, 1955). In some cases of adenomyosis, there is only irregularity of the endometrium, and sometimes filling defects where the uterine wall is unusually thick and may simulate a submucous fibroid. In summary, histologically proven adenomyosis is, therefore, not often evident on hysterography (Sweeney, 1958).

Cavities in the uterine wall demonstrated on hysterography are often normal variants and are not due to cystic glandular hyperplasia, although they are manifestations of adenomyosis in 24% of cases (Slezak & Tillinger, 1976). These authors found that adenomyosis is generally not involved in the pathogenesis of cavities in the lower half of the uterus (Fig. 9.8), and that

adenomyosis does not account for cavities greater than 5 mm in diameter. A spiculated outline to the uterine cavity on hysterography was found by Slezak & Tillinger (1973) to be mainly associated with an atrophic endometrium in the years preceding the menopause and is probably due to mucous glands, while adenomyosis is associated with larger, deeper and more jagged projections into the uterine wall.

Metropathia haemorrhagica

Cystic hyperplasia of the endometrium occurs at any age from puberty to the menopause as part of the syndrome of metropathia haemorrhagica. It is caused by oestrogen acting in the absence of progesterone. Bleeding continues for two to eight weeks, often preceded by amenorrhoea. Histologically, the endometrial glands are hypertrophied, usually giving a 'cystic' appearance, with a hypertrophied stroma. In essence, the picture is one of an exaggerated and prolonged proliferative phase.

More than half the cases of metropathia haemorrhagica have normal appearances on hysterography, while the rest show a hypertrophic, ragged endometrial outline with a polypoid tendency (Bergman & Wehlin, 1958). These prominences may give an irregular crisscross appearance resembling Swiss cheese (di Palma & Beranbaum, 1952) (Fig. 9.9).

It should be remembered that a double contour to the uterine cavity is due to glandular filling in a thickened endometrium occurring in the late secretory phase of the menstrual cycle (Slezak & Tillinger, 1968) (Fig. 9.10).

Intrauterine adhesions

Intrauterine adhesions or synechiae were first described by Hald (1949) and later by Asherman (1950). Single or multiple adhesions, varying in size and shape, were found by Asherman to cause filling defects in the uterus on hysterography and occurred especially after repeated curettage and were associated with amenorrhoea. Bergman (1961) considered that amenorrhoea was associated with either occlusion of the internal os or extensive deformity of the uterine cavity with an atrophic endometrium. Sterility is probably due to mechanical obstruction or defective endometrial function. Most reported cases of intrauterine adhesions follow puerperal curettage, and to a lesser extent postabortal curettage and instrumental abortion, rather than repeated curettage of the non-pregnant uterus. Slightly less than half of all

FIG. 9.9 Hysterosalpingogram in metropathia haemorrhagica, with an irregular endometrium.

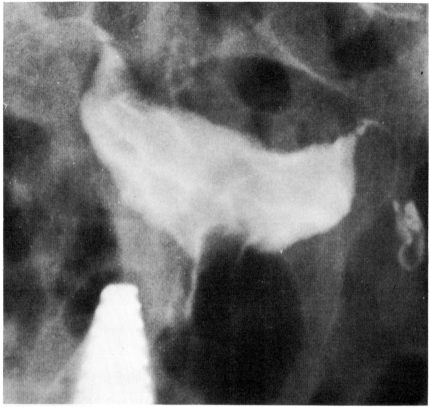

FIG. 9.10 Double contour to uterine cavity due to thickened endometrium in late secretory phase.

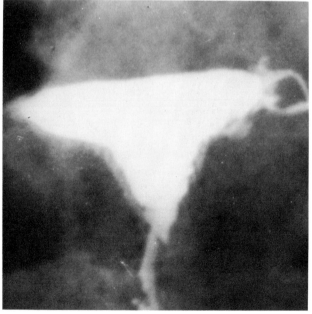

patients undergoing curettage within two months of delivery develop intrauterine adhesions to some degree (Eriksen & Kaestel, 1960). Caesarean section (Cominos & Pantelis, 1969) and myomectomy (Bergman, 1961) are less frequent causes. Jensen & Stromme (1972) found spontaneous resumption of menstruation occurred in more than half the cases of synechiae due to puerperal curettage after eight months or more of total amenorrhoea. It seems that trauma to the basal layer of the endometrium and the myometrium prompts the formation of adhesions between the walls of the uterine cavity.

The radiolucent filling defects seen on hysterography and due to bridging of the uterine cavity may be round, ovoid, linear, branch-like or bizarre in shape. Irregularly shaped straight or angulated filling defects are particularly characteristic of adhesions (Figs. 9.11 to 9.15). Extensive adhesions will distort the uterine cavity, while total obliteration of the cavity may occur in particularly severe

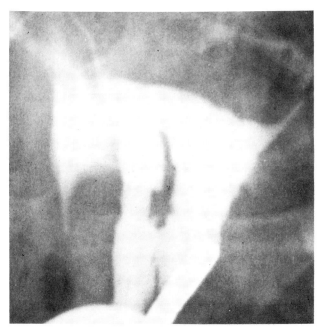

FIG. 9.11 Large intrauterine adhesions, shown on hystero-salpingography.

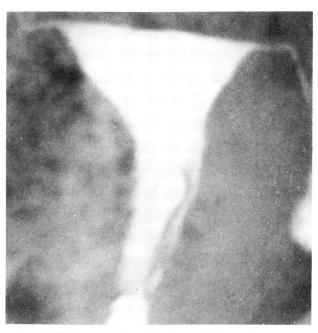

FIG. 9.12 Intrauterine adhesions with long linear configuration.

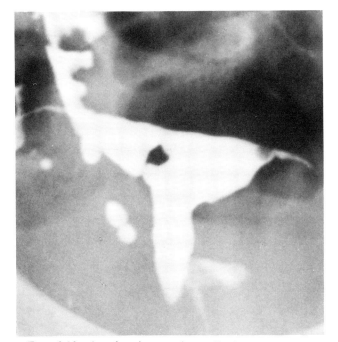

FIG. 9.13 Angular intrauterine adhesions. Persistent appearance throughout series.

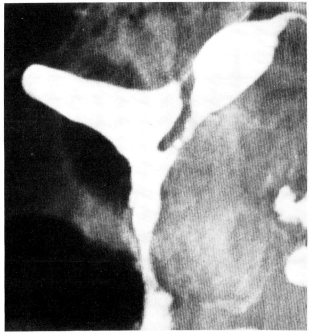

FIG. 9.14 Large filling defect caused by intrauterine adhesion.

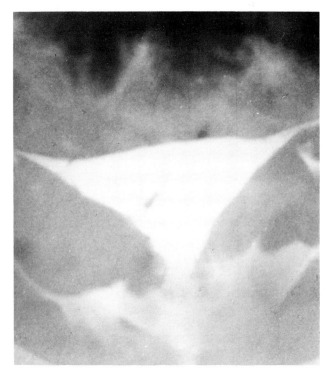

FIG. 9.15 Small, linear filling defect due to intrauterine adhesion.

cases (Fig. 9.16). Altemus *et al.* (1968) have found interstitial and venous intravasation to be a common finding in cases of intrauterine synechiae. Bergman (1961) found bilateral tubal occlusion in 20% and blockage of one uterine tube in 18% of cases, the obstruction usually being at uterine rather than at tubal level. This is a factor to be taken into consideration in the assessment of sterility in patients with intrauterine adhesions. Hysterography is useful in determining the effectiveness of treatment.

The differential diagnosis includes air bubbles, but these are round and inconstant. Although peripheral adhesions may be mistaken for polyps, the persistence of adhesions on injecting more contrast medium is an important point of differentiation. A deformed and contracted uterine cavity is seen in tuberculous endometritis, but tubal abnormalities are consistently found in this disease. Zondek & Rozin (1964) have observed filling defects which resemble adhesions on hysterography although the uterine cavity was normal on hysterotomy.

These defects disappeared following incision of the uterus alone or after denervation, the authors attributing the changes to muscular contraction.

Changes following lower segment Caesarean section

Uterine deformities are demonstrated on hysterography in about 55% of patients who have undergone Caesarean section (Ruiz-Valasco *et al.*, 1964; Zilberman *et al.*, 1968). Lateral and AP views, and sometimes oblique views, are required to fully demonstrate the deformity. The usual appearance is a localized wedge-shaped or convex protrusion directed ventrally (Figs. 9.17 and 9.18) and sometimes laterally, from the isthmus and upper part of the cervical canal with a depth and width of less than 5 mm (Schiøler *et al.*, 1967; Waniorek, 1967). Larger deformities are less commonly found and these may have a sacculated contour. Sometimes deep, duct-like projections occur and these may terminate in a distinct loculation. The defects of the uterine contour are the result of cicatrization with subsequent scar retraction.

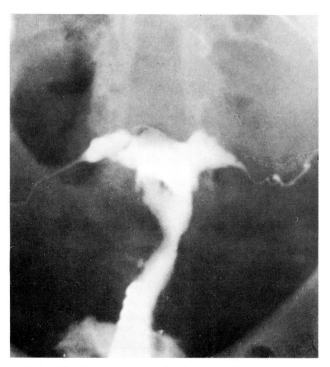

FIG. 9.16 Severe uterine adhesions resulting in marked deformity of uterine cavity with filling defects.

It has been claimed that prominent scar deformities are most likely to occur in association with local infection, when women have had more than one Caesarean section, in patients who had Caesarean section before the onset of labour (Schiøler *et al.*, 1967) and in primiparae over the age of thirty years (Dubois *et al.*, 1969). The application of numerous sutures because of haemorrhage or tearing is another predisposition to large defects (Waniorek, 1967). While safe vaginal delivery may be anticipated with the smaller, well defined deformities, the larger defects indicate a weak or even dehiscent scar and repeat Caesarean section is then advisable in subsequent pregnancies.

Thin longitudinal filling defects have been observed running from the fundus to the cervix in a few cases after Caesarean section (Ruiz-Valasco *et al.*, 1964; Waniorek, 1966), and are probably intrauterine adhesions.

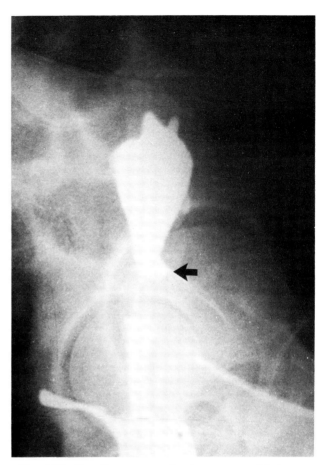

FIG. 9.18 Post-Caesarean section hysterogram. Moderate sized wedge-shaped defect on anterior aspect of isthmus. Courtesy of Dr Graham Russell.

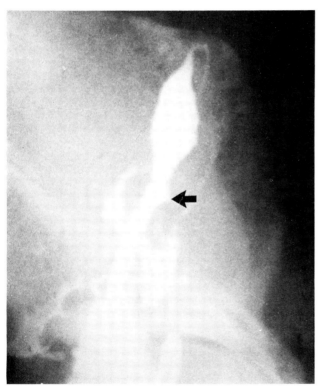

FIG. 9.17 Lateral view of hysterogram showing small anterior defect following lower uterine Caesarean section. Courtesy of Dr Graham Russell.

Vesicouterine fistula is one possible result of breakdown of the uterine incision after Caesarean section. The patient typically has menouria, urinary incontinence being an unusual occurrence. The fistulous communication to the uterus is demonstrable on cystography (Sammour, 1970) and usually extends to the level of the internal os. Occasionally, the vesical fistula may involve both the cervix and the vagina, in which case the patient will be incontinent of urine (Falk & Tancer, 1956).

Ureterouterine fistula is a very rare complication of Caesarean section. IV urography shows narrowing of the lower end of the involved ureter, with hydronephrosis and proximal hydroureter, and leakage of contrast medium into the uterine cavity (el Mahgoub & el Zeniny, 1972; Jequier & Piper, 1973).

Uterine fistula

UTEROVESICAL FISTULA

Other causes of uterovesical fistula, apart from Caesarean section (see above) and other obstetric and gynaecological operations, include neoplastic and inflammatory disease of the bladder and uterus, radiotherapy and urological procedures.

ENTEROUTERINE FISTULA

Fistula formation between the sigmoid colon and uterus usually results from carcinoma arising in either structure (Franco & Clough, 1956). Diverticulitis is a less frequent cause (see Fig. 6.5), and spontaneous or instrumental uterine rupture is a rare aetiology. Barium enema will often delineate a uterosigmoid fistula.

Incompetence of the uterine isthmus

Incompetence of the internal os causes miscarriage during the second trimester and is the result of forceful cervical dilatation before curettage or during criminal abortion, incision of the uterine cervix, forceps or breech extraction before full cervical dilatation and precipitate labour. A congenital weakness of the internal os may be postulated in the absence of any of these predisposing causes.

The width of the internal os normally varies during the menstrual cycle, being wider in the proliferative phase than in the secretory phase. The internal os may or may not be shown on hysterography as a distinct region of transition between the cervix and the body of the uterus in the normal state. When present, it appears as a constriction immediately above the cervix.

Appearances on conventional hysterography which are suspicious of incompetence are a width of 6 mm or more at internal os level and an imperceptible merging of the cervical canal and the cavity of the uterine body (Asplund, 1952) (Fig. 9.19). Leakage of contrast medium around the cannula is not a sign of incompetence.

Rubovits *et al.* (1953) inserted a balloon catheter into the uterine cavity, filled the balloon with 3 to 4 ml of

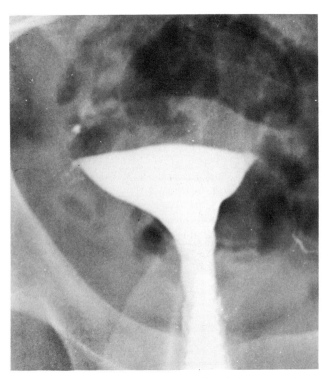

FIG. 9.19 Hysterogram showing wide isthmus merging with uterine body. History of two midtrimester miscarriages.

contrast medium and applied traction to the catheter. Small amounts of contrast medium were then removed and serial radiographs were taken as the balloon was pulled through the isthmus and cervical canal. This method will certainly demonstrate gross incompetence, but there are problems of reproduceability and standardization of the technique.

Mann (1959) introduced a balloon of two parts, a head and neck attached to a hard rubber catheter. The thin balloon at the head is distended with contrast medium and is moulded to the internal uterine contour. After an initial pressure is reached, the neck portion expands below the level of the internal os and outlines the isthmus and cervical canal. Changes in calibre of the delineated isthmus and cervical canal are obtained under conditions of controlled pressure. It is found that marked isthmic hypotonia correlates closely with impaired function of the isthmus during pregnancy. The finding that dilatation of the normally sphincter-like segment and merging of the isthmus and cervical canal without definite junction

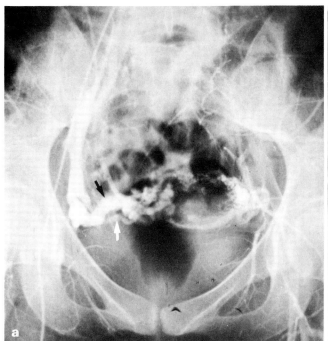

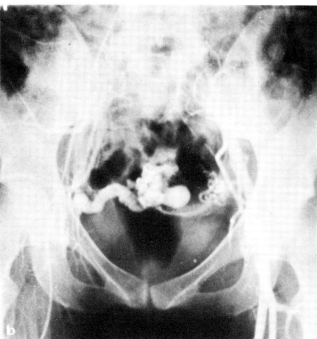

FIG. 9.20 Aortogram in 30-year-old women with uterine haemorrhage.

(a) Circoid arteriovenous malformation of uterus with enlargement of right uterine artery (white arrow) and early filling of enlarged right uterine vein (black arrow).

(b) Late arterial phase. Dense opacification of right uterine vein and iliac vein. Multiple tortuous uterine vessels are still opacified. From *Acta Radiologica Diagnostica* (1975), **16**, 43–48.

was diagnostic of isthmic incompetence was confirmed by Brünner & Ulrich (1966).

Arteriovenous malformations of the uterus

Congenital arteriovenous malformations of the uterus present in women of childbearing age with haemorrhage per vaginam which is spontaneous, is associated with menstruation or follows curettage. On vaginal palpation, the uterus is soft and enlarged, often pulsatile, and there may be an audible bruit. Greatly dilated and tortuous vessels are found in the uterus and parametrium at laparotomy. Pathologically, the vascular lesions are usually 'circoid' in type, being composed of multiple arteriovenous fistulas within a conglomeration of dilated vascular channels, while in some cases the vessels are either large and 'cavernous' or smaller than in the circoid type (Salm, 1959).

Angiography will demonstrate the presence and extent of uterine arteriovenous malformations. In reported cases (Liggins, 1964; Frencken & Landman, 1965; Bottomley & Whitehouse, 1975), the internal iliac arteries were dilated, and the enlarged uterine arteries supplied a large plexus of convoluted vessels within the uterus and parametrium in which the contrast medium remained for several seconds before passing into large veins (Figs. 9.20 and 9.21). At the same time, venous filling occurred while the arteries were still delineated by contrast medium, indicative of arteriovenous shunting. The ovarian arteries may also supply the vascular malformations, and it is important that the aortic catheter is inserted sufficiently high to delineate the ovarian arteries.

Regions of necrotic villi in the placenta during uterine pregnancy (Borell & Fernström, 1958) and retained placenta following abdominal pregnancy (Smulewicz *et al.*, 1971) may be associated with arteriovenous shunts of the uterine and parametrium. A traumatic fistula

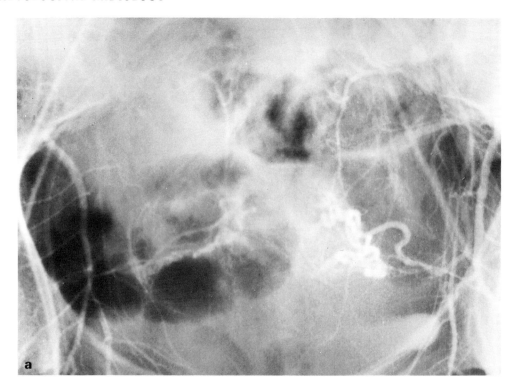

between a uterine artery and vein may occur after Caesarean section (Howard, 1968) and after hysterectomy (Morley & Lindenauer, 1968). The presence of arteriovenous shunts with carcinoma of the cervix and choriocarcinoma has been described in Chapter 7.

FIG. 9.21 Aortogram in 18-year-old women with uterine haemorrhage.

(a) Arterial phase, enlarged and tortuous left uterine artery supplies circoid arteriovenous malformation of left parametrium and left side of uterus.

(b) Persistent filling of the malformation after the arterial phase. Left uterine vein is opacified (arrow).

(c) Further vaginal haemorrhage occurred 7 months after ligation of left uterine artery. Repeat angiogram shows left ovarian artery (black arrows) and right uterine artery (white arrows) now supply the arteriovenous malformation. From *Acta Radiologica Diagnostica* (1975), **16**, 43–48.

REFERENCES

Vulva

COMAS M. R., MORRIS C. H. & AVERETTE H. E. (1969) Lymphography and vulvar carcinoma. *Obst. Gynec.*, **33**, 177–181.

DIXON J. A. & MITCHELL W. A. (1970) Venographic and surgical observations in vulvar varicose veins. *Surg. Gynec. Obst.*, **131**, 458–464.

HAGEN S. & BJØRN-HANSEN R. (1971) Lymphography in the treatment of carcinoma of the vulva. *Acta Radiol. (Diag.)*, *11*, 609–618.

LEA THOMAS M., FLETCHER E. W. L., ANDRESS M. R. & COCKETT F. B. (1967) The venous connections of vulvar varices. *Clin. Radiol.*, **18**, 313–317.

PARRY-JONES E. (1963) Lymphatics of the vulva. *J. Obst. Gynaec. Br. Emp.*, **70**, 751–765.

REYMOND R. D., HAZRA T. A., EDLOW D. W. & BAWAB M. S. (1972) Haemangiopericytoma of vulva with metastasis to bone 14 years later. *Brit. J. Radiol.*, **45**, 765–768.

Vagina

CHASSOR MOIR J. (1973) Vesico-vaginal fistulae as seen in Britain. *J. Obst. Gynaec. Br. Cwth.*, **80**, 598–602.

GRAY L. A. (1969) Urethrovaginal fistulas. *Amer. J. Obst. Gynec.*, **101**, 28–36.

KATZEN P. & TRACHTMAN B. (1954) Diagnosis of vaginal ectopic ureter by vaginogram. *J. Urol.*, **72**, 808–811.

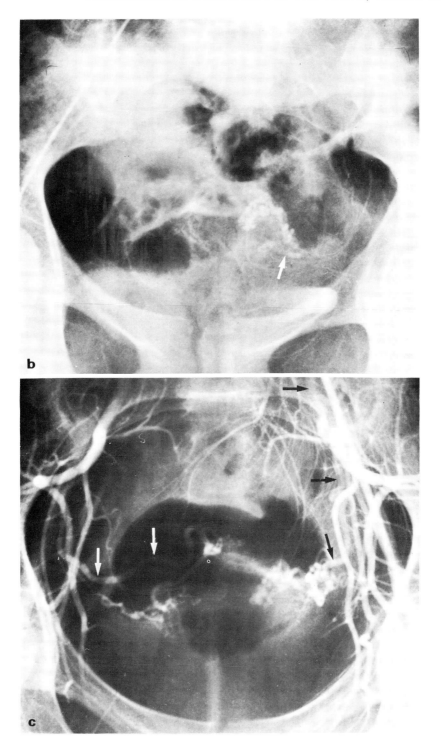

LAWSON J. (1972) Vesical fistulae into the vaginal vault. *Brit. J. Urol.*, **44**, 623–631.

NAVANI S. & TESSIER P. A. (1970) A primary vaginal stone. *Brit. J. Radiol.*, **43**, 222–223.

WESOLOWSKI D. P. & MEANEY T. F. (1977) Use of a vaginal tampon in the diagnosis of vesicovaginal fistulae. *Radiology*, **122**, 262.

Uterus

ALTEMUS R., CHARLES D. & STOCK R. J. (1968) Hysterography used in the diagnosis of intrauterine trauma. *Amer. J. Roentgenol.*, **104**, 865–869.

ARMENIA C. S. (1967) Sequential relationship between endometrial polyps and carcinoma of the endometrium. *Obst. Gynec.*, **30**, 524–529.

ASHERMAN J. G. (1950) Traumatic intrauterine adhesions. *J. Obst. Gynaec. Br. Emp.*, **57**, 892–896.

ASPLUND J. (1952) The uterine cervix and isthmus under normal and pathological conditions. *Acta Radiol. Suppl.*, 91.

BÉCLÈRE C. (1965) Hysterosalpingography in the diagnosis of functional uterine haemorrhages. *Gynec. Prac.*, **16**, 17–42.

BERGMAN P. (1961) Traumatic intrauterine lesions. *Acta Obst. Gynaec. Scand.*, **40**, Suppl. 4.

BERGMAN P. & WEHLIN L. (1958) The hysterographic appearance of cystic glandular hyperplasia. *Acta Radiol.*, **50**, 255–260.

BORELL U. & FERNSTRÖM I. (1958) Arteriovenous fistulae of the uterus and adnexa. *Acta Radiol.*, **49**, 1–16.

BOTTOMLEY J. P. & WHITEHOUSE G. H. (1975) Congenital arteriovenous malformations of the uterus demonstrated by angiography. *Acta Radiol. (Diag.)*, **16**, 43–48.

BRÜNNER. S. & ULRICH J. (1966) Roentgenologic changes in uterine isthmus insufficiency. *Amer. J. Roentgenol.*, **98**, 239–243.

COMINOS A. & PANTELIS Z. (1969) Treatment of intrauterine adhesions. *Amer. J. Obst. Gynec.*, **105**, 862–866.

DUBOIS R., FLIPO B., MONICER, J. C., GUIOT P. & DELECOUR M. (1969) Hysterography of the uterus subject to Caesarean section. *J. Radiol. Electr.*, **50**, 887–891.

DUFRESNE M. R., GERIN-LAJOIE L. & MALTAIS R. (1959) Problems in hysterosalpingography. *J. Amer. Med. Assoc.*, **170**, 1169–1171.

EL MAHGOUB S. & EL ZENINY A. (1972) Ureterouterine fistula after caesarean section. *Amer. J. Obst. Gynec.*, **110**, 881–882.

ERIKSEN J. & KAESTEL C. (1960) The incidence of uterine atresia after postpartum curettage. *Danish Med. Bull.*, **7**, 50–54.

FALK H. C. & TANCER M. L. (1956) Management of vesical fistulas after caesarean section. *Amer. J. Obst. Gynec.*, **71**, 97–105.

FODA M. S., YOUSSEF A. F., SHAFEEK M. A. & KASSEM K. A. (1962) Hysterography in diagnosis of abnormalities of the uterus. II acquired structural abnormalities. *Brit. J. Radiol.*, **35**, 783–795.

FRANCO F. O. & CLOUGH D. M. (1956) Parietal entero-uterine fistula. *Amer. J. Surg.*, **91**, 377–380.

FRENCKEN V. A. M. & LANDMAN G. H. M. (1965) Circoid aneurysm of the uterus: specific arteriographic diagnosis. *Amer. J. Roentgenol.*, **95**, 775–781.

HALD H. (1949) On uterine atresia consequent to curettage. *Acta Obst. Gynaec. Scandinav.*, **28**, 169–174.

HOWARD L. R. (1968) Iatrogenic arteriovenous sinus of a uterine artery and vein. *Obst. Gynec.*, **31**, 255–257.

JENSEN P. A. & STROMME W. B. (1972) Amenorrhoea secondary to puerperal curettage (Asherman's syndrome). *Amer. J. Obst. Gynec.*, **113**, 151–157.

JEQUIER A. M. & PIPER J. V. (1973) Uretero-uterine fistula after lower segment Caesarean section. *J. Obst. Gynaec. Br. Cwth.*, **80**, 276–279.

LIGGINS G. C. (1964) Uterine arteriovenous fistula. *Obst. Gynec.*, **23**, 214–217.

MANN E. C. (1959) Habitual abortion. A report in two parts, on 160 patients. *Amer. J. Obst. Gynec.*, **77**, 706–718.

MARSHAK R. H. & ELIASOPH J. (1955) The roentgen findings in adenomyosis. *Radiology*, **65**, 846–851.

MORLEY G. W. & LINDENAUER S. M. (1968) Arteriovenous fistula following pelvic operations. *Obst. Gynec.*, **31**, 722–726.

NOVAK E. R. (1954) Relationship of endometrial hyperplasia and adenocarcinoma of the uterine fundus. *J. Amer. Med. Assoc.*, **154**, 217–220.

DI PALMA S. & BERANBAUM S. L. (1952) The roentgenographic diagnosis of endometritis hyperplastica ovarialis. *Amer. J. Obst. Gynec.*, **64**, 162–167.

PETERSON W. F. & NOVAK E. R. (1956) Endometrial polyps. *Obst. Gynec.*, **8**, 40–49.

RUBOVITS F. G., COOPERMAN N. R. & LASH A. F. (1953) Habitual abortion: a radiographic technique to demonstrate the incompetent internal os of the cervix. *Amer. J. Obst. Gynec.*, **66**, 269–280.

RUIZ-VALASCO V., GUERRERO R., MORALES A. & GAMITZ R. (1964) Post-Caesarean section hysterographic control. *Obst. Gynec.*, **32**, 153–157.

SALM R. (1959) Diffuse cavernous haemangioma of the uterus. *J. Path. Bull.*, **77**, 111–129.

SAMMOUR M. B. (1970) Cystouterine fistula following Caesarean section with discharge of menstrual blood per urethram. *Amer. J. Obst. Gynec.*, **107**, 321–322.

SCHIØLER H., EIKEN M., ØVLISEN B. & TRALLE D. (1967) Hysterographic changes following transverse lower segment Caesarean section. *Acta Radiol. (Diag.)*, **6**, 145–155.

SLEZAK P. & TILLINGER K-G. (1968) The occurrence and significance of a double outlined uterine cavity in the hysterographic picture. *Radiology*, **90**, 756–760.

SLEZAK P. & TILLINGER K-G. (1973) Significance of spiculated outline of uterine cavity on hysterography. *Radiology*, **107**, 527–531.

SLEZAK P. & TILLINGER K-G. (1975) Hysterographic evidence of polypoid filling defects in the uterine cavity. *Radiology*, **115**, 79–83.

SLEZAK P. & TILLINGER K-G. (1976) The incidence and clinical importance of hysterographic evidence of cavities in the uterine wall. *Radiology*, **118**, 581–586.

SMULEWICZ J. J., TAFRESHI M., CAGAN S. H. & HEDJAZI M. (1971) Retained placenta following term abdominal pregnancy disclosed by angiography. *Amer. J. Obst. Gynec.*, **109**, 1220–1224.

SWEENEY W. J. (1958) Hysterosalpingography. I Accuracy of preoperative hysterosalpingograms. *Obst. Gynec.*, **11**, 640–645.

WANIOREK A. (1966) Hysterography after Caesarean section. *Amer. J. Obst. Gynec.*, **94**, 42–49.

WANIOREK A. (1967) Hysterography after Caesarean section for evaluation of suturing technique. *Obst. Gynec.*, **29**, 192–199.

ZILBERMAN A., SHARF M. & POLISHUK W. Z. (1968) Evaluation of Caesarean section scar by hysterography. *Obst. Gynec.*, **32**, 163–157.

ZONDEK B. & ROZIN S. (1964) Filling defects in the hysterogram simulating intrauterine synechiae which disappear after denervation. *Amer. J. Obst. Gynec.*, **88**, 123–127.

CHAPTER 10

Miscellaneous Conditions of the Fallopian Tubes; Endometriosis

THE FALLOPIAN TUBES

Salpingitis (and its possible sequelae of hydrosalpinx, pyosalpinx and tubo-ovarian abscess), tuberculous salpingitis, and diverticulosis of the Fallopian tubes are described in Chapter 6.

Tubal calcification

Most calcifications related to the Fallopian tubes are due to tuberculosis. Salpingoliths are rare and have been associated with chronic salpingitis (Kulka, 1942) and with pyosalpinx (Katz & Manfredmia, 1960).

Tumours of the Fallopian tubes

POLYPS

Smooth, rounded polyps, 1 mm or more in diameter, are occasionally found in the Fallopian tubes. The larger polyps are seen in the fimbrial ends of the tubes, but most are situated without the dilated intramural portion of the Fallopian tube. In the majority of cases in the series of Fernström & Lagenhöf (1964) there was bilateral involvement by intramural polyps but rarely more than one polyp in each tube. These polyps consist of endometrial tissue and there is a possibility that they may be associated with endometriosis.

TERATOMAS

Teratomas are an uncommon occurrence, most of them projecting into the lumen of the isthmus or ampulla. They range in size from 0.7 to 20 cm, with an average diameter of 5.7 cm. The majority are cystic in nature while the rest are solid, some are pedunculated, but none reported in the literature have shown malignant change (Mazzorella *et al.*, 1972). Bone occurs in a third of tubal teratomas, while only 7% show tooth formation.

CARCINOMA

Primary malignant tumours of the Fallopian tubes are uncommon, most being adenocarcinomas while occasionally a sarcoma, endothelioma, lymphosarcoma or mixed tumour is found. Carcinomas of the Fallopian tube usually arise between 45 and 55 years of age and present with a history of vaginal discharge, pelvic pain and adnexal enlargement. Hydrosalpinx, sometimes intermittent, is a common finding. Most tumours occur in the distal third of the Fallopian tube, which is closed towards its fimbrial end. The findings on hysterosalpingography are irregular, polypoidal masses within dilated and obstructed Fallopian tubes (Antonowitsch, 1950; Regner, 1967). Fogh (1969) considers that hysterosalpingography neither establishes a positive diagnosis of tubal carcinoma nor permits exclusion of the disease. There is some anxiety that hysterosalpingography may cause dissemination of tumour cells, although this is unproven.

Tubal pregnancy

Hysterosalpingography is contraindicated in ectopic pregnancy because of the potential risk of the procedure causing dislodgement of the mole and haemorrhage. Contrast medium will delineate the mole within the occluded tube and enter the intervillous spaces (Ekengren & Ryden, 1954). Ultrasonography has proved to be an accurate method of diagnosing a tubal pregnancy (Chapter 14).

Stein (1942) found that tubal pregnancies often appeared on pelvic pneumography, nowadays a discarded technique in this context, as a cone-shaped density with its apex arising from the uterine horn and the ipsilateral ovary seen as a separate oval structure or as part of the adnexal mass. On angiography (Fernström, 1955), the tubal branch of the uterine artery often gives off several branches, some of which become straight and arched, while the placental sinuses are seen as irregular opacities from the fifth week of pregnancy.

There is a high incidence of occlusion developing in the residual Fallopian tube following unilateral salpingectomy for tubal pregnancy, presumably a result of fibrosis secondary to bleeding into the pelvic peritoneal cavity (Cook & Butt, 1953). This secondary damage may account in part for the high recurrence rate of ectopic pregnancy, although the original causative pelvic inflammatory disease is also a contributing factor to this incidence. Hysterosalpingography should therefore be performed after surgery for ectopic pregnancy to exclude damage to the residual tube and to anticipate the risk of a second similar event.

Some gynaecologists pursue a conservative surgical approach in the treatment of tubal pregnancy, having found that the chances of a successful pregnancy increase more after tubal section than after radical salpingectomy (Kucera et al., 1969). A technique has been devised whereby the Fallopian tubes are irrigated by means of a balloon catheter inserted into the uterine cavity following tubal section (Vuovinen et al., 1972). Contrast medium is introduced at the time of tubal irrigation to monitor progress and to determine the effectiveness of the irrigation regimen in producing patent Fallopian tubes.

Plastic operations on the Fallopian tubes

Hysterosalpingography plays an important role in the preoperative assessment and postoperative evaluation of

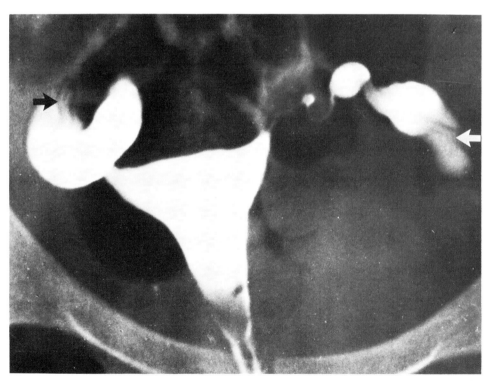

FIG. 10.1 Failed Mulligan's prostheses (arrows). Recurrence of bilateral hydrosalpinges shown by postoperative hysterosalpingography.

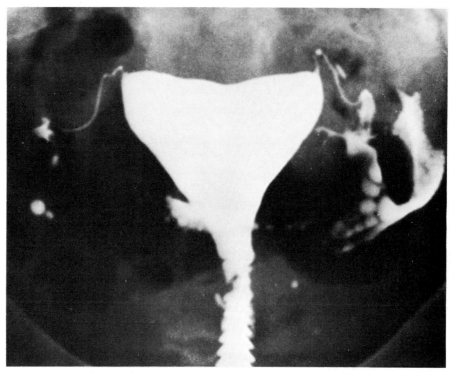

FIG. 10.2 Lipiodol hysterosalpingogram. Resection of distal portions of Fallopian tubes and salpingostomy following bilateral tubal ligation.

surgical procedures aimed at restoring patency to occluded Fallopian tubes.

SALPINGOLYSIS

Many peritubal adhesions are flimsy and are easily divided, although dense and numerous adhesions may be impossible to sever at operation.

SALPINGOSTOMY

The standard operative treatment of hydrosalpinx is resection of the distal end of the occluded Fallopian tube and the creation of a new ostium, with eversion and suturing of the divided edges to form a cuff. An alternative has been the removal of a small portion of the wall of the occluded tube with the creation of an aperture in close proximity to the ovary, a procedure which is rarely associated with success.

Once the ostia is restored, patency must be maintained by preventing recurrence of adhesions. Polythene splints have been inserted into the tubal lumen with the ends running out through the abdominal wall or cervix, with the risk of ascending infection, or the cornual end was allowed to remain within the uterine cavity. These earlier splints have been replaced by the Mulligan Silastic hood which is sutured into place to cover the newly formed fimbriated end. The hood is left in position for at least six months before it is removed by a second operation. Unless there has been proper case selection and meticulous surgical technique, occluding adhesions are likely to form around the hood (Fig. 10.1).

RESECTION AND ANASTOMOSIS

Resection of the middle portion of the Fallopian tube and subsequent splinting of the anastomosis by a plastic catheter is often a successful technique for reconstituting the tubes after ligation (Fig. 10.2). Fibrous occlusion is likely to occur after this procedure when there has been salpingitis.

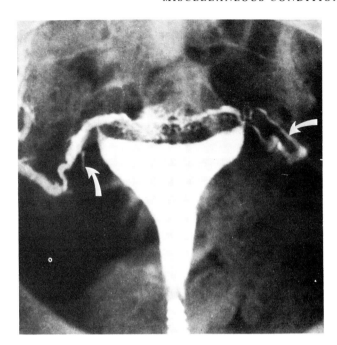

CORNUAL RESECTION AND REIMPLANTATION

Occlusion of the uterotubal junction may be treated by resection of the isthmus and the creation of a tunnel in the uterine wall through which the proximal end of the Fallopian tube is then inserted and sutured in position. A catheter is used as a splint to maintain the anastomosis.

Tubal sterilization techniques

There are various methods for occluding the Fallopian tubes as a method of contraception including ligation of the tube with or without excision of a segment, detachment of the tube from the uterus by cornual excision, excision or burying the fimbriated ends of the tubes. In recent years, occlusive tantanum or vanadium clips applied to the isthmus portions of the tubes and division of the tubes by electrocoagulation 1.5 to 2 cm from the

Fig. 10.3 Hysterosalpingogram after successful tubal electrocoagulation. Both tubes are occluded (arrows) but there is marked venous intravasation from the uterus.

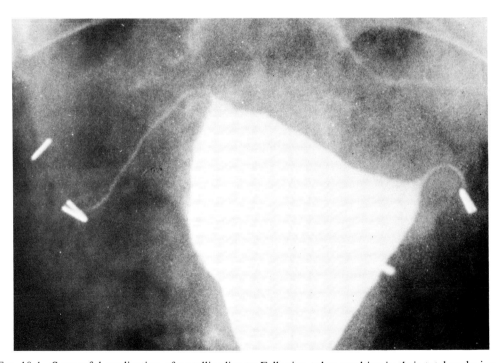

Fig. 10.4 Successful application of metallic clips to Fallopian tubes resulting in their total occlusion.

cornua during laparotomy or through a laparoscope have become popular methods. Tubal electrocoagulation through a laparoscope may result in injury, sometimes with perforation of the small intestine (Levinson *et al.*, 1973).

It may be considered necessary to assess the result of the application of clips, and particularly of electrocoagulation, by hysterosalpingography (Figs 10.3, 10.4 and 10.5). Jordan *et al.* (1971) suggest that the hysterosalpingogram to confirm tubal occlusion be performed no earlier than twelve weeks after electrocoagulation, because fibrosis at the point of occlusion may be incomplete before this time and the contrast medium under pressure may result in a sinus at this point. Hysterosalpingography is also a useful investigation prior to reconstructive tubal surgery following a previous operative tubal occlusion.

ENDOMETRIOSIS

Endometriosis is the presence of endometrial tissue (epithelial, glandular and stromal elements) in situations other than the lining of the uterine cavity. It is a disorder of the reproductive years, usually presenting in the fourth decade.

The pelvic cavity is the prime site of endometriosis, but the disease is variable in extent. Ovarian involvement is particularly common, with typically bilateral cysts filled with thick, dark brown fluid – the so-called 'chocolate cysts'. Haemorrhage into the peritoneal cavity is associated with these ovarian cysts and leads to the formation of prominent adhesions. Elsewhere in the pelvic cavity, especially in the pouch of Douglas, nodules of endometriosis are also found in combination with fibrosis from recurrent bleeding. The surfaces of the uterus and Fallopian tubes as well as the uterosacral ligaments, the rectovaginal septum, posterior fornix of the vagina, urinary bladder and ureters, rectosigmoid and small intestine are also sites of endometriosis. Adenomyosis is considered in Chapter 9.

The symptoms of endometriosis include pelvic pain and dyspareunia which are worse around the time of

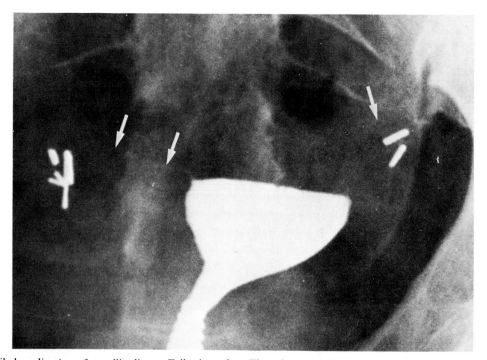

FIG. 10.5   Failed application of metallic clips to Fallopian tubes. The tubes are only faintly opacified at hysterosalpingography, but are above the clips.

menstruation, dysmenorrhoea and secondary infertility. Approximately a quarter of patients with endometriosis have no recognizable symptoms, and the severity of the symptoms does not directly relate to the extent of the disease. On examination, fixed retroversion of the uterus, nodular thickening of the pelvic floor and rectovaginal septum, and bilateral adnexal masses are common findings in severe cases of pelvic endometriosis. Laparoscopy is useful in the assessment and confirmation of endometriosis. Treatment consists of hormone therapy, especially with progestogens, and conservational surgery. Malignant change rarely occurs in endometriosis. Many theories have been propounded to account for endometriosis, especially concerning the possibility of metaplasia in cells related to the pelvic peritoneum.

Radiological investigation

PLAIN RADIOGRAPHS

There are usually no abnormal plain radiographic findings, but visible pelvic masses may be present. Ascites has rarely been associated with ovarian endometriosis (Bernstein, 1961).

HYSTEROSALPINGOGRAPHY

Severe pelvic endometriosis will result in fixity of the uterus, particularly in retroflexion. Adhesions may also cause lateral deviation and rotation of the uterus. The Fallopian tubes may appear normal, but there is often some dilatation of the ampullae with perifimbrial adhesions causing loculation and impaired peritoneal spillage of contrast medium (Fig. 10.6). These appearances should particularly suggest the diagnosis of endometriosis in cases of secondary infertility, but are indistinguishable from pelvic inflammatory disease. Endometriosis in the younger age group may be associated with congenital anomalies of the genital tract, such as uterine hypoplasia.

PELVIC PNEUMOGRAPHY

Although this technique has been largely replaced by laparoscopy, observations have been made on the pneumographic appearances of pelvic endometriosis (Theander & Wehlin, 1968). The uterine displacement may be seen, the common backward retraction of the uterus being most readily visible on the lateral view. Retrouterine adhesions may obliterate the posterior uterine border. Marked anteflexion results from expan-

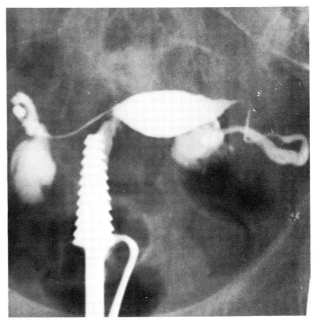

FIG. 10.6 Hysterosalpingogram in secondary infertility shows lateral deviation of uterus and bilateral periampullary loculation of contrast medium. Pelvic endometriosis confirmed by laparoscopy.

sion of retrouterine endometriotic masses. The ovaries appear enlarged because of the development of cysts, whose outlines are visible, and later because of adhesions which give an indistinct ovarian outline. The pouch of Douglas often shows changes, ranging from small aggregations of endometrial tissue to complete obliteration by adhesions. Similar, but usually less extensive, changes may occur in the vesicouterine recess. Pelvic pneumography has been recommended by Borglin *et al.* (1972) as a method for assessing the effect of progestogen therapy on the adnexal and serosal lesions of endometriosis.

ANGIOGRAPHY

Theander & Haeger (1964) have demonstrated deviation and narrowing of the femoral vein and slight displacement of the femoral artery on angiography when inguinal endometriosis has extended to the upper part of the thigh.

Endometriosis involving the intestinal tract

Probably 18–25% of women with pelvic endometriosis

have some degree of intestinal involvement by endometriosis (Jenkinson & Brown, 1943).

RECTOSIGMOID ENDOMETRIOSIS

The rectum and sigmoid colon are the most frequently involved portions of the intestine. Symptoms of involvement of the rectosigmoid segment by endometriosis include constipation, pelvic and rectal pain and diarrhoea, exacerbated by menstruation. In some cases there are no symptoms. Rectal bleeding is not a feature of endometriosis of the large bowel, and its presence should raise the suspicion of other pathology, particularly carcinoma.

Small implantations on the rectum and sigmoid colon may merely produce some local irritability on barium enema examination (Marshak, 1947). Infiltration and obliteration of the pouch of Douglas cause angulation of the anterior wall of the rectum and a blunt transverse ridge, 2 to 4 cm wide, projecting into the rectal lumen on its anterior aspect (Theander & Wehlin, 1961) – the so-called 'shelf tumour' (Lilja & Probst, 1966).

Extensive intramuscular and submucosal lesions may produce constrictive lesions 2 to 7 cm in length on barium

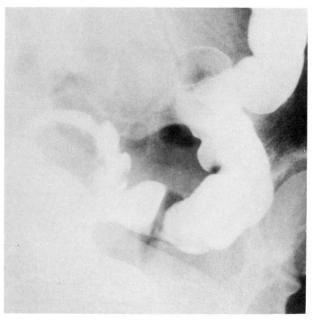

FIG. 10.8   Barium enema shows a stricture of the sigmoid segment due to endometriosis. Courtesy of Dr Keith Simpkins.

enema, but more often involvement of the bowel wall will produce a polypoid mass, mainly due to reactive muscular hypertrophy (Spjut & Perkins, 1959) (Figs 10.7 and 10.8). There may be a considerable degree of obstruction, and swelling of the lesion may occur during menstruation. The mucosa remains intact in endometriosis of the bowel, an important point of differentiation from carcinoma, although the mucosal folds may be crowded together. The transition from abnormal to normal portions of the bowel is either gradual or abrupt when there is a constrictive lesion. Local tenderness in the area of involvement may be appreciated during the barium enema (Culver et al., 1958).

SMALL INTESTINE AND CAECUM

Involvement of the small intestine by endometriosis usually affects the terminal 10 cm of the ileum (Melody, 1956) and may or may not be associated with direct adhesive compression by pelvic endometriosis (Venable, 1972). Symptoms of intestinal obstruction are sometimes exacerbated at the time of menstruation. The mechanism of obstruction is usually due to kinking by adhesions (McGuff et al., 1948) but endometriosis of the muscular

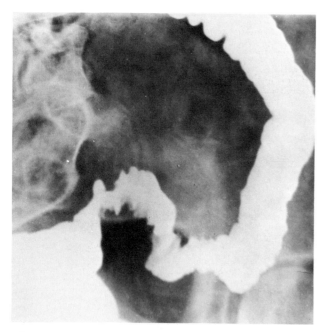

FIG. 10.7   Endometriosis causing narrowing of the rectosigmoid junction on barium enema.

layer may cause stenosis, perhaps with nodules protruding into the intestinal lumen (Venable, 1972).

Constriction and kinking seldom occur with caecal involvement, nodulation with preservation of the mucosa being the rule (Felson & Wiot, 1969), although intussusception may take place.

Endometriosis affecting the urinary tract

THE URETERS

Klempner (1952) found ureterohydronephrosis in more than 40% of patients with pelvic inflammatory disease or endometriosis, while Ball & Platt (1962) recorded a 1.2% incidence of ureteral involvement by endometriosis.

Involvement of the ureter by endometriosis may be intrinsic, affecting the muscular layer and lamina propria and sometimes the mucosa, or extrinsic with ureteral obstructions being secondary to external pressure by endometriosis within the pelvic cavity extending into the adventitia and surrounding connective tissue of the ureter. The prime sites of extrinsic endometriosis of the ureter are the rectovaginal septum and ovarian fossa (Yates-Bell *et al.*, 1972). Extrinsic endometriosis affects

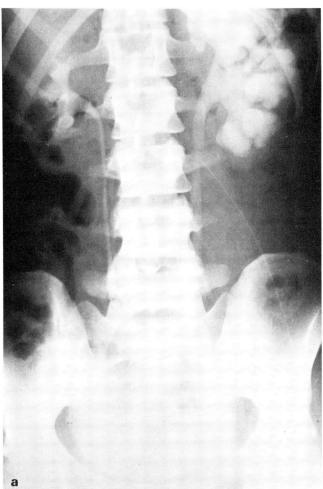 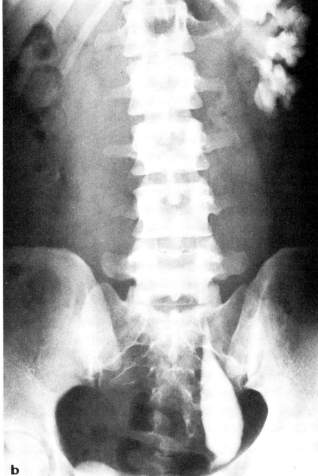

FIG. 10.9   Endometriosis involving lower end of left ureter. (a) Left sided hydronephrosis and hydroureter on intravenous urography.

(b) Smooth stricture at lower end of left ureter shown by retrograde pyeloureterogram.

the ureter four times as frequently as intrinsic endometriosis. Usually only one ureter is affected, but sometimes endometriosis involves both ureters. A history of
flank pain during menstrual periods should suggest the
diagnosis of ureteral endometriosis, especially in women
in the late reproductive years. Endometriosis, intrinsic or
extrinsic in type, causes ureteral obstruction which is
below the level of the pelvic brim in all cases, with ureteral
dilatation and hydronephrosis above a segment of distal
ureteral narrowing demonstrable by IV urography and
retrograde ureteral catheterization. There is usually
smooth tapering of the ureteral lumen in the narrowed
segment (Berlin et al., 1964) (Fig. 10.9) but sometimes a
rounded filling defect is seen (Stanley et al., 1965) on
radiological studies. Although endometrial masses may
decrease in size on progestogen therapy, there is usually
persistence of the ureteral obstruction (Stiehm et al.,
1972).

THE BLADDER

Vesical involvement occurs in 1.1% of patients with endometriosis (Abeshouse & Abeshouse, 1960) and is usually,
but not always, a result of contiguous pelvic endometriosis. The symptoms are frequency, dysuria and
suprapubic pain which are usually related to the
menstrual periods. Extravesical pressure deformities
have been observed on IV urography, and there may
be simultaneous involvement of the lower ureter by the
endometriosis (Stanley et al, 1965).

THE KIDNEYS

The occurrence of endometrial tissue in the kidney is
very rare, but has caused haematuria and a flank mass
in occasional cases. IV urography has shown renal mass
lesions which are found at surgery to be cystic and filled
with old blood (Marshall, 1943; Maslow & Leamer,
1950).

Intrathoracic endometriosis

Endometriosis of the diaphragm cannot be seen on chest
radiographs (Anderson & Forrest, 1973), but recurrent
spontaneous pneumothorax concomitant with the menstrual period should suggest the presence of diaphragmatic endometriosis (Davies, 1968). Such cases are over
25 years of age, the majority being in the fourth decade,
clinical evidence of pelvic endometriosis is found in half
the patients, and pneumothorax does not occur during

every period (Lillington et al., 1969). The right side alone
is affected in the vast majority of cases, although bilateral
catamenial pneumothoraces have been described by Laws
et al. (1977).

Recurrent haemorrhagic pleural effusion is another
manifestation of intrathoracic endometriosis (Charles,
1957), again with a predilection to the right pleural
cavity.

The simultaneous appearance of sarcoma in endometriosis of the pleura and pelvis has been described in
one case with recurrent haemothoraces by Labay &
Feiner (1971).

Lattes et al. (1956) found a solitary nodule in the right
middle lobe, presenting with haemoptysis, and subsequently shown to be due to localized pulmonary
endometriosis. Cyclic haemoptysis is a rare manifestation
of intrathoracic endometriosis.

REFERENCES

Fallopian tubes

ANTONOWITSCH E. (1950) Roentgen diagnosis of primary tubal
carcinoma. Fortschr. a. d. Geb. d. Röntgenstrahlen, **73**, 189–
194.
COOK D. G. & BUTT J. G. (1953) Hysterosalpingography
studies following ectopic pregnancy. Amer. J. Obst. Gynec.,
66, 626–636.
EKENGREN K. & RYDEN A. B. V. (1954) The diagnostic value of
hysterosalpingography in tubal pregnancy. Acta Radiol., **41**,
247–255.
FERNSTRÖM I. (1955) Arteriography of the uterine artery. Acta
Radiol. Suppl. 122.
FERNSTRÖM I. & LAGENHÖF B. (1964) Polyps in the intramural
parts of the Fallopian tubes. J. Obst. Gynaec. Br. Cwth., **71**,
681–691.
FOGH I. (1969) Primary carcinoma of the Fallopian tube. Cancer,
23, 1332–1346.
JORDAN J. A., EDWARDS R. L., PEARSON J. & MASKERY P. J. K.
(1971) Laparoscopic sterilization and follow-up hysterosal-
pingogram. J. Obst. Gynaec. Br. Cwth., **78**, 460–466.
KATZ I. & MANFREDMIA G. A. (1960) Salpingolithiasis. Amer. J.
Roentgenol., **84**, 907–912.
KUCERA E., MACKU F., NOVAK J. & ANDRASOVA V. (1969)
Fertility after operations of extrauterine pregnancy. Internat.
J. Fertil., **14**, 127–129.
KULKA E. W. (1942) True bone formation in the Fallopian tube.
Amer. J. Obst. Gynec., **44**, 384–398.
LEVINSON C. J., SCHWARTZ S. F. & SALTZSTEIN E. C. (1973)
Complication of laparoscopic tubal cauterization – small
bowel performation. Obst. Gynec., **41**, 253–263.

MAZZORELLA P., OKAGAKI T. & RICHANT R. M. (1972) Teratoma of the uterine tube. *Obst. Gynec.*, **39**, 381–388.

REGNER H. (1967) Primary carcinoma of the Fallopian tubes. *Acta Radiol. (Diag.)*, **6**, 204–208.

STEIN I. F. (1942) Gynecographic aid in the diagnosis of ectopic pregnancy. *Amer. J. Obst. Gynec.*, **43**, 400–409.

VUOVINGEN P., PIETILÄ P., NUMMI S. & LAITINEN J. (1972) Modified hysterosalpingography in post-operative examination after tubal pregnancy. *Brit. J. Radiol.*, **43**, 429–431.

Endometriosis

ABESHOUSE B. S. & ABESHOUSE G. (1960) Endometriosis of the urinary tract. *J. Internat. Coll. Surgeons*, **34**, 43–63.

ANDERSON L. S. & FORREST J. V. (1973) Tumors of the diaphragm. *Amer. J. Roentgenol.*, **119**, 259–265.

BALL T. L. & PLATT M. A. (1962) Urological complications of endometriosis. *Amer. J. Obst. Gynec.*, **84**, 1516–1521.

BERLIN L., WALDMAN I., WHITE F. H. & McLAIN C. R. (1964) Endometriosis of the ureter. *Amer. J. Roentgenol.*, **92**, 351–354.

BERNSTEIN J. S. (1961) Massive ascites due to endometriosis. *Amer. J. Digest. Dis.*, **6**, 1–5.

BORGLIN N. E., THEADER G. & WEHLIN L. (1972) Roentgenographic observations on the effect of pseudo-pregnancy in endometriosis. *J. Obst. Gynaec. Br. Cwth.*, **72**, 544–556.

CHARLES D. (1957) Endometriosis and hemorrhagic pleural effusion. *Obst. Gynec.*, **10**, 309–312.

CULVER G. J., PERIERA R. M. & SEIBEL R. (1958) Radiographic features of rectosigmoid endometriosis. *Amer. J. Obst. Gynec.*, **76**, 1176–1184.

DAVIES R. (1968) Recurring spontaneous pneumothorax concomitant with menstruation. *Thorax*, **23**, 370–373.

FELSON B. & WIOT J. F. (1969) Some interesting right lower quadrant entities. *Radiol. Clin. N. Amer.*, **7**, 83–95.

JENKINSON E. L. & BROWN W. H. (1943) Endometriosis: Study of 117 cases with special reference to constricting lesions of rectum and sigmoid colon. *J. Amer. Med. Assoc.*, **122**, 349–354.

KLEMPNER E. (1952) Gynecological lesions and ureterohydronephrosis. *Amer. J. Obst. Gynec.*, **64**, 1232–1241.

LABAY G. R. & FEINER F. (1971) Malignant pleural endometriosis. *Amer. J. Obst. Gynec.*, **110**, 478–480.

LATTES R., SHEPARD F., TOVELL H. & WYLIE R. (1956) A clinical and pathologic study of endometriosis of the lung. *Surg. Gynec. Obst.*, **103**, 552–558.

LAWS H. L., FOX L. S. & YOUNGER J. B. (1977) Bilateral catamenial pneumothorax. *Arch. Surg.*, **112**, 627–628.

LILJA B. & PROBST F. (1966) Intestinal endometriosis. *Acta Radiol. (Diag.)*, **4**, 545–556.

LILLINGTON E. A., MITCHELL S. P. & WOOD G. A. (1969) Catamenial pneumothorax. *J. Amer. Med. Assoc.*, **219**, 1328–1332.

McGUFF P., DOCKERTY M. B., WAUGH J. M. & RANDALL L. M. (1948) Endometriosis as a cause of intestinal obstruction. *Surg. Gynec. Obst.*, **86**, 273–288.

MARSHAK R. H. (1947) Extrinsic lesions affecting the rectosigmoid. *Amer. J. Roentgenol.*, **58**, 439–451.

MARSHALL V. F. (1943) Occurrence of endometrial tissue in the kidney. *J. Urol.*, **50**, 652–654.

MASLOW L. A. & LEAMER A. (1950) Endometriosis of the kidney. *J. Urol.*, **64**, 564–568.

MELODY G. F. (1956) Endometriosis causing obstruction of the ileum. *Obst. Gynec.*, **8**, 468–472.

SPJUT H. J. & PERKINS D. E. (1959) Endometriosis of the sigmoid colon and rectum. *Amer. J. Roentgenol.*, **82**, 1070–1075.

STANLEY K. E., UTZ D. C. & DOCKERTY M. B. (1965) Clinically significant endometriosis of the urinary tract. *Surg. Gynec. Obst.*, **120**, 491–498.

STIEHM W. D., BECKER J. A. & WEISS R. M. (1972) Ureteral endometriosis. *Radiology*, **102**, 563–564.

THEANDER G. & HAEGER K. (1964) Angiography in the diagnosis of inguinal endometriosis. *Acta Radiol. (Diag.)*, **2**, 100–104.

THEANDER G. & WEHLIN L. (1961) Deformation of the rectosigmoid junction in pelvic endometriosis. *Acta Radiol.*, **55**, 241–248.

THEANDER G. & WEHLIN L. (1968) The radiology of pelvic endometriosis. *Clin. Radiol.*, **19**, 19–32.

VENABLE J. H. (1972) Endometriosis of the ileum: four cases with obstruction. *Amer. J. Obst. Gynec.*, **113**, 1054–1055.

YATES-BELL A. J., MOLLAND E. A. & PRYOR J. P. (1972) Endometriosis of the ureter. *Brit. J. Urol.*, **44**, 58–67.

CHAPTER 11

Complications of Hysterectomy and Radiotherapy

Abdominal hysterectomy is a frequently performed operation for benign uterine conditions, such as multiple fibroids. Usually the whole of the uterus is removed, subtotal hysterectomy with retention of the uterine cervix being out of favour with most gynaecologists. The Fallopian tubes and ovaries may be removed at the same time as hysterectomy, often in the presence of endometriosis, pelvic inflammatory disease or coexistent ovarian lesions. The uterus may also be removed by the vaginal route, usually as part of a procedure for correcting prolapse.

The Wertheim or radical hysterectomy consists of removal of the uterus, Fallopian tubes and ovaries, the pelvic lymph nodes and at least half of the vagina. This form of treatment is performed for Stage I and II carcinoma of the cervix. The extensive nature of the surgery is associated with more frequent and more severe complications than are encountered with total hysterectomy.

Taussig's operation consists of the extraperitoneal removal of all pelvic lymph nodes after carcinoma of the cervix has been treated by a full course of radiotherapy.

Pelvic exenteration involves removal of the bladder, uterus and adnexa, vagina and sometimes the rectum. The ureters are transplanted into the colon. This severe surgery is occasionally performed for advanced carcinoma of the uterine cervix or body, vagina or vulva, and is associated with a very high postoperative mortality.

RADIOLOGICAL MANIFESTATIONS OF COMPLICATIONS OF HYSTERECTOMY

Haematoma

The usual site for haematoma formation after a hysterectomy is between the upper end of the vaginal stump and the pelvic peritoneum. Plain radiographs show a soft tissue pelvic mass, while IV urography may demonstrate the mass indenting the bladder. Occasionally, the ureters may be deviated or compressed by the haematoma (Fig. 11.1).

Pelvic sepsis

There is a grave risk of suppuration occurring in a postoperative pelvic haematoma. The abscess thus formed may spontaneously discharge into the vagina, through the abdominal incision, or into the rectum. Adnexal abscesses may develop after vaginal hysterectomy (Ledger *et al.*, 1969). Postoperative pelvic sepsis occurred in nearly 9% of cases after radical hysterectomy in the large series of Green *et al.* (1962).

Pelvic abscesses may form soft tissue masses with similar effects to haematomas on the urinary tract (Fig. 11.2). A loss of definition of pelvic structures may occur in the presence of bleeding and sepsis, with local paralytic ileus resulting from pelvic peritoneal infection. It is rare for generalized peritonitis to develop after hysterectomy, but on plain radiographs this complication will cause

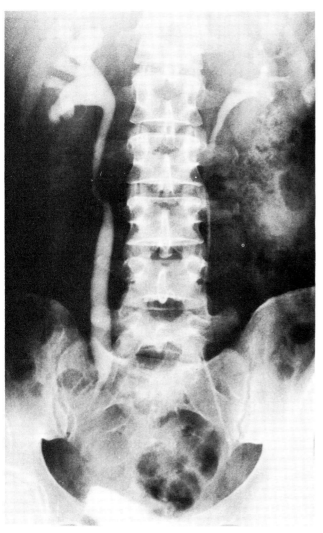

FIG. 11.1 Intravenous urogram showing large pelvic haematoma, post hysterectomy, causing soft tissue mass to compress bladder and causing right hydroureter and hydronephrosis.

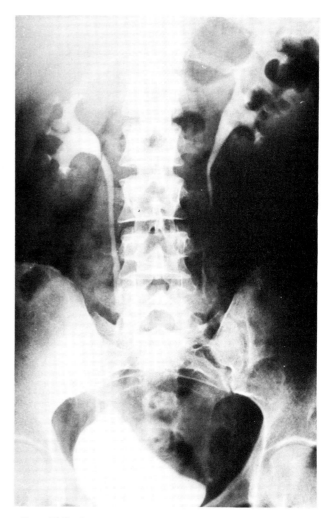

FIG. 11.2 Intravenous urogram 1 month after vaginal hysterectomy. Left-sided pelvic mass indenting bladder. A pelvic abscess was subsequently drained. From *Clinical Radiology* (1977), **28**, 201–210.

some widespread ileus with multiple short fluid levels and some separation of the moderately distended bowel loops by exudate.

URINARY TRACT COMPLICATIONS

It is not surprising that gynaecology produces more damage to the urinary tract than any other branch of surgery, considering the high incidence of malignant disease in the female genital tract and the frequency of difficult surgical procedures deep within the pelvic cavity, sometimes associated with preoperative radiotherapy. Urinary tract complications are especially likely to occur after radical hysterectomy. The main investigative tool in the appraisal of these complications is the intravenous urogram.

Pre-operative IV urography

Because the urinary tract is at risk, it is logical and reasonable to perform urography routinely before surgery in those situations where operative difficulties are likely to arise (Whitehouse, 1977):

1. Pelvic inflammatory disease, extensive endometriosis and large pelvic masses may be the cause of significant ureteral obstruction and displacement.

2. In patients with carcinoma of the cervix or uterine body, a useful baseline is provided in case complications occur during surgery. Urography will also show whether or not the urinary tract is directly involved by the malignant process.

3. Pre-operative urinary infection may be associated with hydroureter and hydronephrosis, or with congenital anomalies of the urinary tract.

Schwartz *et al.* (1964) found preoperative urographic abnormalities in 16% of patients who subsequently underwent hysterectomy for benign conditions. Most of these abnormalities were ureteral deviation and obstruction secondary to a pelvic mass. St Martin *et al.* (1953) found a 10.8% incidence of hydronephrosis and hydroureter in a large series of patients scheduled for major gynaecological surgery, excluding radical hysterectomy, with a failure to return to normal in less than 1% of the total after operation. In the series of Morrison (1960) with preoperative urograms, sixteen of 110 patients (14.5%) had dilatation of the upper urinary tract attributable to large fibroids, ovarian masses and endometriosis, with a return to normality in all but two cases following hysterectomy. Solomons *et al.* (1960) found that 20.5% had various degrees of ureteral obstruction before hysterectomy for benign conditions, but 90.2% reverted to normal after the operation. It may take up to a year for the ureters to revert to normal after hysterectomy, the persistance of ureteral dilatation in the few cases suggesting ureteral involvement by other factors besides extrinsic compression.

Ureteral complications

Green *et al.* (1962) found a 12.5% incidence of ureteral complications with radical hysterectomy, which compares with a 0.02 to 3% incidence in hysterectomy for benign conditions (Freda & Tacchi, 1962). Vaginal hysterectomy has a slightly higher incidence of ureteral damage, 0.12 to 4.76% in various series, than abdominal hysterectomy (van Nagall & Roddick, 1972).

The ureter is in danger at several points during hysterectomy (Benson & Hinman, 1955): (1) The highest and least dangerous point is where the ureter crosses the iliac vessels. (2) In the ovarian fossa where the ureter comes into close proximity with the adnexa. (3) Most commonly where the ureter is crossed by the uterine vessels. (4) The base of the bladder, which may be the site of incisional damage or kinking of the ureter.

Causes of ureteral injury include cutting, ligation, clamping, kinking, needle puncture and necrosis. Inadequate exposure due to a limited incision and poor muscle relaxation, poorly applied haemostasis and careless dissection predispose to ureteral injury. The blood supply of the ureter is mainly adventitial, so that wide stripping of the ureter from the peritoneum and its bed, or Waldeyer's sheath, may endanger the ureteral vascularity and nerve supply.

Many ureteral injuries are not recognized at the time of operation but become manifested later with the onset of symptoms which often include flank or loin pain, pyrexia, urinary infection or the leakage of urine. The occurrence of these symptoms in the postoperative period demands urgent IV urography. It seems likely that some injuries are never detected, while subsequent urography may reveal previously unsuspected ureteral obstruction or a non-functioning kidney. Other radiological evidence of ureteral injury includes extravasation of contrast medium during urography or retrograde pyelography, or a large retroperitoneal soft tissue mass due to extravasation of urine.

Postoperative renal function and ureteral obstruction may be accurately assessed by the use of isotope venography (Koskela *et al.*, 1969; Mogensen *et al.*, 1973).

TRANSIENT HYDROURETER AND HYDRONEPHROSIS

Talbert *et al.* (1965) found that dilatation of the upper urinary tract was invariably seen on urography within 24 hours of radical hysterectomy, becoming maximal in three weeks but usually resolving completely within three months (Fig. 11.3). Green *et al.* (1962) found a 24% incidence of this transient ureteral obstruction after radical hysterectomy, while the occurrence after hysterectomy for benign disease is of the order of 1% (Solomons *et al.*, 1960) to 3.75% (Morrison, 1960).

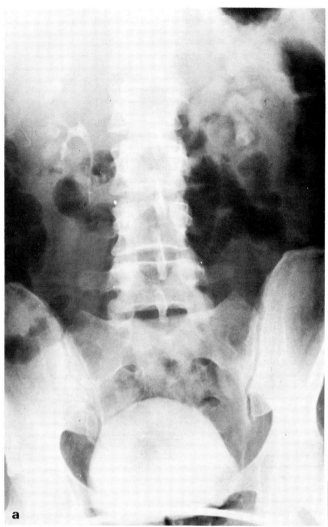

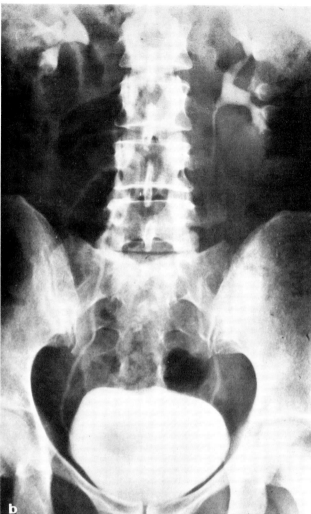

FIG. 11.3 (a) Left hydronephrosis and hydroureter after hysterectomy.

(b) Normal appearances 6 months later. From *Clinical Radiology* (1977), **28**, 201–210.

Local mural and periureteral oedema is one factor which may cause this temporary ureteral obstruction. Separation of the lower ureter from Waldeyer's sheath in the radical procedure may endanger ureteral vascularity and cause deprivation of nerve supply, leading to transient ureteral narrowing or occasionally to permanent stricture.

Kinking of the pelvic portion of one or both ureters has been associated with hysterectomy and bilateral salpingo-oophrectomy, but any resultant back pressure changes tend to resolve spontaneously during the ensuing months (Morrison, 1960).

URETERAL STRICTURE

Ureteral stricture is probably the most frequent irreversible result of ureteral injury. Like other ureteral complications, stricture formation is especially common after radical hysterectomy, due to irreversible denervation and

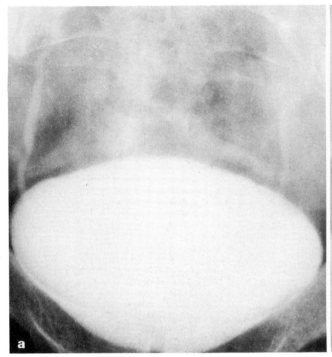

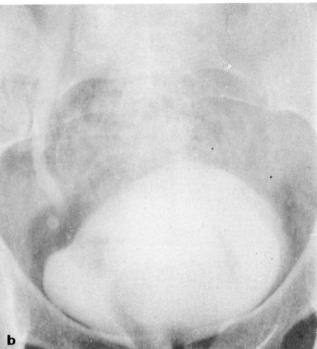

FIG. 11.4 (a) Normal appearances on urography before hysterectomy.

(b) Stricture of lower end of right ureter 1 year later.

devascularization of the distal ureter with subsequent fibrosis. It may also result from attempts at direct repair of a severed ureter. Ureteral stenoses are of varying lengths and occur below the level of the pelvic brim (Fig. 11.4). The incidence of stricture after radical hysterectomy varies between 1 and 2.8% (Green *et al.*, 1962), and is 1 to 1.5% after hysterectomy for benign disease (Freda & Tacchi, 1962; Solomons *et al.*, 1960).

While ureteral stricture after radiation treatment for carcinoma of the cervix is variably reported as occurring in 0.26–1.6% of cases, the incidence rises to 1.6–7.5% after combined radical hysterectomy and radiotherapy (Shingleton *et al.*, 1969). An even higher incidence of stricture formation was found by Shingleton & Palumbo (1968) in cases where indwelling ureteral catheters were used and postoperative radiotherapy was given. Discontinuation of either of these practices resulted in a much lower incidence of ureteral strictures and fistula formation. These same authors found that ureteral strictures occurred between one and four years after radiotherapy alone, and within the first few months after radical hysterectomy or when surgery was combined with radiotherapy.

URETEROVAGINAL FISTULA

A fistula into the vagina may develop secondary to ureteral severence or vascular compromise. Green *et al.* (1962) had an 8.5% incidence of ureterovaginal fistula following radical hysterectomy, while the overall incidence after all hysterectomies is reported as 0.4 to 1% (Carter, 1954). Mack (1969) found that radical surgery combined with radiotherapy had a 10.4% incidence of ureterovaginal fistula, while radiotherapy alone gave a 0.45% incidence.

Patients with ureterovaginal fistula present with urinary incontinence, usually in the second postoperative week, often preceded by flank pain and fever. On examination a mass may be found above and lateral to the vaginal apex.

IV urography very often shows ureteral dilatation,

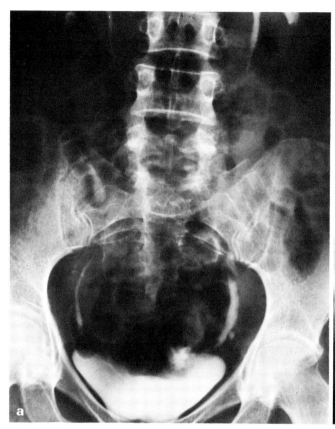

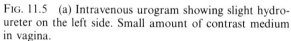

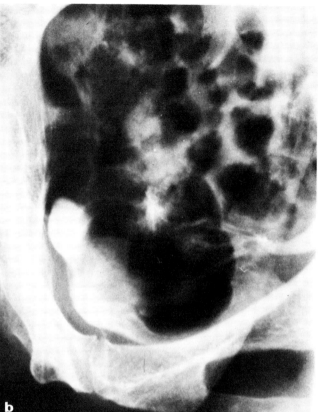

FIG. 11.5   (a) Intravenous urogram showing slight hydro-ureter on the left side. Small amount of contrast medium in vagina.

(b) Site of ureterovaginal fistula shown on oblique view. From *Clinical Radiology* (1977), **28**, 201–210.

perhaps with associated hydronephrosis on the ipsilateral side as the ureterovaginal fistula (Fig. 11.5). The ureteral obstruction is secondary to either compression from extravasated urine or to stenosis from the surgical trauma. The vagina is well delineated by contrast medium although it may be impossible, even with oblique views, to show the actual fistula. If urography is normal, then it may be concluded with reasonable certainty that there is no ureterovaginal fistula.

Vaginography may be used to demonstrate a uretero-vaginal fistula (Wolfson, 1964). It is usually impossible to directly catheterize the involved ureter from either the vaginal or vesical approach.

Spontaneous healing of a ureterovaginal fistula occasionally occurs, but a hydronephrosis or non-functioning kidney often remains in such cases (Fig. 11.6).

URETERAL SEVERENCE

This serious complication is often, but not always, recognized at the time of the operation. A uretero-vaginal fistula, ureteral obstruction, or a communication with the pelvic cavity may result.

Attempted retrograde catheterization may show the catheter to lie outside the normal line of the ureter. The extravasation of large quantities of urine into the space may cause a large soft tissue retroperitoneal mass on plain radiographs. IV urography may show extravasation of contrast medium as an ill-defined opacity developing at the level of the pelvic ureter and spreading within

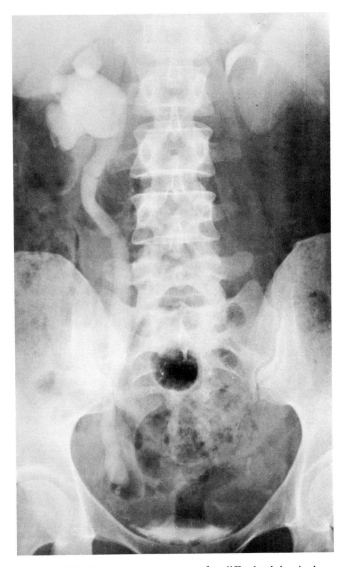

FIG. 11.6 Intravenous urogram of a difficult abdominal hysterectomy. Postoperative leakage of urine per vaginam, which resolved spontaneously. Persistent obstruction of right ureter with hydronephrosis. From *Clinical Radiology* (1977), **28**, 201–210.

the retroperitoneal space (Fig. 11.7). There may be ureteral obstruction or a non-functioning kidney. The inadvertent division or elective partial resection of the ureter should be treated by reimplantation of the ureter into the bladder. An end-to-end anastomosis after ureteral severence is very often followed by the development of ureterovaginal fistula or ureteral stricture (Fig. 11.8).

Bladder complications

VESICOVAGINAL FISTULA

Total abdominal or vaginal hysterectomy accounts for a third of all vesicovaginal fistulae, gynaecological injury causing 80% of the total and the rest being due to obstetric damage (Chassar Moir, 1973). Vesicovaginal fistula occurs in 0.4% of vaginal hysterectomies (Radman, 1961) and in 2.2% of cases after radical hysterectomy (Green *et al.*, 1962). The vesical floor may be damaged on separation of the bladder from the anterior part of the cervix and vagina, which is especially likely if the normal anatomy is distorted by adhesions and endometriosis. Indiscriminate ligation may result in ischaemic necrosis and subsequent sloughing of the bladder wall, forming a fistula into the vagina, usually at about the seventh postoperative day. Overdistension of the bladder, due to postoperative urinary retention, may be a contributing factor. Postoperative radiotherapy may also lead to tissue necrosis and a subsequent vesicovaginal fistula some time later. Recurrent carcinoma is another cause of postoperative vesicovaginal fistula.

On IV urography the kidneys and ureters are normal in the absence of pre-existing radiological disease unless the lower ureters are involved by inflammatory reaction associated with the fistula, in which case there may be ureteral dilatation, hydronephrosis or a nonfunctioning kidney. The vagina should be outlined by contrast medium on urography and there may be poor distensibility of the bladder if the fistula is large (Fig. 11.9). Cystography may delineate the fistula, and is often useful when the communication has not been shown on urography (Fig. 11.9). Vaginography has been sucessfully used to demonstrate vesicovaginal fistulae (Wolfson, 1964).

POSTOPERATIVE BLADDER CALCULI

Green *et al.* (1962) have found a 1.4% incidence of bladder calculi following radical hysterectomy (Fig. 11.10), and attribute this to the indwelling bladder catheter which is maintained for the first six or eight postoperative weeks. However, this is not always a prerequisite, the denervation of the bladder and the high

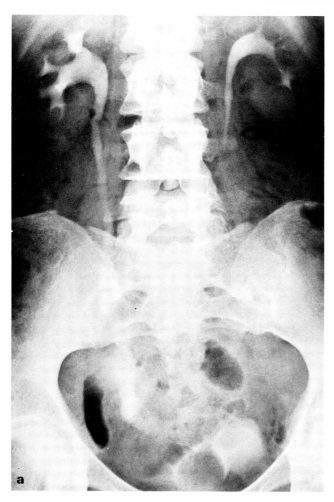

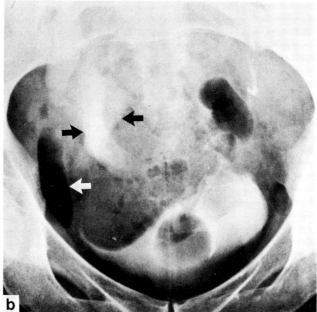

FIG. 11.7 (a) and (b) Intravenous urogram after ureteral severence showing right-sided hydroureter and mild hydronephrosis. Extravasation of contrast medium (black arrows). Pelvic soft tissue contains some gas (white arrow) due to abscess developing secondary to pelvic infection and extravasation of urine.

incidence of urinary infection after radical hysterectomy being other predispositions to stone formation. Vesical calculi are sometimes seen in vesicovaginal fistulae (Lawson, 1972).

URINARY RETENTION AND OTHER POSTOPERATIVE SYMPTOMS

Urinary retention is common after hysterectomy, especially following the radical procedure, but is usually a transient phenomenon, although it is sometimes persistent (Fraser, 1966). In the immediate postoperative period vaginal hysterectomy is more likely to cause retention than abdominal hysterectomy. Cystometric studies have shown that a state of hypertonic bladder dysfunc-

tion results from vaginal hysterectomy and persists to a lesser degree after the return of clinically normal function (Roman-Lopez & Barclay, 1973). Severance of the nerves to the bladder from the sacral plexus during radical hysterectomy is associated with a high incidence of impaired bladder sensation and other urinary symptoms, including difficulty in micturition and incontinence of urine (Smith et al., 1969). There is often reversal or improvement of these symptoms within a year. Ureteral reflux has sometimes been found for a year or so after radical hysterectomy (Mallik, 1961).

Stress incontinence often develops after radical hysterectomy, but symptoms clear within the first year in the majority of cases, probably as a result of recovery of normal bladder function and tone and the development of scar tissue beneath the bladder neck.

The combination of frequency and urgency of micturition, dysuria and retropubic discomfort arising after hysterectomy may be due to development of the 'urethral syndrome'. In most cases there is no evidence of urinary infection to account for these symptoms. Smith *et al.* (1970) found urethral narrowing on cystoscopy in more than half the cases. They postulate that the aetiology of the urethral syndrome is an obstruction of the urethra secondary to periurethral fibrosis which occurs following the hysterectomy. Another factor is oestrogen deficiency, which is associated with a tendency to stricture formation in the distal urethra. Many of the cases of Smith *et al.* (1969) were improved by urethral dilatation alone or in combination with oestrogen supplements. Jackson (1976) has described cystographic appearances in the urethral syndrome. He found a crenated appearance to the bladder base, and often elevation of the bladder base with hypertrophy of the bladder neck. Paraurethral glandular hyperplasia and periurethral calcification were not uncommon findings. There was further thickening and rigidity of the bladder neck in long standing cases, with hypertrophy of the detrusor muscle secondary to this obstruction.

GASTROINTESTINAL COMPLICATIONS

POSTOPERATIVE ILEUS

Flatulent distention of the colon is very common after hysterectomy. Severe paralytic ileus and concomitant gross abdominal distention is not frequent, being reported by Green *et al.* (1962) in 1% of cases after radical hysterectomy, and respectively in 3.1% and 0.5% of abdominal and vaginal hysterectomies (Crisp & Satterspiel, 1965). The typical radiological features are small and large bowel dilatation with fluid levels (Fig. 11.11).

INTESTINAL OBSTRUCTION

Obstruction due to adhesions is especially likely to occur when hysterectomy is complicated by pelvic inflammatory disease or endometriosis. The level of the obstruction is usually in the ileum. Intestinal dilatation and fluid levels are seen proximal to the obstruction.

ACUTE GASTRIC DILATATION

Gastric dilatation is a very rare complication of hysterectomy, and may be associated with paralytic ileus. The patient is very ill, vomits copious amounts of fluid, and has a grossly distended and atonic stomach.

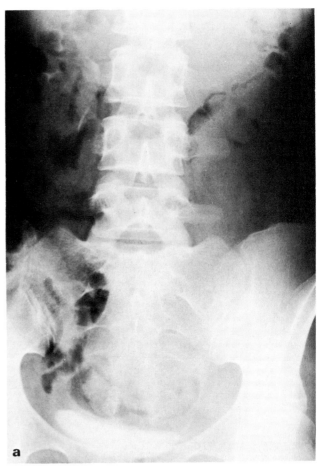

FIG. 11.8   Left ureter had been severed at hysterectomy and repaired by end-to-end anastomosis.
   (a) Postoperative intravenous urogram shows very little excretion by left kidney. Pelvic soft tissue mass is seen.

STRESS ULCERS OF THE STOMACH

These ulcers usually take the form of multiple shallow erosions. While 'stress' is a common factor, severe infection, intestinal obstruction and extensive pelvic surgery may be present, often in combination (Dunn & Nash, 1964).

INTESTINAL FISTULAE

Rectovaginal fistulae occurred in less than 0.2% of radical hysterectomies in the experience of Green *et al.* (1962). The rectosigmoid may be damaged when the uterus is

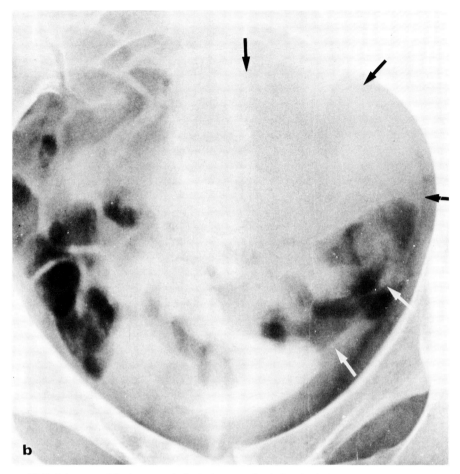

(b) Pelvic mass (black arrows) deviating poorly defined pelvic portion of left ureter (white arrows). From *Clinical Radiology* (1977), **28**, 201–210.

adherent to it because of chronic pelvic inflammatory disease or endometriosis.

Intestinal fistulae have been found to follow pelvic exenteration in 13.6% of cases (Clark *et al.*, 1962). Most occur in the immediate postoperative period, on average eighteen days after surgery and are due to breakdown of anastomoses, infection or previous radiotherapy. Those fistulae which develop later are usually due to recurrence of the carcinoma. Both small and large bowel fistulae drain via the incision or into the vagina.

The formation of a fistula from the small intestine or colon will be demonstrated by barium follow-through and barium enema examination respectively.

VENOUS THROMBOSIS

Venous thrombosis was found by Crisp & Satterspiel (1965) after 1.7% of abdominal and 0.5% of vaginal hysterectomies but by Jeffcoate & Tindall (1965) in 3.3% and 3.1% respectively. Käsar (1967) noted a 6.4% incidence of venous thrombosis after radical hysterectomy. These quoted series are probably an underestimation of the true incidence of venous thrombosis, as none of them give the overall incidence found on leg venography. The peak occurrence is in the second postoperative week, and the elderly and obese are especially prone to this complication. The most frequent

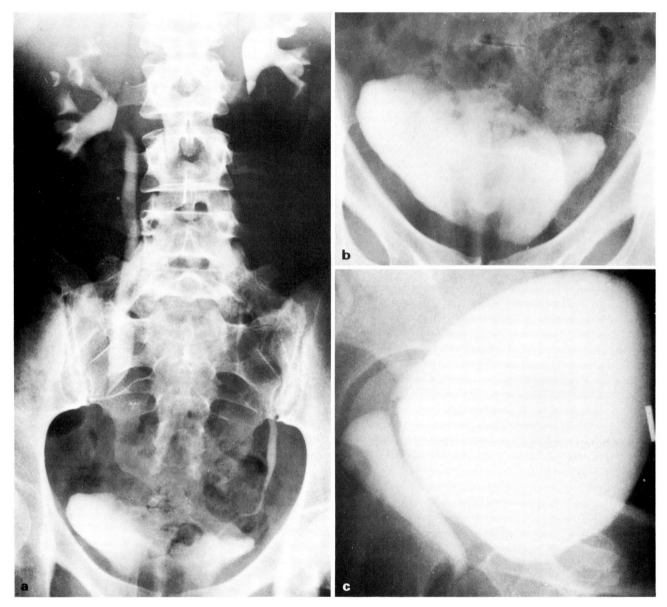

FIG. 11.9 (a) Intravenous urogram after radical hysterectomy showing postoperative vesicovaginal fistula, and right-sided hydroureter with contrast medium in bladder.

(b) Later radiograph shows marked vaginal pooling through opacified bladder.

(c) Lateral radiograph of cystogram showing vesicovaginal fistula.

From *Clinical Radiology* (1977), **28,** 201–210.

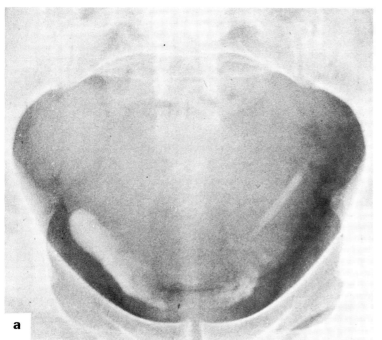

a

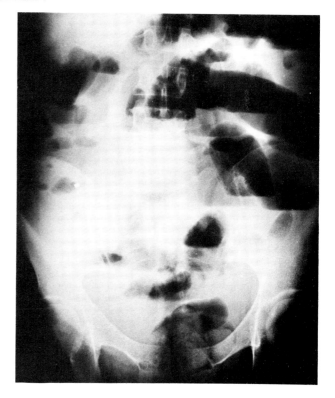

FIG. 11.11 Paralytic ileus after total hysterectomy. Generalized dilatation of small intestine and colon, with multiple fluid levels.

FIG. 11.10 (a) Preoperative intravenous urogram. No bladder abnormality seen on plain radiograph or after opacification.

(b) Two large bladder calculi, seen 2½ years after radical hysterectomy.

From *Clinical Radiology* (1977), **28**, 201–210.

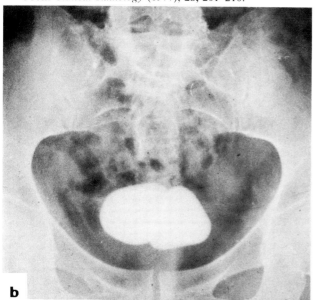

b

site of thrombosis on venography is the ileofemoral vein, especially on the left side where the left common iliac vein may be impinged by the right common iliac artery (Crockett, 1968).

ARTERIOVENOUS FISTULA

Several cases have been described where a fistula has occurred between the ipsilateral uterine artery and vein (Wideman *et al.*, 1959; Field *et al.*, 1963). Morley & Lindenauer (1968) have described the arteriographic appearances of such a case; the left internal iliac artery and uterine artery were dilated and tortuous, the latter terminating in a saccular aneurysm which drained into multiple dilated veins with rapid opacification of the left iliac vein. Transfixion and ligation of the uterine vessels *en masse*, with the accidental passage of a needle through the uterine artery and vein, is likely to be the cause of the arteriovenous fistula.

LYMPHATIC CHANGES AFTER RADICAL HYSTERECTOMY

Lymphography will show one of two possible patterns after lymphadenectomy (Chiappa *et al.*, 1965; Jackson, 1968):

1. Small collateral lymphatic vessels run from the inguinal nodes and pass laterally across the iliac fossa and hip, while others course medially to unite with the lymph pathways of the opposite side or run upwards over the pelvic inlet to rejoin the main lymphatic pathways at a higher level. Lymphaticovenous anastomoses also develop after lymphadenectomy.

2. Opacified lymph vessels and sometimes even lymph nodes may persist within the pelvic cavity. These structures have either been left at surgery or represent regeneration of resected lymphatics.

LYMPHOCYSTS

Lymphocysts occur where there is efficient clearance of lymph nodes from the pelvic cavity, but only a small proportion cause symptoms. Lymph continues to flow from transected distal lymphatic vessels into actual or potential spaces which are formed after the removal of lymph nodes and connective tissue. The incidence of lymphocyst formation after radical hysterectomy is 29%

(Dodd *et al.*, 1970). The diagnosis is usually made within six months of surgery, when the patient complains of lower abdominal swelling; oedema of the external genitalia and leg, constipation and frequency of micturition are due to compression of the various pelvic structures by the lymphocyst.

Abdominal radiographs may show soft tissue masses protruding into the pelvic cavity from the lateral pelvic walls, occasionally with displacement of pelvic phleboliths. Rarely, and usually when intestinal radiation necrosis is present, a fistula may communicate between the lymphocyst and an adjacent loop of bowel so that intestinal gas or contrast medium may enter an extraluminal pocket. IV urography often shows the ureters to be displaced medially and anteriorly, and sometimes ureteral obstruction is present. The bladder may be compressed by a lymphocyst. Displacement and compression of the sigmoid segment, and even frank obstruction, may be seen on barium enema. Compression of the pelvic veins is often visible on venography. The direct puncture, aspiration and contrast delineation of a lymphocyst must be avoided at all costs because of the risks of infection.

CHEST INFECTION

There is much less chance of developing pneumonia after pelvic surgery than following abdominal operations. Käser found a 2.2% incidence of pneumonia after radical hysterectomy. Mucus impaction of lower lobe bronchi may cause basal collapse (Fig. 11.12).

Pneumoperitoneum

Air rarely enters the peritoneal cavity through an open vaginal vault (Bryant *et al.*, 1961) or through a prolapsed Fallopian tube after vaginal hysterectomy (Tabrisky *et al.*, 1972) to give a pneumoperitoneum.

COMPLICATIONS OF RADIOTHERAPY

Serious and even life-threatening changes sometimes occur in the urinary tract or the intestine as a result of radiotherapy applied to gynaecological malignancy. The risk of complications increases with the extent of the tumour and also depends on the skilful application and dose of the irradiation.

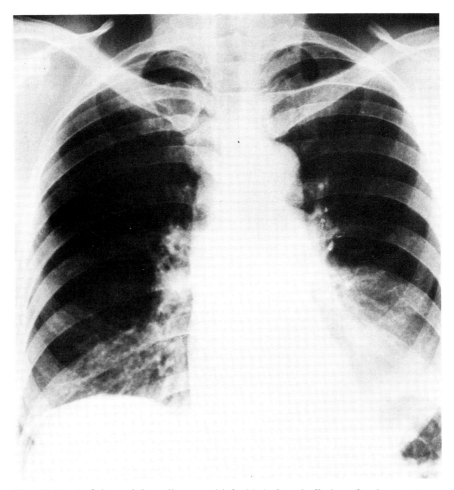

Fig. 11.12 Left lower lobe collapse and left-sided pleural effusion after hysterectomy.

The urinary tract

URETERAL STRICTURE

Radiotherapy results in relief of ureteral obstruction secondary to carcinoma of the cervix in only 10% of cases (Slater & Fletcher, 1971). The ureter is relatively resistant to the effects of irradiation, and stricture developing after radiotherapy is due to recurrent carcinoma in the vast majority of cases. Rhamy & Stander (1962) and Kaplan (1977) estimate the incidence of ureteral stricture secondary to irradiation to be 1% in all patients treated for carcinoma of the cervix and 5.8% of those patients with ureteral obstruction after treatment. The fibrous stricture is smoothly tapered and is situated 4 to 6 cm from the distal end of the ureter as it passes through the broad ligament (Fig. 11.13), and occurs about three years after radiation therapy whereas tumour recurrence causes ureteral obstruction at, on average, a year after treatment.

Initially, transient hydronephrosis due to oedema secondary to irradiation may occur three weeks after the initial radium application for cervical carcinoma (Rhamy & Stander, 1961), and may be sufficient to produce complete obstruction in the presence of pre-existent partial occlusion (Kickham, 1961).

Ureterovaginal fistulae are an uncommon sequence to

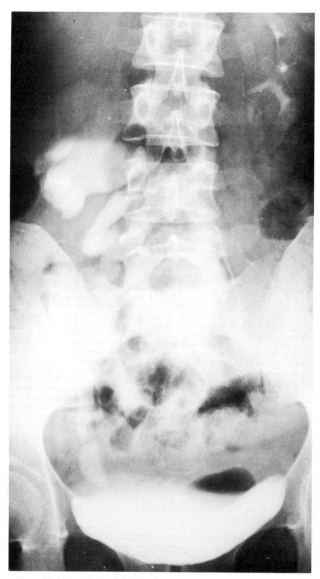

FIG. 11.13 Right-sided hydronephrosis and hydroureter due to postradiotherapy stricture of pelvic portion of right ureter.

radiotherapy, but are more likely to occur when irradiation is combined with hysterectomy.

THE BLADDER

When levels of 6000–7000 R are approached, there is very often a severe acute radiation cystitis. There are no specific radiological findings of radiation cystitis, but usually there is increased irritability and contractibility of the bladder. Occasionally, the bladder capacity becomes small and rarely there is stasis in the pelvic portions of the ureters (Chau *et al.*, 1962).

Chronic radiation reaction in the bladder may develop between one and four years after treatment, and sometimes earlier with high doses. Faulty radiation technique or the presence of an anteflexed uterus increases the incidence of chronic bladder change. Interstitial fibrosis and obliterative endarteritis are frequently found, and ischaemia leads to necrosis with the development of ulcers, fissures and fistulae. As a result, IV urography shows a thick walled, small volume bladder and sometimes bilateral ureteral obstruction. Free vesicoureteral reflux may occur. Rectovesical (Fig. 11.14) and vesicovaginal fistulae (Fig. 11.15) are often the result of poor radiation technique or when radiotherapy is combined

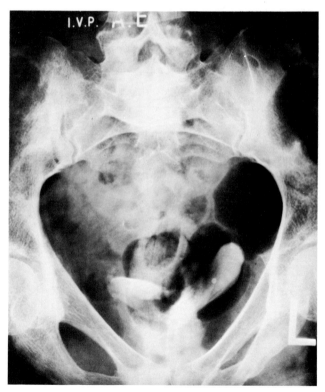

FIG. 11.14 Intravenous urogram showing vesicorectal fistula secondary to radiotherapy for carcinoma of the cervix.

proctocolitis, but occasionally proceeds to ulceration, stricture formation and fistulation. Some 60% of patients who have intestinal symptoms after radiotherapy show some abnormality on barium enema examination (Marshak, 1947). Spasm and serration of the margins are the commonest signs, the latter being due to submucosal oedema and fibrosis which broadens the plicae (Perkins & Spjut, 1962). Multiple ulcerations are common. There is never a clear-cut delineation between involved and unaffected segments of bowel. The presence of mucosal oedema and fibrosis may result in a 'pseudotumour' which is difficult to differentiate radiologically from an advanced infiltrating carcinoma (Kaplan *et al.*, 1965). Stricture formation may lead to complete obstruction to retrograde barium filling, the radiation strictures usually being 3 to 8 cm in length (Perkins & Spjut, 1962).

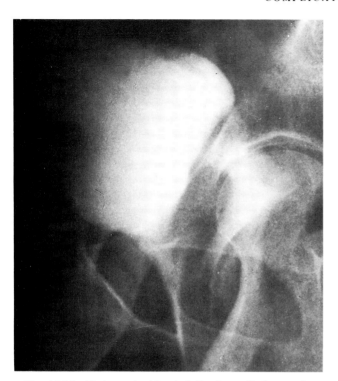

FIG. 11.15   Vesicovaginal fistula following radiotherapy for carcinoma of the cervix. The fistula was secondary to a recurrence of the tumour.

with surgery, and develop between six months and three years after treatment (Everett & Mattingly, 1956), but may be 'inevitable' when there is tumour involving the walls of these structures. The incidence of vesicovaginal fistula after radiotherapy is 1.2% in carcinoma of the cervix (Boronow & Rutledge, 1971). A necrosed area of the bladder wall may undergo calcification, with contrast medium filling the roughened crevices of the calcified area on urography, but no evidence of a filling defect (Mallik, 1962).

Intestinal changes

RECTOSIGMOID

The rectum is damaged in 2.4% of cases when 6000 R are applied to the rectal wall by external irradiation and intracavitary radium (Strickland, 1954) and in 6.3% of cases when at least 6500 R are given (Mason *et al.*, 1970). The damage to the rectosigmoid is usually a self limiting

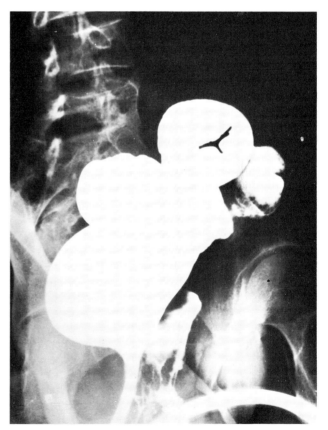

FIG. 11.16   Barium enema showing rectovaginal fistula following radiotherapy for carcinoma of the cervix.

Perforation of a necrotic area may be accompanied by abscess and fistula formation, and the use of water-soluble contrast medium is recommended if there is suspicion of this complication. Rectovaginal fistula will occur when the tumour has spread between these structures, the communication developing within a few months of treatment (Fig. 11.16).

The transverse colon will be in the field when there is irradiation of the retroperitoneal lymph nodes and may be affected by radiation colitis.

SMALL INTESTINE

Damage to the small intestine is a rare complication of pelvic irradiation because of its mobility, occurring in 0.6% of all cervical carcinomas and other gynaecological

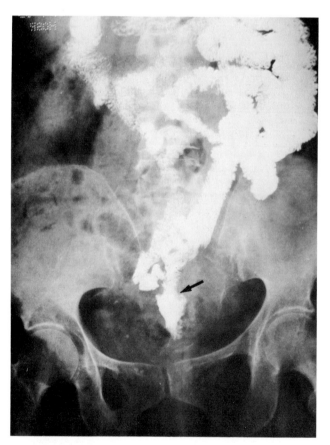

FIG. 11.17. Barium follow-through showing fistula (arrow) between small intestine and vagina following intracavitary and external irradiation for carcinoma of the cervix.

cancers treated by radiotherapy (Graham & Villalba, 1963). Previous surgery and pelvic infection may cause adhesions, the immobilized loops of small intestine then becoming susceptible to radiation damage. At least 4000 R are required to cause appreciable damage to the small intestine.

During the course of radiotherapy, acute injury may cause ileus which is visible on abdominal radiographs. Chronic radiation injury is largely due to endarteritis with vascular occlusion. On barium studies (Mason et al., 1970), thickening of mucosal folds, nodular defects due to submucosal oedema, and dilatation of proximal small bowel are seen. Submucosal oedema and fibrosis result in thickening of the bowel wall with an increased distance between adjacent loops, and rigidity with angulations and impaired peristalsis. Advanced fibrosis will result in stenosis. Thickening and shortening of the mesentery and adhesions cause matting together of several loops of bowel, with mucosal folds being pulled obliquely outside the lumen due to adhesions. Intestinal perforation will cause generalized peritonitis, abscess formation or fistulae to the bladder, colon, skin and vagina (Fig. 11.17) (Graham & Villalba, 1963).

Dencker et al. (1972) have performed mesenteric arteriography in cases of radiation injury to the bowel. Arterial stenosis and occlusion was due to endarteritis, and in some cases the vasa recta in the bowel wall were tortuous and close together at sites of intestinal stenosis and decreased length. Avascularity of the lesion was usually a pronounced feature, although occasionally newly formed capillaries grew into granulation tissue to give an appearance of increased vascularity.

Lymph node changes

There is usually a uniform diminution in the size of lymph nodes following irradiation, although the nodes retain a normal shape and contour. Doses of radiation which are large enough to cause pelvic fibrosis, bladder and rectal injury are likely to cause delayed emptying of lymphatic vessels with extravasation of contrast medium into adjacent tissues, as well as a decrease in the size and number of lymph nodes (Averette & Ferguson, 1963).

Parametrial soft tissue calcification is seen in approximately half the patients with cervical carcinoma treated by the parametrial injection of Au[198] colloid (Deeths & Stanley, 1976).

Bone changes

Fractures of the femoral neck, and less frequently of the pelvis, have been described following radiotherapy for cervical carcinoma. Most cases of hip and pelvic bone radionecrosis occur in orthovoltage therapy and are especially frequent in patients who have undergone re-treatment. Smaller and fewer portals with supravoltage therapy, increased depth dose and shielding of the proximal femur have led to a markedly decreased incidence of bone radionecrosis (Dalinka *et al.*, 1974).

The femoral neck fractures are usually subcapital in situation, and are preceded by an irregular line of osteo-sclerosis (Fig. 11.18), and occasionally by smaller scattered areas of bone absorption before the spontaneous occurrence of the fracture (Stephenson & Cohen, 1956). Increased bone density and areas of rarefaction due to radionecrosis may also be apparent in the femoral head and acetabulum (Gratzek *et al.*, 1945). Osteoporosis may

also predispose to femoral neck fracture after radio-therapy, as an increased incidence has been noted in older patients (Stampfli & Kerr, 1947).

Osteosarcoma, secondary to radiation necrosis, very occasionally occurs after treatment for carcinoma of the cervix (Rushforth, 1974).

REFERENCES

Complications of hysterectomy

BENSON R. C. & HINMAN F. (1955) Urinary tract injuries in obstetrics and gynecology. *Amer. J. Obst. Gynec.*, **70**, 467–485.

BRYANT L. R., HAYDON G. B. & ALTEMEIER W. A. (1961) An unusual complication of radical hysterectomy and pelvic lymphadenectomy. *Surg. Gynec. Obst.*, **113**, 455–457.

CARTER R. G. (1954) Ureterovaginal fistula. *J. Urol.*, **71**, 200–207.

CHASSAR MOIR J. (1973) Vesico-vaginal fistulae as seen in Britain. *J. Obst. Gynaec. Br. Cwth.*, **80**, 598–602.

CHIAPPA S., GALLI G., LUCIANI L. & SEVERINI A. (1965) Considerations on the restoration of the lymphatic circulation after pelvic lymphadenectomy. *Surg. Gynec. Obst.*, **120**, 323–324.

CLARK D. G. C., DANIEL W. W. & BRUNSCHWIG A. (1962) Intestinal fistulas following pelvic exenteration. *Amer. J. Obst. Gynec.*, **84**, 187–191.

COCKETT F. B. (1968) Ilio femoral thrombosis following confinement and hysterectomy. *J. Obst. Gynaec. Br. Cwth.*, **75**, 1316–1319.

CRISP W. E. & SATTERSPIEL E. (1965) The morbidity of hysterectomy. *Surg. Gynec. Obst.*, **120**, 965–969.

DODD G. D., RUTLEDGE F. & WALLACE S. (1970) Post-operative pelvic lymphocysts. *Amer. J. Roentgenol.*, **108**, 312–323.

DUNN L. J. & NASH L. D. (1964) Stress ulcers of the stomach following obstetric and gynecological surgery. *Amer. J. Obst. Gynec.*, **90**, 1288–1292.

FIELD C. A., WELCH J. S. & JOHNSON C. E. (1963) Post hysterectomy arteriovenous fistula involving uterine artery and vein. *Amer. J. Obst. Gynec.*, **87**, 105–108.

FRASER A. C. (1966) The late effects of Wertheim's hysterectomy on the urinary tract. *J. Obst. Gynaec. Br. Cwth.*, **73**, 1002–1007.

FREDA V. C. & TACCHI D. (1962) Ureteral injury discovered after pelvic surgery. *Amer. J. Obst. Gynec.*, **83**, 406–409.

GREEN T. H., MEIGS J. V., ULFELDER H. & CURTIN R. R. (1962) Urologic complications of radical Wertheim's hysterectomy. *Obst. Gynec.*, **20**, 293–312.

JACKSON E. A. (1976) Urethral syndrome in women. *Radiology*, **119**, 287–291.

JACKSON R. J. A. (1968) Observations on changes in the lymphatic circulation which develop after pelvic lymphadenectomy. *J. Obst. Gynaec. Br. Cwth.*, **75**, 521–530.

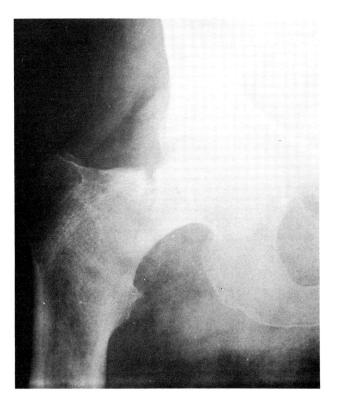

FIG. 11.18 Spontaneous fracture of femoral neck after radiotherapy for carcinoma of the cervix. The fracture has occurred through an area of osteosclerosis.

JEFFCOATE T. N. A. & TINDALL V. R. (1965) Venous thrombosis and embolism in obstetrics and gynaecology. *Aust. N. Z. J. Obst. Gynaec.*, **5**, 119–130.

KÄSER O. (1967) Results of 600 Wertheim operations for cancer of the cervix. *Med. Coll. Virginia Quart.*, **3**, 42–51.

KOSKELA O., KOKKONEN J. & VAHALA J. (1969) Renographic studies of ureteric patency following total hysterectomy. *Acta Obst. Gynaec. Scand.*, **48**, 567–574.

LAWSON J. (1972) Vesical fistulae into the vaginal vault. *Br. J. Urol.*, **44**, 623–631.

LEDGER W. J., CAMPBELL C., TAYLOR D. & WILLSON J. R. (1969) Adnexal abscess as a late complication of pelvic operations. *Surg. Gynec. Obst.*, **129**, 973–978.

MACK W. S. (1969) Urological complications of pelvic surgery. *Br. J. Urol.*, **41**, 641–648.

MALLIK M. K. B. (1961) A study of the urinary bladder following Wertheim hysterectomy with special reference to the incompetence of the urethral and ureteric orifices. *J. Obst. Gynaec. Br. Emp.*, **68**, 945–951.

MOGENSEN P., RØDHO P. & LEFËURE H. (1973) Radioisotope venography in the surgical management of carcinoma of the cervix. *Acta Obst. Gynec. Scand.*, **52**, 109–112.

MORLEY G. W. & LINDENAUER S. M. (1968) Arteriovenous fistula following pelvic operations. *Obst. Gynec.*, **31**, 722–726.

MORRISON J. K. (1960) The ureter and hysterectomy. *J. Obst. Gynaec. Br. Emp.*, **67**, 66–73.

VAN NAGELL J. R. & RODDICK J. W. (1972) Vaginal hysterectomy, the ureter and excretory urography. *Obst. Gynec.*, **39**, 784–786.

RADMAN H. M. (1961) Vesicovaginal fistula. *Amer. J. Obst. Gynec.*, **82**, 1238–1242.

ROMAN-LOPEZ J. J. & BARCLAY D. L. (1973) Bladder dysfunction following Schauta hysterectomy. *Amer. J. Obst. Gynec.*, **115**, 81–90.

ST MARTIN E. C., TRICHEL B. E., CAMPBELL J. H. & LOCKE J. M. (1953) Ureteral injuries in gynaecologic surgery. *J. Urol.*, **70**, 51–57.

SCHWARTZ W. R., HOFMEISTER F. J. & MATTINGLY R. F. (1964) The value of intravenous urograms in pelvic surgery. *Obst. Gynec.*, **23**, 584–588.

SHINGLETON H. M. & PALUMBO L. (1968) Ureteral complications of radical hysterectomy: effects of preoperative radium and ureteral catheters. *Surg. Forum*, **19**, 410–412.

SHINGLETON H. M., FOWLER W. C., PEPPER F. D. & PALUMBO L. (1969) Ureteral strictures following therapy for carcinoma of the cervix. *Cancer*, **24**, 77–83.

SMITH P., ROBERTS M. & SLADE N. (1970) Urinary symptoms following hysterectomy. *Br. J. Urol.*, **42**, 3–9.

SMITH P. H., TURNBULL G. H., CURRIE D. W. & PEEL K. R. (1969) Two urological complications of Wertheim's hysterectomy. *Br. J. Urol.*, **41**, 685–688.

SOLOMONS E., LEVIN E. J., BAUMAN J. & BARON J. (1960) A pyelographic study of ureteric injuries sustained during hysterectomy for benign conditions. *Surg. Gynec. Obst.*, **111**, 41–48.

SYMMONDS R. E. & SHELDON R. S. (1965) Vaginal prolapse after hysterectomy. *Obst. Gynec.*, **25**, 61–67.

TALBERT L. M., PALUMBO L., SHINGLETON H., BREAM C. A. & MCGEE J. A. (1965) Urological complications of radical hysterectomy for carcinoma of the cervix. *Southern Medical Journal*, **58**, 11–17.

TABRISKY J., MALLIN L. P. & SMITH J. A. (1972) Pneumoperitoneum after coitus. A complication due to uterine tube prolapse after vaginal hysterectomy. *Obst. Gynec.*, **40**, 218–220.

WHITEHOUSE G. H. (1977) The radiology of urinary tract abnormalities associated with hysterectomy. *Clin. Radiol.*, **28**, 201–210.

WIDEMAN G. L., GRAVLEE L. C. & JONES W. N. (1959) Arteriovenous aneurysm of the uterine artery and vein following total abdominal hysterectomy. *Amer. J. Obst. Gynec.*, **78**, 200–203.

Wolfson J. J. (1964) Vaginography for demonstration of ureterovaginal, vesicovaginal and rectovaginal fistulas with case reports. *Radiology*, **83**, 438–441.

Complications of radiotherapy

AVERETTE H. E. & FERGUSON J. H. (1963) Lymphographic alterations of pelvic lymphatics after radiotherapy. *J. Amer. Med. Assoc.*, **186**, 554–557.

BORONOW R. C. & RUTLEDGE F. (1971) Vesicovaginal fistula, radiation, and gynecological cancer. *Amer. J. Obst. Gynec.*, **111**, 85–90.

CHAU P. M., FLETCHER G. H. & RUTLEDGE F. N. (1962) Complications of high dose whole pelvic irradiation in female pelvic cancer. *Amer. J. Roentgenol.*, **87**, 22–40.

DALINKA M. K., EDEIKEN J. & FINKELSTEIN J. B. (1974) Complications of radiation therapy: adult bone. *Seminars Roentgenol.*, **9**, 29–40.

DEETHS T. M. & STANLEY R. J. (1976) Parametrial calcification in cervical carcinoma patients treated with radioactive gold. *Amer. J. Roentgenol.*, **127**, 511.

DENCKER H., HOLMDAHL K. H., LUNDERQUIST A., OLIVECRONA H. & TYLEN U. (1972) Mesenteric angiography in patients with radiation injury of the bowel after pelvic irradiation. *Amer. J. Roentgenol.*, **114**, 476–481.

EVERETT H. S. & MATTINGLY R. F. (1956) Vesicovaginal fistula. *Amer. J. Obst. Gynec.*, **72**, 712–724.

GRAHAM J. B. & VILLALBA R. J. (1963) Damage to the small intestine by radiotherapy. *Surg. Gynec. Obst.*, **116**, 665–668.

GRATZEK F. R., HOLMSTROM E. G. & RIGLER L. G. (1945) Postirradiation bone changes. *Amer. J. Roentgenol.*, **53**, 62–76.

KAPLAN A. L. (1977) Postradiation ureteral obstruction. *Obst. Gynec. Survey*, **32**, 1–8.

KAPLAN A. L., HUDGINS P. T. & WALL J. A. (1965) Postradiation pelvic fibrosis simulating recurrent carcinoma. *Amer. J. Obst. Gynec.*, **92**, 117–124.

KICKHAM C. J. E. (1961) Urologic problems in carcinoma of the cervix. *Surg. Gynec. Obst.*, **112**, 27–32.

MALLIK M. K. B. (1962) Radiological appearances of the urinary bladder in carcinoma of the cervix, before and after treatment. *J. Obst. Gynaec. Br. Cwth.*, **69**, 66–70.

MARSHAK R. H. (1947) Extrinsic lesions affecting the recto-sigmoid. *Amer. J. Roentgenol.*, **58**, 439–450.

MASON G. R., DIETRICH P., FRIEDLAND G. W. & HANKS G. E. (1970) The radiological findings in radiation-induced enteritis and colitis. *Clin. Radiol.*, **21**, 232–247.

PERKINS D. E. & SPJUT H. J. (1962) Intestinal stenosis following radiation therapy. *Amer. J. Roentgenol.*, **88**, 953–966.

RHAMY R. K. & STANDER R. W. (1961) Postradiation ureteral stricture. *Surg. Gynec. Obst.*, **113**, 615–622.

RHAMY R. K. & STANDER R. W. (1962) Pyelographic analysis of radiation therapy in carcinoma of the cervix. *Amer. J. Roentgenol.*, **87**, 41–43.

RUSHFORTH G. F. (1974) Osteosarcoma of the pelvis following radiotherapy for carcinoma of the cervix. *Brit. J. Radiol.*, **47**, 149–152.

SLATER J. M. & FLETCHER G. H. (1971) Ureteral strictures after radiation therapy for carcinoma of the uterine cervix. *Amer. J. Roentgenol.*, **111**, 269–272.

STAMPFLI W. P. & KERR H. D. (1947) Fractures of the femoral neck following pelvic irradiation. *Amer. J. Roentgenol.*, **57**, 71–83.

STEPHENSON W. H. & COHEN B. (1956) Post-irradiation fractures of the neck of the femur. *J. Bone Jt. Surg.*, **38B**, 830–845.

STRICKLAND P. (1954) Damage to the rectum in the radium treatment of carcinoma of the cervix. *Brit. J. Radiol.*, **27**, 630–634.

CHAPTER 12

Contraception and Abortion

INTRAUTERINE CONTRACEPTIVE DEVICES

Following the pioneer work of Gräfenberg and the introduction of his pliable ring of coiled silver wire in the 1920s, the use of intrauterine contraceptive devices (IUCDs) was generally regarded with some suspicion for many years. Renewed interest and subsequent widespread use of this form of contraception developed in the 1960's with a plethora of devices of many different shapes and materials. Currently employed IUCDs are made of metal or inert plastic, and may usually be left *in situ* for an indefinite period. The modern standard IUCDs have tails, usually with two strings, which extend down into the vagina. The principal effect of IUCDs is probably an interference with embedding of the blastocyst in the endometrium.

Types of IUCD

LIPPE'S LOOP

The Lippe's loop (Fig. 12.1) is one of the most frequently fitted devices in the United Kingdom (Snowden *et al.*, 1977). It is made of polyethylene impregnated with barium sulphate to permit radiographic visualization. The device is obtainable in various sizes. A satisfactory intrauterine position will result in a general reduction in distance between the loops of the coil, and between the bulbous tip and the first loop.

SAF-T-COIL

The Saf-T-Coil (Fig. 12.2), another popular IUCD, also consists of polyethylene impregnated with barium sulphate.

GRAVIGARD

The Gravigard (Copper 7) (Fig. 12.3) is a frequently used device. It is composed of a polypropylene carrier impregnated with barium and bearing 89 mg of copper. The small size of the Copper 7 causes less discomfort both during and after insertion than the previously mentioned IUCDs. Unfortunately, copper IUCDs have to be renewed every two years because of a high pregnancy rate after this time.

GYNE T

The Gyne T (Copper T) (Fig. 12.4) has a polyethylene carrier supporting 120 mg or 0.25 mm diameter copper wire.

ANTIGON

The Antigon device is made of polyethylene, with a small piece of metal attached to one side which gives it radiographic visibility.

DALKON SHIELD

The Dalkon shield (Fig. 12.5) consists of polyvinyl acetate and is of low radiographic density, although it contains barium sulphate, copper dust and copper sulphate. There are a series of lateral fins surrounding a central membrane (Fig. 12.6). The fins aid retention of the device in the uterine cavity, while the central membrane increases the surface area for interaction between the device and the endometrium. The Dalkon shield has not been manufactured since 1974, following reports from the USA of septic midtrimester abortions. How-

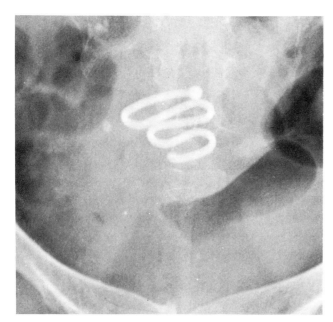

FIG. 12.1 Lippe's loop.

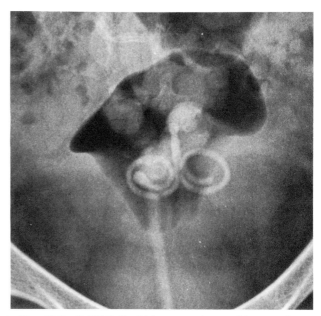

FIG. 12.2 Saf-T-Coil which appears inverted but was in a good position within a retroverted uterus.

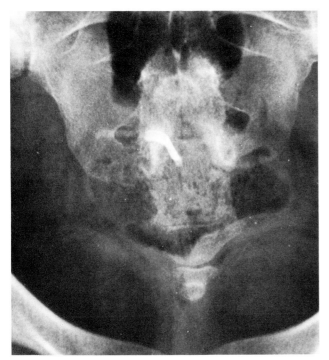

FIG. 12.3 Gravigard (Copper 7) lying in a transverse position.

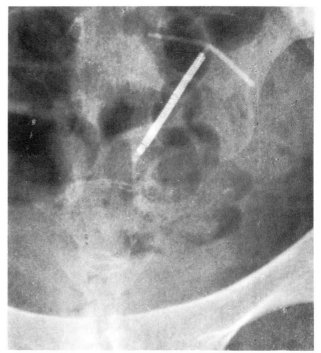

FIG. 12.4 Gyne T (Copper T).

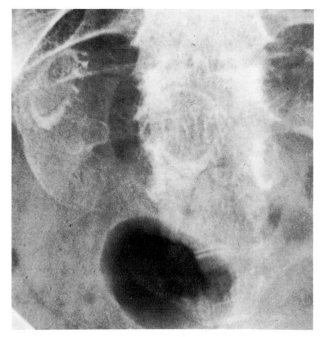

FIG. 12.5   Two Dalkon shields, one inside and the other outside the uterus.

FIG. 12.7   Birnberg bow. Courtesy of Dr John Stewart.

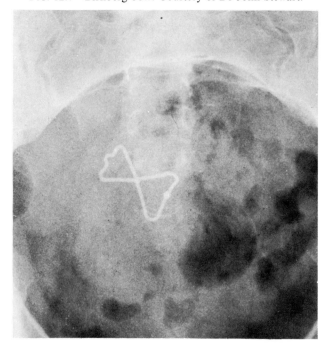

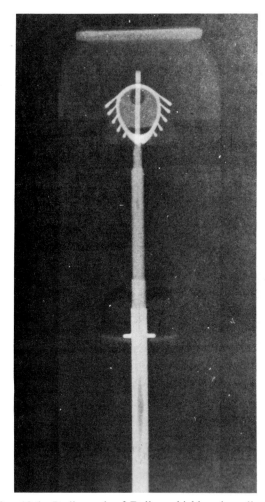

FIG. 12.6   Radiograph of Dalkon shield and applicator.

ever, some women in the United Kingdom are still using this device at the present time.

PROGESTASERT

The Progestasert is a T-shaped unit containing progesterone in its hollow stem. Barium sulphate renders the device radio-opaque. This IUCD requires annual replacement.

BIRNBERG BOW

The Birnberg bow (Fig. 12.7) has been a very popular IUCD, especially in the USA.

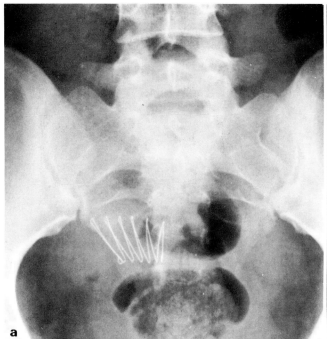

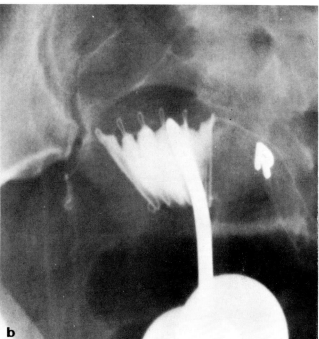

FIG. 12.8 Majzlin spring. (a) Plain radiograph.

(b) Hysterogram shows this IUCD embedded in the uterine wall.

MARGULIES COIL

The Margulies coil, like the Birnberg bow, is made of barium impregnated with polyethylene but has a long intracervical extension.

MAJZLIN SPRING

The Majzlin spring (Fig. 12.8) was mainly used in the USA but has now been banned by the Food and Drug Administration because of the high risk of pelvic infection. The device often becomes embedded in the uterine wall, with a tendency to fragment on its removal.

Complications from IUCDs

MISSING THREADS

A substantial number of women with IUCDs are referred to gynaecological departments with the marker threads missing. The causes of missing threads include expulsion, the incidence of which varies from 2 to 20% and is related to the type of device, and translocation which occurs in 0.05 to 13 per thousand insertions (Gentile & Siegler, 1977). Pregnancy will cause the threads to retract because of uterine enlargement. In most cases of missing threads, however, the IUCD is in the uterus without pregnancy (McArdle, 1978). Rosen (1965) has found that the threads may be retracted into the uterus in 10% of insertions using a Lippe's loop. The packaging of the Gravigard (Copper 7), partly loaded with the thread looped alongside it, may particularly predispose to thread retraction (Sparks, 1977). Ultrasonography is the most reliable and the safest method for investigating missing threads (Meire & Renton, 1977). In addition, ultrasound will diagnose pregnancy within four weeks of conception. A plain radiograph will help to differentiate between expulsion and translocation through the uterine wall if ultrasonography fails to demonstrate the device within the uterus. The use of an intrauterine probe with a hooked end for the retrieval under fluoroscopic control of an IUCD with retracted threads has been described by Diaconis & Weiner (1974). Other, simpler methods are now available.

PREGNANCY

The pregnancy rate with a correctly positioned IUCD is 1 to 4% of women in the first year of insertion, becoming lower in succeeding years, except in the case of copper devices after the second year. Pregnancies associated with an IUCD are especially likely to be extrauterine (Seward *et al.*, 1972) or to result in spontaneous abortion (Baker, 1969). Furthermore, spontaneous abortions occurring in women with an IUCD *in situ*, especially a Dalkon shield, are more likely than usual to be complicated by infection which may be fatal (Cates *et al.*, 1976). In many cases, the IUCD does not impede an otherwise normal pregnancy (Fig. 12.9).

BLEEDING

Persistently heavy menstrual loss and intramenstrual bleeding occur in 41% of women using a Lippe's loop (Willson & Ledger, 1968). Tejiya & Malkani (1969) and Kamal *et al.* (1971) performed hysterography with Lippe's loops in utero, and found that excessive bleeding was especially likely when the uterine cavity was small in relation to the size of the IUCD. However, Adel *et al.* (1971) found that menometrorrhagia was not related to different degrees of moulding of the uterine outline by the Lippe's loop, although pelvic pain or dysmenorrhoea were more frequent with marked moulding (Fig. 12.10).

INFECTION

Pelvic infection seems to be four or five times more likely among IUCD users than other women (British Medical Journal, 1976), and is the main cause of mortality and severe morbidity associated with IUCDs (Scott, 1968). According to Tietze (1968), the inflammation is usually mild and may be an exacerbation of infection which existed prior to insertion. Pelvic abscess may certainly occur with nonperforating IUCDs (Wilson & Dilts, 1972). Elstein (1969) has found a 76% incidence of salpingographic evidence of tubal damage, usually tubal occlusion, in patients who developed symptoms and signs of pelvic inflammatory disease after being fitted with an IUCD.

MALPOSITION AND DISTORTION OF IUCDS

Distortion of an IUCD within the uterine cavity, particularly the Lippe's loop, may affect either end or the whole

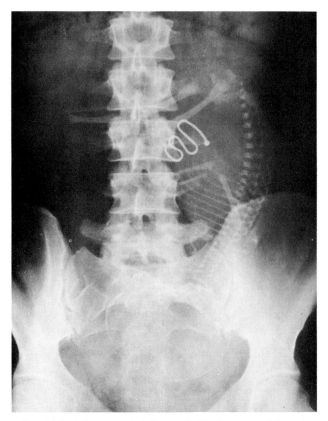

FIG. 12.9   The normal delivery of this fetus was followed by spontaneous expulsion of the Lippe's loop.

length of the device (Fig. 12.11). Sometimes a distorted IUCD may lie within the cervix. The presence of distortion raised the possibility of perforation of the uterine wall, although this is not always the case. The IUCD may lie on its side (Fig. 12.12) or may even be upside down within the uterine cavity.

UTERINE PERFORATION BY AN IUCD

Perforation of the uterine wall by an IUCD occurs at the time of its insertion. The IUCD is completely extruded into the peritoneal cavity in most cases (Fig. 12.13), less often remaining partly embedded in the uterine wall (Figs 12.14 and 12.15). Perforation is usually asymptomatic and pelvic infection is a very rare complication (Schwartz & Markowitz, 1970). The patient often subsequently becomes pregnant or suspicion is aroused by missing

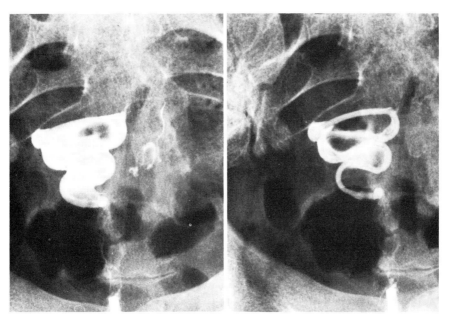

FIG. 12.10 Hysterography showing marked moulding of the uterine outline by a Lippe's loop in a patient with severe dysmenorrhoea. Courtesy of Dr John Stewart.

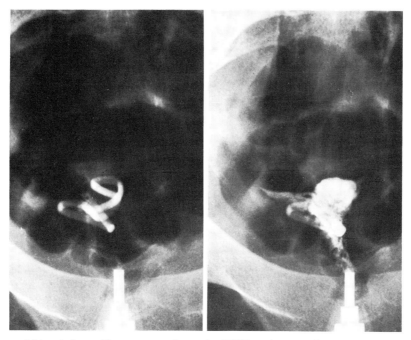

FIG. 12.11 Very distorted Lippe's loop. Hysterogram shows the IUCD to be very distorted and has partially penetrated the endometrium on the right side. Courtesy of Dr John Stewart.

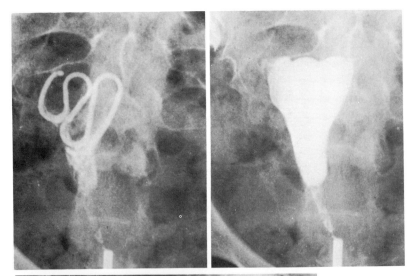

FIG. 12.12 Lippe's loop lies transversely within the uterine cavity. Courtesy of Dr John Stewart.

FIG. 12.13 Total uterine perforation by Lippe's loop demonstrated by hysterography. Courtesy of Dr John Stewart.

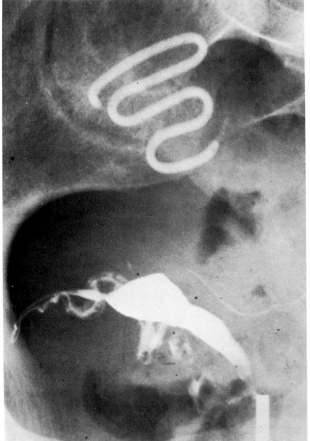

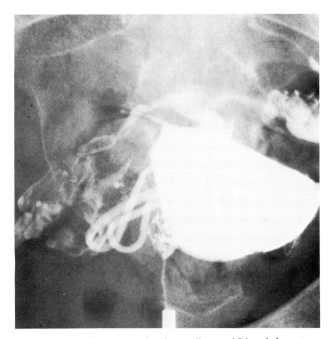

FIG. 12.14 Hysterography shows distorted Lippe's loop to lie almost free of uterus. Courtesy of Dr John Stewart.

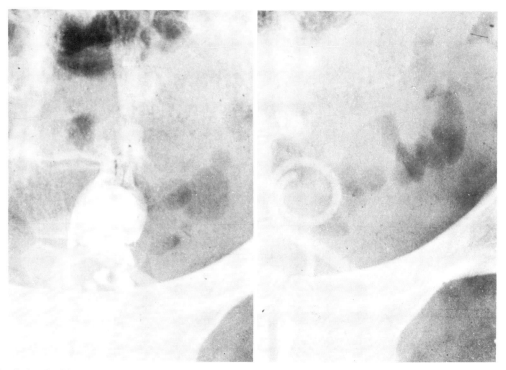

FIG. 12.15 Saf-T-Coil lies in a low transverse position and has perforated the uterine wall. Courtesy of Dr John Stewart.

threads. The practice of inserting an IUCD in the post-partum period when the uterine wall is soft and weak is a definite predisposition to uterine perforation. The type of device has a bearing on the chance of perforation; bows have an incidence of 0.7 per hundred insertions, while spirals and loops respectively have perforation rates of 0.03 and 0.04 per hundred insertions (Tietze, 1968).

Ultrasonography is the method of choice in identifying uterine perforation by an IUCD, although plain radiography may be a valuable supplement in showing the extrauterine site in such cases. An anteroposterior radiograph demonstrates displacement of the IUCD from the expected position in only one third of cases (Shimkin et al., 1969). This is because the extrauterine IUCD often lies either directly anterior to the uterus or in the pouch of Douglas. The value of an additional lateral radiograph is limited by the possibility of uterine anteflexion or retroflexion. Obvious displacement of the device may be present, but may sometimes be only discernible when a follow-up radiograph is taken in equivocal cases. An unusual alignment of an IUCD in the pelvic cavity may

be solely due to the wide variation in uterine position with the IUCD in a satisfactory intrauterine situation. The IUCD itself may lie in an abnormal position within the uterine cavity (Fig. 12.12). Distortion of the IUCD is sometimes seen with uterine perforation (Fig. 12.14). Eisenberg (1972) found that the distance between the bulbous tip on the end of a Lippe's loop was approximately 1 cm from the second loop in cases with uterine perforation, whereas this distance was always 0.5 cm or less in correctly inserted devices (Fig. 12.16).

Hysterography has been widely advocated in the past (Friedman & Pine, 1966) for the demonstration of an extrauterine IUCD, but nowadays has little or no application. Fluoroscopy is of value during the removal of an IUCD by a peritoneoscope (Brooks et al., 1972).

An unusual complication of uterine perforation by the bow or ring (closed loop) type of IUCD is intestinal obstruction (Scott, 1968). The obstruction occurs at ileal level and is either due to herniation of a portion of bowel through an aperture of the IUCD or to volvulus about a point of fixation caused by adhesions to the

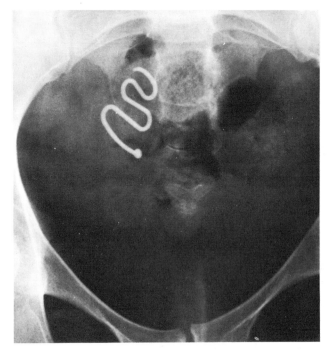

FIG. 12.16   Total intraperitoneal extrusion of Lippe's loop proven at laparoscopy. The bulbous tip of the IUCD is widely separated from the second loop.

device. With either cause, the IUCD may be partially or completely extruded from the uterus (Shimkin *et al.*, 1969). Strangulation of the involved ileal segment is common.

FRAGMENTATION

Fracture of Lippe's loops has been reported in 2.8% of insertions (Last, 1972) and has also occurred with Birnberg bows (Rosenfeld, 1970) and Saf-T-Coils (Provost, 1971). Obviously, plain radiography is useful in detecting the remains of these fragmented devices.

ORAL CONTRACEPTION

Circulatory disorders

There has been increasing concern in recent years regarding the hazards of vascular disorders in women taking oral contraceptives. A survey under the auspices of the Royal College of General Practitioners (1977) found that deaths from circulatory disorders (nonrheumatic heart disease, hypertension and cerebrovascular disorders) were five times as common in women on the Pill than in those using other methods of contraception. The risk of death from cardiovascular disease was confirmed by the Oxford/Family Planning Association Study (Vessey *et al.*, 1977b). In both studies, the deaths from cardiovascular disease were concentrated in women aged 35 years or more and there was a strong association with smoking. However, these surveys related particularly to oral contraceptives containing 50 mg of oestrogen. Preparations containing lower doses of oestrogen may be associated with lower risks (Vessey *et al.*, 1977b). The progestogenic component of the Pill is also important, the risk of hypertension increasing with the dose of norethisterone acetate although there is a decrease in the incidence of benign breast disease (Royal College of General Practitioners, 1977). In 1967, the Medical Research Council drew attention to the risk of developing venous thrombosis and pulmonary embolism. This hazard is apparently related to the dose of oestrogen (Inman *et al.*, 1970). Venous thrombosis may occur at other sites than the pelvis and lower limbs (Figs 12.17 and 12.18).

Bergeron & Wood (1969) studied the cerebral angiograms of women aged 20–44 years with symptoms of cerebral ischaemia. Eight of the nine patients who had angiographically demonstrated arterial occlusion had been taking oral contraceptives. The middle cerebral artery was occluded in five cases, while the branches of that artery were thrombosed in all but one case. A history of significant headaches was present well in advance of the ischaemic episode.

Brodelius *et al.* (1971) found, in a review of venograms of patients with acute deep venous thrombosis of the leg, that the thrombosis originated most often in the ileofemoral vein if the patient was taking oral contraceptives but usually arose in the calf veins in women not on the Pill.

Ischaemic colitis and enteritis

Kilpatrick *et al.* (1968) described two cases of ischaemic colitis occurring in women on the Pill. The history was classically of abdominal pain of acute onset followed by bloody diarrhoea and abdominal tenderness. Barium enema examination in both cases showed the typical findings of lumenal narrowing and intramural 'thumb

FIG. 12.17 Venous phase of right carotid arteriogram in a 40-year-old woman who presented with fits and had been taking oral contraceptives. Thrombosis of superior saggital sinus and some cortical veins. Courtesy of Dr J. Occleshaw.

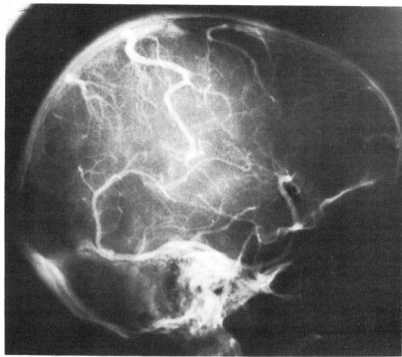

FIG. 12.18 Spontaneous axillary vein thrombosis in 22-year-old taking oral contraceptives.

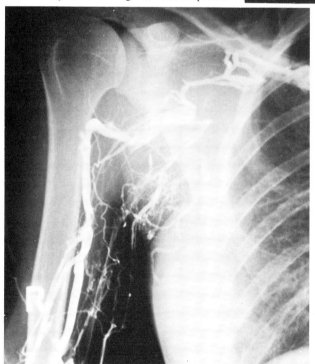

print' filling defects. Unlike the usual left sided situation of ischaemic colitis, the abnormality affected the ascending segment and hepatic flexure in these two cases.

Small bowel ischaemia, with a high morbidity and mortality rate, has been found in oral contraceptive users. It is secondary to either mesenteric artery or mesenteric vein thrombosis, the former being the most common (Hoyle *et al.*, 1977). The symptoms are variable and are usually slow in onset. A narrowed segment of small intestine may be subsequently identified on barium follow-through.

Liver tumours

Baum *et al.* (1973) reported seven cases of benign hepatomas (hepatic adenomas) occurring in women who had been on oral contraceptives for between six months and five years. They described the angiographic findings of a clearly defined margin and a peripheral arterial supply with approximately parallel centrally penetrating arteries (Fig. 12.19). These tumours did not show the vascular pooling, arteriovenous shunting and portal vein invasion which are seen with malignant hepatomas. The

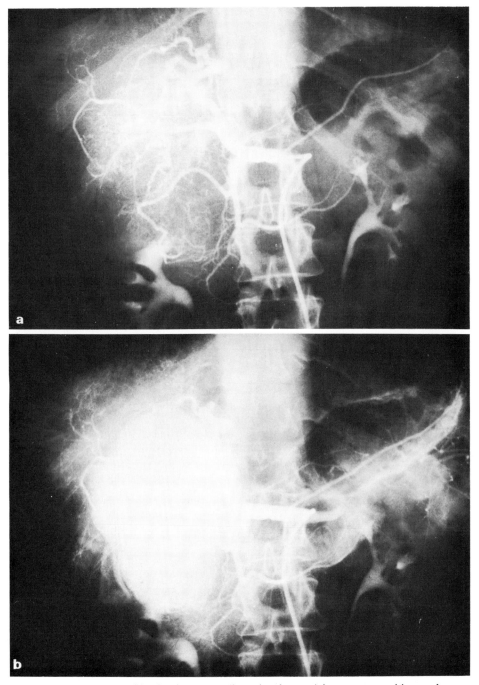

FIG. 12.19   Hepatic angiogram of benign hepatoma (hepatic adenoma) in a woman taking oral contraceptives.
(a) The large well-defined mass in the liver has a rich arterial blood supply, without features of malignancy.
(b) Generalized dense opacification of adenoma in capillary phase. Courtesy of Dr Heather Nunnerly.

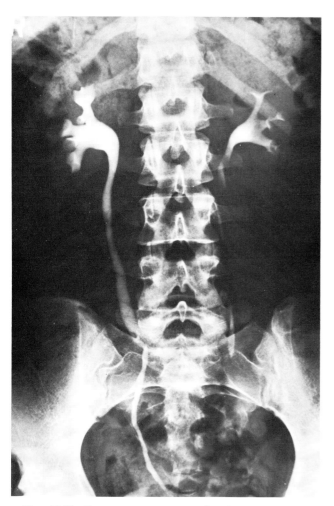

FIG. 12.20 Intravenous urogram of nulliparous woman with no history of urinary infection, but currently taking oral contraceptives. Dilatation of right urinary tract down to pelvic brim level, where the ureter is indented by iliac vessels.

United Kingdom than in the USA (Vessey *et al.*, 1977a). Spontaneous regression of the tumour after withdrawal of oral contraceptives may or may not occur. Ultrasonography may possibly be of use in screening long term users of oral contraceptives for liver tumours.

Urinary tract changes

Guyer & Delaney (1974) have found overdistention of the upper urinary tract on the IV urograms of 17% of women. The right ureter and calyces were affected in most of these cases, the overdistension being especially pronounced and most frequent when there was history of past pregnancies and previous urinary infection. It also appears that oral contraceptives play an aetiological role, usually in combination with a history of urinary infection and previous pregnancy. In a few cases, oral contraception alone has been associated with upper urinary tract dilatation, usually on the right side (Guyer & Delaney, 1970) (Fig. 12.20). Presumably this dilatation is due to hormonal influences causing hypotonicity of the ureters, as in pregnancy, with compression at pelvic level from the ovarian vein (Clarke, 1964) or iliac vessels (Dure-Smith, 1970) causing the changes to be most often on the right side. The resultant stasis predisposes to urinary infection, whereupon the overdistensibility may become permanent due to inflammatory damage to the ureteral wall (Spiro & Fry, 1970).

ABORTION

Criminal abortion

A wide variety of objects have been used to provoke an abortion (Fig. 12.21). When the instrument is long and pointed it may readily perforate the uterine wall, although blunt objects such as urethral catheters have been found to perforate the uterus and lie free within the peritoneal cavity or to be walled off in an abscess cavity (Zakin *et al.*, 1955). Rarely, a catheter may enter a pelvic blood vessel, a case having been described where a twelve inch catheter actually migrated upwards into the chest (Powell, 1956). The urinary tract may also be damaged by a perforating device, such as a pencil, perhaps resulting in a vesicovaginal fistula (Thomas, 1944).

Highly irritant abortifacients, such as vinegar or Dettol, may cause severe changes where they are inadvertently introduced into the bladder – the so-called 'abortion

survey of Christopherson & Mays (1977) showed that pain and haemoperitoneum were the commonest clinical findings in liver tumours developing with oral contraception. Most are histologically benign, being either hepatic adenomas or focal nodular hyperplasia, but some cases of hepatocellular carcinoma were also found which suggests that the benign lesion may progress to malignant change. The incidence of hepatic tumours in patients on the Pill seems to be much less frequently found in the

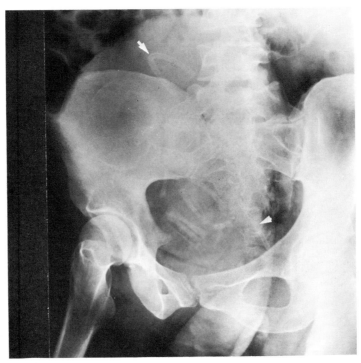

FIG. 12.21   Radiograph of a 6-month gestation showing rubber catheter (arrows) and fetus in uterus; taken 9 weeks after attempted abortion.

bladder' (Kinder, 1959). An initial acute cystitis and pelvic cellulitis causes haematuria, dysuria and much pain. Urography will subsequently show bilateral hydronephrosis and hydroureter with an irregular contracted bladder, while free vesicoureteral reflux may be demonstrated by cystography.

The most life-threatening hazard of criminal abortion is air embolism. This is due to air being introduced through a tube or nozzle inserted into friable vessels of the vascular pregnant uterus. Radiographs are inevitably not taken because of the precipitate death of the patient. Ritvo & Nikolaidis (1962) have described the postmortem radiographic appearances, with air-fluid levels in the right side of the heart and air in the veins of the pelvis, abdomen, chest and neck.

Surgical abortion

The intra-amniotic injection of hypertonic saline via an abdominal amniocentesis is a popular method of abortion after the first trimester. The injection of water-soluble contrast medium through the needle under fluoroscopic control confirms the placement of the needle in the amniotic sac and prevents an intraplacental or intravascular injection. The inadvertent intravascular injection of hypertonic saline results in shock and in some instances death.

When unsuspected severe damage occurs to the uterine cervix during cervical dilatation, the bladder has been lacerated due to the very high negative pressure used to evacuate the uterus by means of vacuum curettage (Rous et al., 1971).

REFERENCES

Intrauterine contraceptive devices

ADEL S-K., GHENEIM M. A. & SOBRERO A. J. (1971) Hysterography study of long-term effects of intrauterine contraceptive devices. *Fertil. Steril.*, **22**, 651–662.
BAKER J. W. (1969) Serious complications of intrauterine contraceptive devices. *Med. J. Austral.*, **1**, 1126–1131.

BRITISH MEDICAL JOURNAL (1976) Editorial: Risk of pelvic infection associated with intrauterine devices. *Brit. Med. J.*, **2**, 717–718.

BROOKS P. G., BERCI G., LAWRENCE A., SLIPYOU P. & WADE M. E. (1972) Removal of intra-abdominal intrauterine contraceptive devices through a peritoneoscope with the use of intraoperative fluoroscopy to aid localization. *Amer. J. Obst. Gynec.*, **113**, 104–106.

CATES W., ORY H. W., ROCHAT R. W. & TYLER C. W. (1976) The intrauterine device and deaths from spontaneous abortion. *New Engl. J. Med.*, **295**, 1155–1159.

CLARKE J. C. (1964) The right ovarian vein syndrome. In *Clinical Urology*, 2nd edn, ed. J. C. Emmet. Saunders, Philadelphia.

DIACONIS J. N. & WEINER C. I. (1974) Intrauterine device extraction: a safe method utilizing fluoroscopy. *Radiology*, **111**, 479–480.

DURE-SMITH P. (1970) Pregnancy dilatation of the urinary tract. *Radiology*, **96**, 545–550.

EISENBERG R. L. (1972) The widened loop sign of Lippe's loop perforations. *Amer. J. Roentgenol.*, **116**, 847–852.

ELSTEIN M. (1969) The effects of pelvic inflammation associated with the IUD. A salpingographic study. *Internat. J. Fertil.*, **14**, 275–279.

FRIEDMAN P. J. & PINE H. L. (1966) Radiographic localization of the ectopic intrauterine contraceptive device. *Obst. Gynec.*, **27**, 814–819.

GENTILE G. P. & SIEGLER A. M. (1977) The misplaced or missing IUCD. *Obst. Gynec. Survey*, **32**, 627–641.

KAMAL I., HEFNAWI F., GHONGIM M., TALAAT M. & ABDALLA M. (1971) Dimensional and architectural disproportion between the intrauterine device and the uterine cavity. A cause for bleeding. *Fertil. Steril.*, **22**, 514–521.

LAST P. A. (1972) Fracture of the Lippe's loop in utero. *J. Obst. Gynaec. Br. Cwth.*, **79**, 190–191.

MCARDLE C. R. (1978) Ultrasonic localization of missing intrauterine contraceptive devices. *Obst. Gynec.*, **51**, 330–333.

MEIRE H. B. & RENTON P. (1977) Missing tails. *Br. Med. J.*, **1**, 713.

PROVOST R. W. (1971) Fragmented intrauterine devices. *Obst. Gynec.*, **37**, 484.

ROSEN E. (1965) Intrauterine contraceptive devices. *Amer. J. Obst. Gynec.*, **93**, 896–897.

ROSENFELD P. A. (1970) Fragmented bows. *Obst. Gynec.*, **36**, 166.

SCHWARTZ F. G. & MARKOWITZ A. M. (1970) Serious sequelae of intrauterine contraceptive devices. *J. Amer. Med. Assoc.*, **211**, 959–960.

SCOTT R. B. (1968) A survey of deaths and critical illnesses in association with the use of intrauterine devices. *Internat. J. Fertil.*, **13**, 297–300.

SEWARD P. N., ISRAEL R. & BALLARD C. A. (1972) Ectopic pregnancy and intrauterine contraception. *Obst. Gynec.*, **40**, 214–217.

SHIMKIN P. M., SIEGEL H. A. & SEAMAN W. B. (1969). Radiographic aspects of perforated intrauterine contraceptive devices. *Radiology*, **92**, 353–358.

SNOWDON R., WILLIAMS M. & HAWKINS D. (1977) *The IUD. A Practical Guide.* Croom Helm, London.

SPARKS R. A. (1977) Problems with IUCD tails. *Br. Med. J.*, **2**, 1351–1352.

SPIRO F. I. & FRY I. K. (1970) Ureteric dilatation in non-pregnant women. *Proc. Roy. Soc. Med*, **63**, 462–466.

TEJIYA S. & MALKANI P. K. (1969) Clinical significance of correlation between size of uterine cavity and IUCD. *Amer. J. Obst. Gynec.*, **103**, 620–627.

TIETZE C. (1968) Contraception with intrauterine devices. *Amer. J. Obst. Gynec.*, **96**, 1043–1054.

WILLSON J. R. & LEDGER W. J. (1978) Complications associated with the use of intrauterine contraceptive devices in women of middle and upper socioeconomic class. *Amer. J. Obst. Gynec.*, **100**, 649–661.

WILSON E. A. & DILTS P. V. (1972) Unusual complications of an intrauterine contraceptive device. *Amer. J. Obst. Gynec.*, **112**, 237–238.

Oral contraception

BAUM J. K., HOLTZ F., BOOKSTEIN J. J. & KLEIN E. W. (1973) Possible association between benign hepatomas and oral contraceptives. *Lancet*, **2**, 926–929.

BERGERON R. T. & WOOD E. H. (1969) Oral contraception and cerebrovascular complications. *Radiology*, **92**, 231–242.

BRODELIUS A., LÖRINC P. & NYLANDER G. (1971) Localization of acute deep venous thrombosis in women taking oral contraceptives. *Radiology*, **101**, 297–300.

CHRISTOPHERSON W. M. & MAYS E. T. (1977) Liver tumours and contraceptive steroids: Experience with the first one hundred registry patients. *J. Nat. Cancer Institute*, **58**, 167–171.

GUYER P. B. & DELANEY D. J. (1970) Ureteral dilatation and oral contraceptives. *Brit. Med. J.*, **4**, 588–590.

GUYER P. B. & DELANEY D. J. (1974) Over-distensibility of the female upper urinary tract. *Clin. Radiol.*, **25**, 367–377.

HOYLE M., KENNEDY A., PRIOR A. L. & THOMAS G. E. (1977) Small bowel ischaemia and infarction in young women taking oral contraceptives and progestional agents. *Brit. J. Surg.*, **64**, 533–537.

INMAN W. H. W., VESSEY M. P., WESTERHOLM B. & ENGELUND A. (1970) Thromboembolic disease and the steroidal content of oral contraceptives. A report to the Committee on Safety of Drugs. *Brit. Med. J.*, **2**, 203–209.

KILPATRIC Z. M., SILVERMAN J. F., BETANCOURT E., FARMAN J. & LAWSON J. P. (1968) Vascular occlusion of the colon and oral contraceptives. *New Engl. J. Med.*, **278**, 438–440.

MEDICAL RESEARCH COUNCIL (1967) Risk of thromboembolic disease in women taking oral contraceptives. *Brit. Med. J.*, **2**, 355–359.

ROYAL COLLEGE OF GENERAL PRACTITIONERS (1977) Mortality among oral contraceptive users. *Lancet*, **2**, 727–730.

VESSEY M. P. (1978) Contraceptive methods: risks and benefits. *Brit. Med. J.*, **2**, 721–722.

VESSEY M. P., KAY C. R., BALDWIN J. A., CLARKE J. A. & MACLEOD I. B. (1977a) Oral contraceptives and benign liver tumours. *Brit. Med. J.*, **1**, 1964–1965.

VESSEY M. P., McPHERSON K. & JOHNSON B. (1977b) Mortality among women participating in the Oxford/Family Planning Association contraceptive study. *Lancet*, **2**, 731–733.

Abortion

KINDER C. H. (1959) Abortion bladder: The late effects of introducing abortifacients into the bladder. *Brit. J. Urol.*, **31**, 89–94.

POWELL M. M. (1956) Catheter migration from uterus to lung, perforating the diaphragm. *Dis. Chest.*, **30**, 583–584.

RITVO M. & NIKOLAIDIS D. (1962) Roentgen diagnosis of air embolism due to criminal abortion. *Amer. J. Roentgenol.*, **88**, 119–124.

ROUS S. N., MAJOR F. & GORDON M. (1971) Rupture of the bladder secondary to uterine vacuum curettage. *J. Urol.*, **106**, 685–686.

THOMAS R. C. (1944) Vesicovaginal fistula, foreign body and calculi in bladder following attempted criminal abortion, and normal labour. *J. Obst. Gynaec. Br. Emp.*, **51**, 350–352.

ZAKIN D., GODSICK W. H. & SEGAL B. (1955) Foreign bodies lost in the pelvic during attempted abortion with special reference to urethral catheters. *Amer. J. Obst. Gynec.*, **70**, 233–251.

CHAPTER 13

The Lower Urinary Tract in Gynaecology

There are many aspects of the female bladder and urethra which are likely to come to the attention of the gynaecologist, and some of these are also of interest to the radiologist. Some congenital anomalies, the effects of pelvic lesions, and injuries sustained by the lower urinary tract as a result of treatment of gynaecological conditions are discussed in other chapters.

URINARY INCONTINENCE

Continuous urinary incontinence may result from an ectopic ureter which opens into the vagina or the introitus, and from a fistulous communication between the lower urinary tract and the vagina. The International Continence Society (1976) defined genuine *stress incontinence* as an involuntary loss of urine when the intravesical pressure exceeds the maximum urethral pressure but in the absence of detrusor activity. *Urge incontinence*, on the other hand, is the involuntary loss of urine associated with a desire to void, and is due either to the presence or absence of uninhibited detrusor contractions. *Reflex incontinence* is an involuntary loss of urine due to abnormal reflex activity in the spinal cord in the absence of the sensation usually associated with the desire to micturate. *Overflow incontinence* is an involuntary loss of urine when the intravesical pressure exceeds the maximum urethral pressure due to an elevation of intravesical pressure associated with bladder distention but absent detrusor activity. Continence is a complex multifactorial mechanism and the distinction between the various forms of incontinence is often difficult.

Stress urinary incontinence

Genuine stress incontinence is associated with a deficient urethral closure mechanism, usually with an insufficient suspension of the bladder neck and proximal urethra, in contradistinction to urge incontinence which is usually due to detrusor hyper-reflexia or instability. Unlike detrusor instability, genuine stress incontinence is usually not a cause of nocturia. Stress incontinence is a very frequent condition, 95% of those affected being multiparous women (Green, 1968). Obstetric injury is therefore a prime factor in stress incontinence, but other influences include postmenopausal soft tissue atrophy and long term gravitational stresses which may be related to obesity and chronic pulmonary disease. Although many patients have varying degrees of uterovaginal prolapse, the presence of prolapse is not necessarily associated with stress incontinence.

RADIOLOGICAL INVESTIGATION

Intravenous urography

This is indicated when outflow obstruction is suspected, and when there is a history of continuous incontinence or recurrent urinary tract infection. The morphology of the bladder outlet cannot be assessed by this technique.

Cystourethrography

The cystourethrographic features of the normal state and those found in stress incontinence have been described by, amongst others, Roberts (1952). He observed that normally, the bladder base forms a straight line in the lateral view with the patient at rest and lies just above and

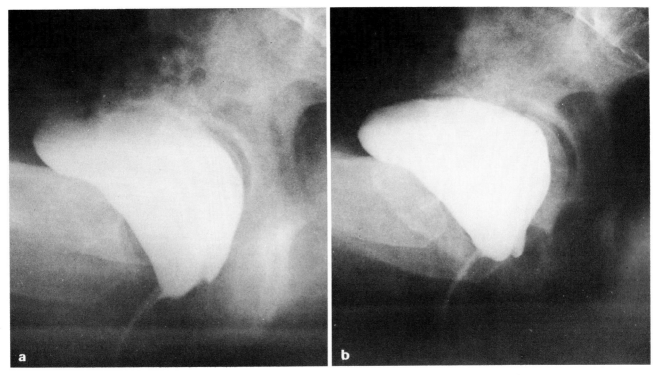

FIG. 13.1 Lateral view of cystourethrogram in stress incontinence. Bladder filled with diodone and bladder catheter opacified with neohydriol.

(a) Prolapse of bladder base on straining with loss of urethrovesical angle.

(b) Repeat cystogram with vaginal pessary. Less descent of bladder base on straining and restoration of urethrovesical angle.

parallel to a line joining the lower border of the symphysis pubis to the lower end of the sacrum. Roberts used a soft rubber bladder catheter containing contrast medium to delineate the course of the urethra and its relationship to the bladder base. The urethra was then found to be straight and the posterior urethrovesical angle was approximately 100° at rest. On 'bearing down', the bladder and urethra descended slightly but retained a normal relationship one to another. Normally during micturition the bladder base and proximal urethra swung downwards and backwards, the posterior urethrovesical angle disappearing so that the urethra and bladder base came into line. Obliteration of the urethrovesical angle was described by Roberts as being the most characteristic anatomical change associated with stress incontinence (Fig. 13.1). Even if the angle was present at rest, it disappeared on straining. Funnelling of the urethrovesical

junction was usually associated with loss of the posterior urethrovesical angle. In the presence of prolapse without stress incontinence the posterior urethrovesical angle was maintained no matter how much the descent of the bladder base (Fig. 13.2).

The use of a catheter may be criticized because of the inevitable distortion of the bladder neck which it causes, and because the true path of the urethra is not necessarily followed when the latter is delineated by a catheter. Hodgkinson (1953) used a metallic bead chain to delineate the urethra during cystourethrography and claimed that this method gave freedom from urethral distortion and allowed measurement of the length of the urethra.

Warrell (1960) claimed that if the bladder was overdistended, or if the contrast medium was cold, there may be irritation of the bladder neck with dilatation of the proximal urethra and flattening of the posterior urethro-

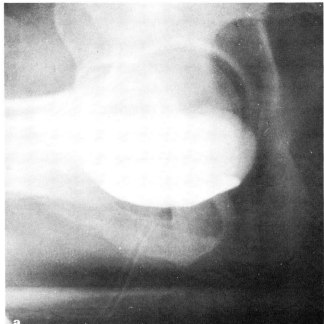

FIG. 13.2 Cystourethrogram in prolapse without stress incontinence.
(a) At rest.

(b) On straining there is marked descent of the bladder base but preservation of the urethrovesical angle.

vesical angle. Sodium iodide solution is no longer used, although it was the cystographic contrast medium employed by Roberts, because it may cause irritation with increased detrusor tone and loss of the urethrovesical angle. Hoffman & Ulrich (1966) found that the extent of depression of the bladder base is in itself of no significance, but considered that funnelling often occurred in stress incontinence and genital prolapse when these are found in isolation or in combination, and that the size of the posterior urethrovesical angle was not of paramount importance in the diagnosis of stress incontinence. Greenwald et al. (1967) found that many of the abnormalities described in bead chain cystourethrography occurred in most parous patients with pelvic relaxation but who were continent. Loss of the urethrovesical angle has been shown to be an almost constant finding in stress incontinence, due to an open bladder neck, but it is also seen on bladder contraction and with detrusor incontinence (Bates et al., 1973). In general, therefore, it is currently believed that the static anatomi-

cal relationships shown on cystography alone are a poor method of evaluating functional problems (Graber, 1977).

Ardran et al. (1956) performed cystourethrograms without urethral delineation by catheters or other appliances. They found that the internal meatus of women without any disorder of micturition and at rest was often delineated by a small projecting 'beak' of contrast medium 2 to 5 mm in length at the junction of the base and anterior border of the bladder. The vagina was delineated by barium paste and on straining both the bladder base and the vagina usually moved downwards and forwards in the asymptomatic patient. Sometimes the movement of the bladder base was so great as to form a cystocoele. The small 'beak' of contrast medium in the internal meatus became more pronounced on straining and the angle between the anterior border and the bladder base became more acute. Contrast medium entered the urethra to a varying degree on straining in patients with stress incontinence, returning to the bladder on cessation of the strain. A posterior urethrovesical angle of less than 180° was usually found at the beginning of micturition in patients with or without stress incontinence. The external sphincter closed first and the contents of the proximal two-thirds of the urethra returned to the bladder by progressive obliteration of the lumen whether or not stress incontinence was present.

Frewen (1971), performing urethrography with a modified Foley catheter, has consistently demonstrated dilatation of the urethrovesical junction and upper urethra independent of micturition in cases of stress incontinence.

Cinecystography may give information on prolapse and urethral distortion and allows the demonstration of incontinence. However, the crucial diagnostic difficulty is the recognition and exclusion of patients with abnormalities of bladder function. Patients with bladder contraction associated with leakage cannot be assessed by either static or cine cystography (Bates et al., 1973). While these patients can usually be distinguished by symptoms of urgency, they sometimes present with a history of leakage on coughing without urgency, thus closely resembling true stress incontinence due to sphincter weakness. It has become clear that problems of stress and urge incontinence would be best investigated by a combined synchronous recording of urodynamic data provided by pressure and flow studies combined with visualization of the urethrodynamics relating to the proximal urethral closure mechanisms and urethral distortion (Bates et al., 1970).

Videocystourethrography (VCU)

VCU (Bates et al., 1970; Stanton, 1978) is a combination of supine cystometry and radiographic screening of the bladder and urethra during voiding, recorded with a sound commentary on video tape (Fig. 13.3). This method is used in the diagnosis of urinary incontinence, voiding difficulties and retention.

A 12F bladder catheter is inserted while the patient lies supine on a radiographic screening table (Fig. 13.4). The residual urine volume is measured and the bladder is then filled with contrast medium, such as diodone 25%, by gravity at a rate of 100 ml/min, with the filling rate being measured by a weighing transducer. A fluid-filled catheter, 1 mm in diameter, is then placed alongside the filling catheter and is connected to a pressure transducer to measure the intravesical pressure. The rectal (abdominal) pressure is measured by means of a 2 mm fluid-filled catheter inserted a short distance into the rectum. The electronic subtraction of the rectal pressure from the intravesical pressure gives the detrusor pressure, which is an exact index of detrusor activity. Initial sensation and the full bladder capacity are noted during the filling phase. When the bladder is full, the filling catheter is removed and the patient is stood upright and screened in the erect oblique position, when it is noted whether or not there is any leakage or descent of the bladder base. The patient is next asked to void and then to interrupt her stream. The peak flow rate and volume voided are recorded by a uroflowmeter, and the maximum voiding pressure and ability to 'milk back' are noted during the manœuvres. Voiding is then resumed and the patient is rescreened to detect any residual urine. Difficulty in voiding in the erect position is overcome by transferring the patient to an adjacent side room, with the pressure lines in situ and still connected to the transducers, and she then micturates in privacy while seated on a commode with the uroflowmeter still in place.

Using a television camera positioned above the recorder, and a mixing device, three out of the six recorded channels are placed alongside the radiographic image of the bladder on a television monitor. This combined picture, with a sound commentary, is recorded on videotape for subsequent replay.

Provocative tests for detrusor irritability are carried out and include rapid filling, passive postural change and coughing and filling in the erect position.

FIG. 13.3   Videocystourethrography. Simultaneous recording of bladder and rectal pressure changes during supine cystometry, combined with a display of bladder filling volume, is shown on the left-hand side of the polygraph trace. The bladder and rectal pressures during voiding, with the voiding rate and volume, are recorded on the right side of the race. A television camera selects three parameters (intravesical pressure, detrusor pressure and voiding rate) which are added to the radiographic image of the bladder and recorded with sound commentary on videotape. Courtesy of S. L. Stanton, and Harper & Row Inc.

FIG. 13.4   Videocystourethrography showing patient lying on radiographic screening table. Grass recorder with television camera and stand with transducers. Courtesy of S. L. Stanton, and Harper & Row Inc.

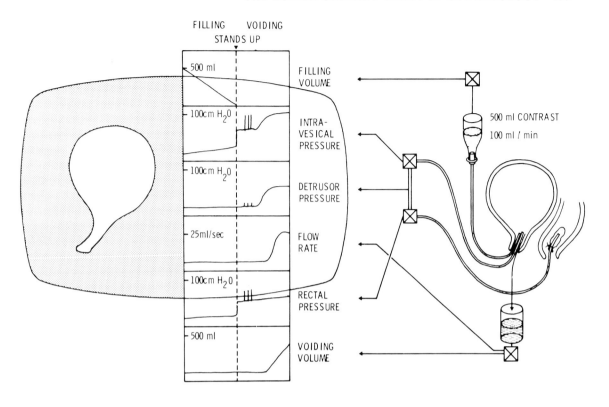

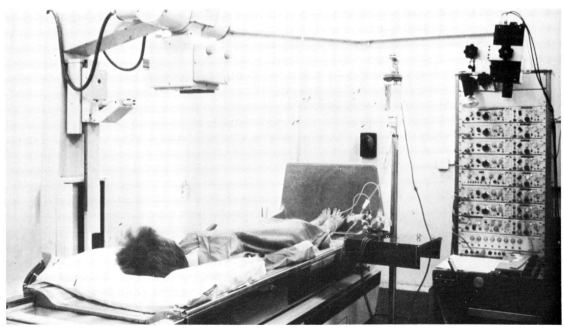

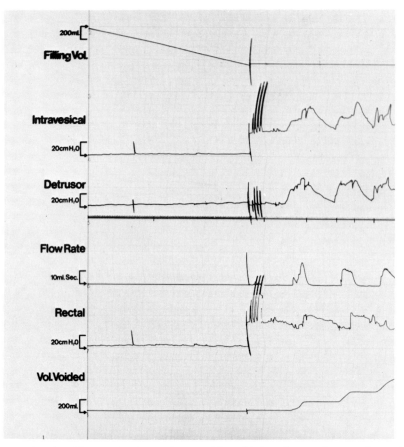

FIG. 13.5   A normal trace, showing filling and voiding phases, with multiple voluntary interruptions of micturition. Courtesy of S. L. Stanton, and Harper & Row Inc.

The total screening time is about one minute and each examination takes about twenty minutes. The radiation dose to the ovaries is approximately 700 R/min.

The criteria for normal bladder function (Stanton, 1978) are:

1. A residual urine of less than 50 ml.
2. First sensation recorded at 150–200 ml capacity.
3. Strong desire to micturate at 450–500 ml capacity.
4. A detrusor pressure rise on filling, standing or coughing of up to 15 cm of water.
5. No loss of urine and only slight descent of the bladder base on coughing.
6. A rise of detrusor pressure on voiding which does not exceed 70 cm of water, with a peak flow rate of more than 200 ml/sec (Fig. 13.5).
7. Ability to stop voiding on instruction. The urinary stream is interrupted at midurethral level. Fluid proximal to this point is 'milked back' into the bladder. The bladder neck gradually closes as the detrusor pressure falls to the premicturition level. Fluid distal to the midurethra is voided.
8. No significant residual urine on completion of voiding.

The diagnosis of urethral sphincter dysfunction (genuine stress incontinence) is made by an open bladder neck at rest or on coughing without a detrusor contrac-

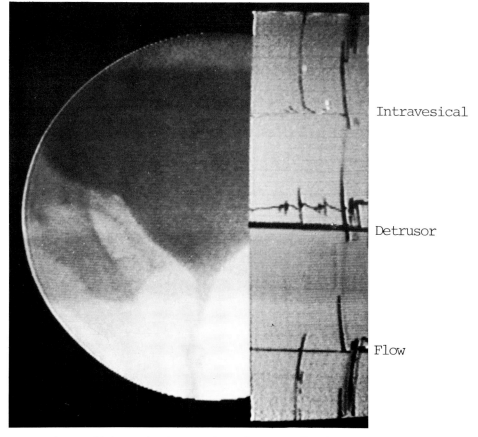

Intravesical

Detrusor

Flow

FIG. 13.6   Videocystourethrographic image showing stress incontinence on effort due to urethral sphincter incompetence. On the left-hand side the image of the bladder is shown with the bladder neck open and escape of contrast medium via the urethra. On the right-hand side there is a momentary rise of intravesical pressure in response to coughing but little change in detrusor pressure. Courtesy of S. L. Stanton.

tion or abnormal pressure rise, either without loss of urine or with actual leakage (Fig. 13.6).

In detrusor instability there is a rise of detrusor pressure or an uninhibited detrusor contraction of more than 15 cm of water on provocative testing. If there are dominant symptoms of urgency, frequency and enuresis then 10 cm may be taken as the upper limit. Leakage of urine may occur if urethral sphincter dysfunction is present, depending on the ultimate rise in detrusor pressure. Abnormal pressure changes are shown during filling, standing erect and on coughing (Fig. 13.7).

Difficulties in voiding, sometimes with retention, may occur because of some neuromuscular dysfunction or some structural abnormality involving the urethra. Some of these causes may be differentiated by electromyography of the periurethral striated muscle. Other dynamic methods of assessing lower urinary tract disorders in the female are reviewed by Stanton (1978).

Surgical treatment of prolapse and stress incontinence

While good results are usually obtained following the surgical correction of stress incontinence, incontinence due to detrusor instability is associated with a poor response. The aims of surgery are: (1) to elevate and restore the bladder neck and proximal urethra to their original position, (2) to prevent funnelling of the bladder

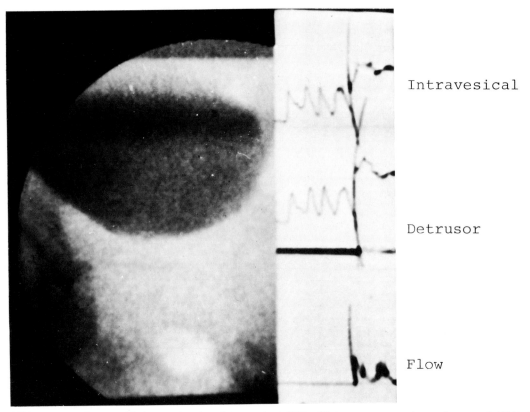

Intravesical

Detrusor

Flow

FIG. 13.7 Videocystourethrographic image showing detrusor instability. Detrusor pressure trace shows uninhibited detrusor contractions occurring during filling and an abnormal pressure rise on standing. Courtesy of S. L. Stanton.

neck, by increasing the bulk of supporting tissue around this area and (3) to increase urethral resistance. Suprapubic urethrovesical suspensory operations are more effective in correcting stress incontinence than those operations which are performed through the vagina.

Anterior colporrhaphy is often used for the correction of genital prolapse in the absence of incontinence. Bailey (1963), using a modified Manchester colporrhaphy with a suburethral bolster in some cases, found the cystographic anatomy to be restored to near normality. In some cases, there was a deterioration after two years, especially when there was obesity or chronic constipation. The urethral length is increased by 0.5–2.5 cm after urethro-colporrhaphy (Mitrani *et al.*, 1971).

The urethra and bladder are rarely injured, although a ureter is occasionally damaged and subsequently obstructed following anterior colporrhaphy. Simmons & Baker (1963) stressed the infrequency of ureteral damage demonstrated by postoperative intravenous urography.

Urethrovesical slings consisting of fascia, muscle or synthetic materials are used to treat stress incontinence by the elevation of the urethrovesical junction. Elevation and fixation of the vesical neck is also achieved by suturing the bladder neck and proximal urethra to anterior or antero-lateral structures such as the cartilage of the symphysis pubis, the periosteum of the pubic ramus (Marshall-Marchetti-Krantz operation), the rectus sheath (Pereyra technique), or to the ileopectinal ligament (Burch operation).

The Marshall-Marchetti technique is a frequently performed operation. Marchetti (1949) has described the cystographic appearance after urethrovesical suspension operations. The bladder base is elevated compared to the preoperative position but is still slightly lower in the

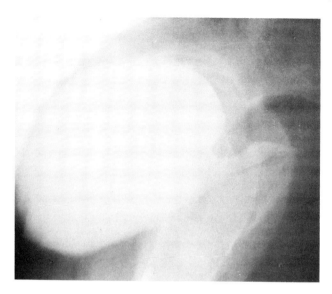

erect posture than in the recumbent position even though the patient is now continent. The bladder neck and urethra should be closely approximated to the superior surface of the symphysis pubis without any distortion of their contour or lumen. However, Stanton *et al.* (1978) consider that some distortion of the bladder neck occurs after colposuspension and that it is difficult to be sure where the bladder neck lies on radiological screening. Excessive elevation of the bladder neck may obstruct the bladder outlet, resulting in urinary retention (Fig. 13.8). Hoodin *et al.* (1967) also claim that excessive elevation also produces elongation and angulation of the intra-vesical ureter with resultant ureteral obstruction. Occasionally the bladder and urethra may be injured during their dissection, and the ureters are rarely injured by the incorrect placement of sutures.

Osteitis pubis is a postoperative complication in 3.2%

Fig. 13.8 Overcorrection of elevation of bladder base and proximal urethra by Marshall–Marchetti operation, shown on micturating cystourethrogram.

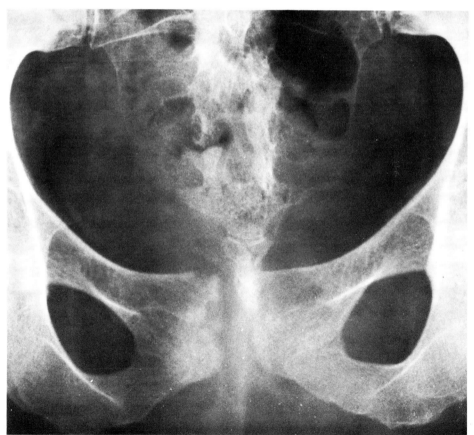

FIG. 13.9 Osteitis pubis following vesicourethral suspension. There is irregular absorption of the bone ends at the symphysis pubis, with underlying sclerosis and rarefaction.

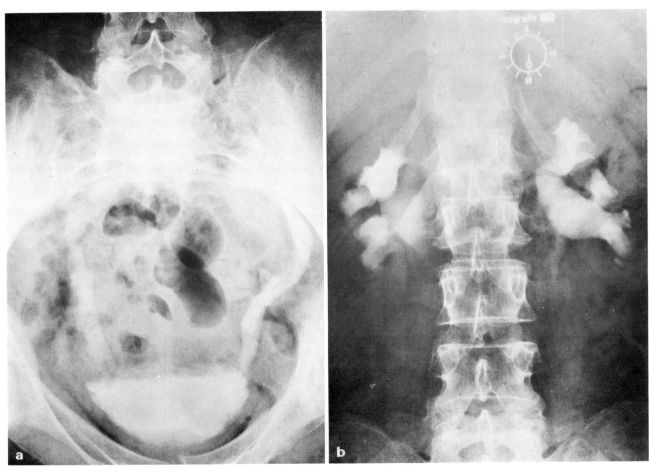

FIG. 13.10 Intravenous urography in patient with severe prolapse of the bladder.
(a) Dilatation of whole length of ureters (supine position).

(b) Bilateral hydronephrosis (supine position).

of cases following vesicourethral suspension (O'Leary, 1964), and is probably the result of the adjacent operative trauma and infection (Fig. 13.9). Local bone rarefaction and irregular destruction of the articular surfaces of the symphysis pubic occur within a few months of the operation. The process is self limiting with healing which results in obliteration of the joint space within two or three years.

Ureteral obstruction associated with uterine prolapse

The possibility of ureteral obstruction being caused by uterine prolapse has been recognized since the early part of the last century. Lang & Montgomery (1952) found a 38% incidence of ureteral obstruction associated with uterine prolapse with a cystocoele, while Klempner (1952) detected ureterohydronephrosis on IV urography in 25% of cases of uterine prolapse, with a higher incidence and greater severity the more pronounced the prolapse. Elkin *et al.* (1974) also observed that the majority of patients with ureteral obstruction had a third degree prolapse of the uterus. Urinary tract infection was present in three-quarters of Elkin's cases, a much higher incidence than in Klempner's series. Elkin *et al.* found that ureteral dilatation was bilateral in the majority of their cases,

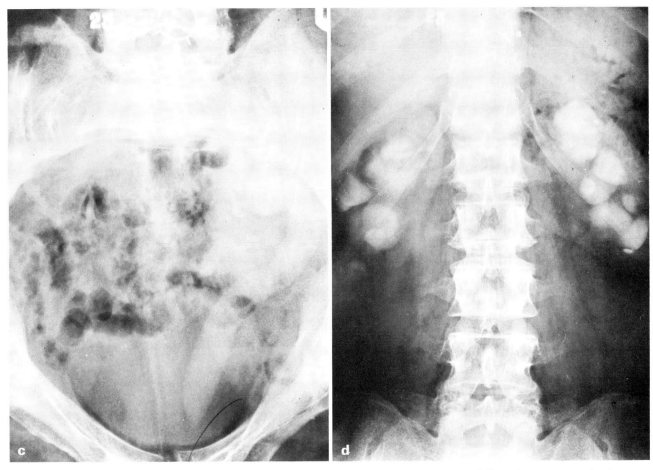

(c) Descent and further dilatation of both ureters with patient standing. Right ureter not clearly seen.

(b) Increase in degree of bilateral hydronephrosis, also on standing.

although associated dilatation of the renal pelvis had less tendency to bilaterality. Adequate surgical treatment of the prolapse led to a definite reduction of ureteral obstruction. Cystocoeles are an expected finding on IV urography, and prone and erect radiographs accentuate the extent of caudal displacement of the lower portions of the ureters (Fig. 13.10). The ureteral obstruction may only become apparent on prone and/or erect radiographs.

Various theories, including kinking of the lower ureters by the downward displacement of the broad ligament with prolapse (Lieberthal & Frankenthal, 1941) and kinking and compression of the ureters by uterine vessels (Brettauer & Rubin, 1923) have postulated the cause of

this ureteral obstruction. It seems most likely that caudal displacement of the trigone in patients with severe prolapse results in mechanical deformity and narrowing of the ureteral meati with resultant obstruction to ureteral emptying (Elkin *et al.*, 1974). IV urography should be considered in all women with complete procidentia, because of the particular risk of ureteral obstruction, rather than being routinely employed in all cases with lesser degrees of uterine prolapse (Stabler, 1977).

Some other aspects of the female urethra

The abnormalities of the lower urinary tract which are associated with intersex states have been described in

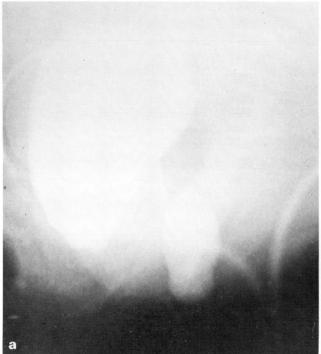
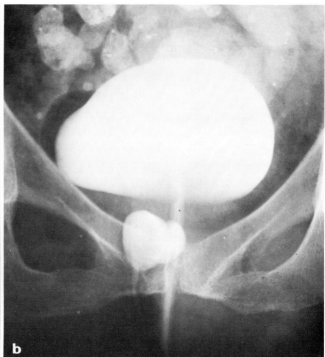

FIG. 13.11 Urethral diverticulum.
  (a) Lateral cystogram with urethral catheter *in situ*. Large calculus shown in urethral diverticulum.

(b) Anteroposterior view also shows relationship of calculus in urethral diverticulum to urethra.

Chapter 5. The so-called 'urethral syndrome' is discussed in Chapter 11.

Strictures of the urethra may result from obstetric and surgical injury, while gonococcal urethritis may cause an inflammatory stricture. Congenital strictures and obstructing valves occasionally occur in the female urethra.

Calculi of the female urethra are very uncommon, often being associated with a stricture or diverticulum of the urethra, but may arise from encrustation of a foreign body which has been inserted into the urethra.

Urethral coitus is sometimes practised in women with a rigid hymen or vaginal atresia. Micturating cystography shows good urinary control but a wide bladder neck and a dilated urethra (Borski & Mittemeyer, 1971).

Urethral diverticulum usually arises from infection and obstruction of a urethral gland which subsequently ruptures into the urethral lumen. Diverticula may occur anywhere along the urethra, but the majority arise in the middle third of the urethra, usually on the vaginal aspect. They are usually one to 2.5 cm in diameter, but may be as large as 8 cm (Spraitz & Welsh, 1965). The condition usually presents in the third and fourth decades with frequency and dysuria as the commonest symptoms although urgency of micturition and dyspareunia are sometimes presenting cmplaints. On examination, a mass may be found on the anterior vaginal wall. IV urography may show elevation of the bladder base when the diverticulum originates from the proximal portion of the urethra (Dretler *et al.*, 1972). Micturating cystourethrography will often delineate a diverticulum (Spence & Duckett, 1970) but retrograde urethrography has been advocated by many as the investigation of choice (Davis & Robinson, 1970). The diverticulum often expands during retrograde filling of the urethra, and the distensibility may be well shown on cine radiography (Kittredge *et al.*, 1966). Direct catheterization of the diverticulum is often impossible (Wharton & Telinde, 1956). There is a 10%

incidence of calculi in diverticula (Wharton & Kearns, 1950) (Fig. 13.11). Carcinoma occasionally arises in a urethral diverticulum and has been demonstrated by urethrography as an irregular filling defect within the diverticulum (Falkner, 1957).

REFERENCES

Ardran G. M., Simmons C. A. & Stewart J. H. (1956) The closure of the female urethra. *J. Obst. Gynaec. Br. Emp.*, **63**, 26–35.

Bailey K. V. (1963) A clinical investigation into uterine prolapse with stress incontinence. *J. Obst. Gynaec. Br. Cwth.*, **70**, 947–958.

Bates C. P., Loose H. & Stanton L. R. (1973) The objective study of incontinence after repair operations. *Surg. Gynec. Obst.*, **136**, 17–22.

Bates C. P., Whiteside C. G. & Turner-Warwick R. (1970) Synchronous cine/pressure/flow/cysto-urethrography with special reference to stress and urge incontinence. *Brit. J. Urol.*, **42**, 714–723.

Borski A. A. & Mittemeyer B. T. (1971) Urethral coitus – maximum urethral dilatation. *J. Urol.*, **105**, 400–402.

Brettauer J. & Rubin I. C. (1923) Hydroureter and hydronephrosis; a frequent secondary finding in cases of prolapse of the uterus and bladder. *Amer. J. Obst. Gynec.*, **6**, 672–696.

Davis B. L. & Robinson D. G. (1970) Diverticula of the female urethra: assay of 120 cases. *J. Urol.*, **104**, 850–853.

Davis H. J. & Telinde R. W. (1958) Urethral diverticula: an essay of 121 cases. *J. Urol.*, **80**, 34–39.

Dretler S. P., Vermillion C. D. & McCullough D. L. (1972) The roentgenographic diagnosis of female urethral diverticula. *J. Urol.*, **107**, 72–77.

Elkin M., Goldman S. M. & Meng C. H. (1974) Urethral obstruction in patients with uterine prolapse. *Radiology*, **110**, 289–294.

Faulkner J. W. (1957) Primary carcinoma in a diverticulum of the female urethra. *J. Urol.*, **82**, 337–340.

Frewen W. R. (1971) Foley catheter urethrography in stress incontinence. *J. Obst. Gynaec. Br. Cwth.*, **78**, 660–663.

Graber E. A. (1977) Stress incontinence in women. *Obst. Gynec. Survey*, **32**, 565–577.

Green T. H. (1968) The problem of urinary stress incontinence in the female. *Obst. Gynec. Survey*, **23**, 603–634.

Greenwald S. W., Thornbury J. R. & Dunn L. J. (1967) Cystourethrography as a diagnostic aid in stress incontinence. *Obst. Gynec.*, **29**, 324–327.

Hodgkinson C. P. (1953) Relationship of the female urethra and bladder in urinary stress incontinence. *Amer. J. Obst. Gynec.*, **65**, 560–573.

Hoffmann J. & Ulrich J. (1966) Cystourethrography and female urinary stress incontinence. *Acta Radiol. (Diag.)*, **4**, 1–13.

Hoodin A. O., Malin J. M. & Evans A. T. (1967) Unusual complication of urethrovesical suspension for treatment of stress incontinence. *J. Urol.*, **98**, 479–481.

International Continence Society (1976) First report on the standardisation of terminology of lower urinary tract function. *Brit. J. Urol.*, **48**, 39–41.

Kittredge R. D., Bienstock M. & Finby N. (1966) Urethral diverticula in women. *Amer. J. Roentgenol.*, **98**, 200–207.

Klempner E. (1952) Gynecological lesions and ureterohydronephrosis. *Amer. J. Obst. Gynec.*, **64**, 1232–1241.

Lieberthal F. & Frankenthal L. (1941) The mechanism of ureteral obstruction in prolapse of the uterus. *Surg. Gynec. Obst.*, **73**, 828–832.

Long J. P. & Montgomery J. B. (1952) The incidence of ureteral obstruction in benign and malignant gynecological lesions. *Amer. J. Obst. Gynec.*, **59**, 552–562.

Marchetti A. A. (1949) The female bladder and urethra before and after correction for stress incontinence. *Amer. J. Obst. Gynec.*, **58**, 1145–1154.

Mitrani A., Sharf M., Zilberman A. & Singer J. (1971) Urethral length in urinary stress incontinence. *J. Obst. Gynaec. Br. Cwth.*, **78**, 664–666.

O'Leary J. A. (1964) Osteitis pubis following vesicourethral suspension. *Obst. Gynec.*, **24**, 73–77.

Roberts H. (1952) Cystourethrography in women. *Brit. J. Radiol.*, **25**, 253–259.

Simmons S. C. & Baker H. R. W. (1963) Investigation of the renal tract following repair operations. *J. Obst. Gynaec. Br. Cwth.*, **70**, 968–970.

Spence H. M. & Duckett J. W. (1970) Diverticulum of the female urethra. *J. Urol.*, **104**, 432–437.

Spraitz A. F. & Welsh J. S. (1965) Diverticulum of the female urethra. *Amer. J. Obst. Gynec.*, **91**, 1013–1016.

Stabler J. (1977) Uterine prolapse and urinary tract obstruction. *Brit. J. Radiol.*, **50**, 493–498.

Stanton S. L. (1978) Preoperative investigation and diagnosis. *Clin. Obst. Gynec.*, **21**, 705–721.

Stanton S. L., Cardozo L., Williams J. E., Ritchie D. & Allan V. (1978) Clinical and urodynamic features of failed incontinence surgery in the female. *Obst. Gynec.*, **51**, 515–520.

Warrell D. W. (1960) Pitfalls in cystourethrography. *J. Obst. Gynaec. Br. Emp.*, **67**, 508.

Wharton L. R. & Kearns W. (1950) Diverticula of the female urethra. *J. Urol.*, **63**, 1063–1076.

Wharton L. R. & Telinde R. W. (1956) Urethral diverticulum. *Obst. Gynec.*, **7**, 503–509.

CHAPTER 14

Ultrasound in Gynaecological Diagnosis

by C. H. Wright

The introduction of grey scale signal processing and focussed transducers has resulted in widespread clinical usage of ultrasound as a diagnostic imaging procedure. This has been reflected in the extensive literature of the last four years documenting the increasing value and accuracy of ultrasonic assessment of the normal and diseased female pelvis. The increased resolution of current equipment allows almost routine delineation of the pelvic organs and musculature. Grey scale processing gives previously unavailable detail of the echo texture of both normal and abnormal structures, and an appreciation of changes in echo pattern not demonstrable with bistable imaging. The more recent introduction of digital processing of the ultrasound signal promises not only increased stability of the equipment, but also the facility to manipulate and enhance subtle textural changes.

Where clinical suspicion of a pelvic mass or pelvic pathology exists, or where the clinical examination is difficult due to obesity, ultrasonic examination provides an initial non-invasive means of confirming the presence or absence of a pelvic mass, and frequently a definitive diagnosis, excluding or indicating the need for further examination.

TECHNIQUE

A full bladder is necessary for the examination. The bladder should not be overdistended, as this may result in distortion of the pelvic anatomy, and patient discomfort. If necessary, a catheter should be inserted to ensure adequate bladder filling at the time of examination. Routine saggital and transverse sections are obtained at 1 cm intervals. Compound scans are valuable initially to establish the pelvic anatomy and any abnormality that may be present. It is also useful to continue the transverse scan round to the gluteal regions to demonstrate the exact position of the iliac wings and ilio-psoas muscles where asymmetry of the pelvic anatomy is suspected.

When examining a suspected abnormality in greater detail, sector or single sweep scans are indicated. Compound scanning may obscure the fine echo pattern of the abnormality and cause loss of definition of anatomical detail, such as separation of the lesion from the pelvic or uterine wall. It may be useful to empty the bladder and re-examine the patient when there is difficulty in differentiating the bladder from a cystic or transonic mass. This may also be useful in demonstrating fixity of the pelvic structures.

With modern equipment a 3.5 MHz transducer should be employed if possible. This provides more detailed visualization of the pelvic anatomy and improved characterization of the tissue echo pattern. In the more obese patient a 2.25 MHz transducer may be necessary and will usually provide adequate detail, without the need to use a 1.65 MHz transducer. Use of a transducer of this frequency may, however, be necessary in the extremely obese patient or where the uterus is acutely retroflexed. Due to the variability of the control parameters of present equipment, no specific gain settings can be recommended, but must be tailored to fit the individual patient.

An adequate examination should show uniform diffuse echoes from within the uterus. The examination should be recorded on hard copy (preferably an 8 × 10 inch single emulsion film) to provide a permanent record of the examination. The display format is governed by individual preference, a 'white on black' format does seem to demonstrate more fully changes in the echo pattern of both normal and abnormal pelvic structures.

NORMAL PELVIC ANATOMY

On saggital scans the vaginal canal is demonstrated posterior to the bladder as a uniform echogenic line without the transonic vaginal walls (Fig. 14.1). The bladder wall shows a dense echogenic line of specular reflection. The uterus is demonstrated posterior to the bladder and a uniformly fine echo pattern to the myometrium should be obtained. The endometrial cavity may be visualized as a thin echogenic line within the uterus. This is not necessarily obtained with every examination, and is more frequently seen at the time of menstruation. It may normally be visualized at other times in the menstrual cycle but does show cyclical changes, being more prominent at the time of menstruation. During the secretory phase the endometrium shows a more transonic appearance surrounding the central echogenic cavity (Hall *et al.*, 1979). The normal uterus measures approximately $7.5 \times 5 \times 3$ cm but may measure up to 10 cm in length and 5 cm in width.

The normal ovaries can now routinely be visualized in a high percentage of cases (Fig. 14.2). Normal measurement of the ovaries is $1 \times 2 \times 3$ cm. An ovary measuring more than 2 cm in any of two dimensions should be considered enlarged (Zemlyn, 1974). The ovaries are more easily defined on a transverse scan than on a saggital scan. Follicular and luteal cysts may be visualized within an ovary. The Fallopian tubes and suspensory ligaments are occasionally visualized as thin transonic structures measuring not more than 1 cm (Sample *et al.*, 1977).

The gas-containing rectosigmoid may be demonstrated as a dense echogenic area between the uterus and the pelvic walls, and identified by a lack of through transmission. Overlying bowel may obscure the adnexal areas or cause confusing echoes which may be mistaken for a

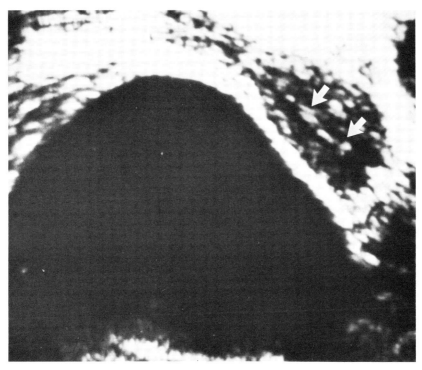

FIG. 14.1   Saggital scan of the normal uterus and vaginal canal. The endometrial cavity is visualized as a thin echogenic line.

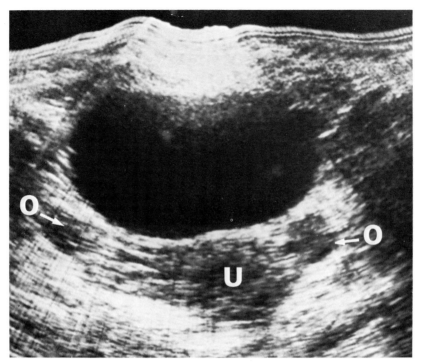

FIG. 14.2 Transverse scan demonstrating the uterus (U) and normal ovaries (O).

fluid collection or a complex mass. It is often helpful to re-examine the patient within half an hour in such circumstances, when the lack of constancy of the appearance will confirm the presence of a pseudo-mass due to bowel. If this is not possible, or confusion still exists, the patient should be re-examined the following day.

CONGENITAL ABNORMALITIES OF THE GENITAL TRACT

Abnormalities of the uterus

Development of the Müllerian and Wolffian ducts are closely linked embryologically and associated anomalies are common. Estimates of the association between unilateral renal agenesis and genital tract abnormalities in the female vary from 48% to 90%. A suspected or known congenital abnormality of the urogenital tract should thus lead to a complete ultrasonic evaluation of the pelvis and renal areas (Fig. 14.3). Development of the ovaries from the genital ridge occurs separately and normal ovaries are usually present in association with a congenital uterine or vaginal abnormality. Abnormalities of uterine development are difficult, if not impossible, to identify in the immature uterus unless gross. In the adolescent or adult patient, the presence of a unicornuate uterus may be suspected from its eccentric location and small size. A bicornuate uterus has a bilobed appearance with an increase in the transverse diameter. A septum may be identified between the two horns. If occlusion of one of the horns is present, asymmetry will be demonstrated with distension of the obstructed horn. The appearances vary according to the nature of the contained fluid. A haematometra demonstrates a transonic appearance, with a diffuse fine echo pattern due to inspissated blood. If infection is present a complex echo pattern may be identified due to the cellular debris in the infected cavity (Fried *et al.*, 1978). If pregnancy occurs within a bicornuate uterus the non-pregnant horn may be demonstrated as a localized protruberance of the lower uterine segment with a uniform echo pattern similar to that of the wall of the pregnant horn. This may be difficult to distinguish from a subserous fibroid, but size, position, echo pattern and an associated endometrial reaction may assist in making the differentiation. In both cases serial examinations will be indicated.

Abnormalities of the vagina

Septation abnormalities of the vagina may similarly be difficult to identify, unless associated with obstruction, although their presence may be inferred from an increased AP diameter of the vaginal image (Haller *et al.*, 1977). Where obstruction of one of the septal elements has occurred, a palpable para-vaginal mass is identified, and is associated with painful menses following the menarche (Vinstein & Franken, 1972). In the case of an imperforate hymen the clinical history and findings are more characteristic. In both circumstances, the distended vagina is identified ultrasonically by its midline position posterior to the bladder and its elongate shape (Fig. 14.3b). The haematocolpos shows a transonic appearance with posterior echo enhancement. With inspissation and resorption of the water content of the altered blood a fine diffuse echo pattern is noted. Ultrasound may also

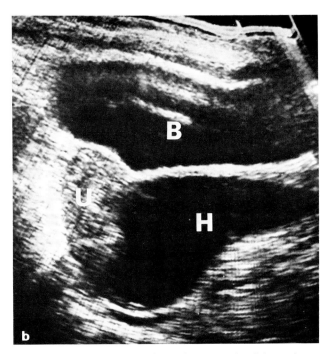

FIG. 14.3 (a) Intravenous urogram showing absent left kidney. No definite pelvic kidney is identified.

(b) Saggital scan showing septation anomaly of the vagina with marked distension of the obstructed horn: U, uterus; B, bladder; H, haematocolpos.

demonstrate the presence of an associated haematometra and haematosalpinx.

Ultrasonic demonstration of a pelvic kidney

A further congenital abnormality which may be diagnosed ultrasonographically is that of a pelvic kidney. This may be an incidental finding, or may have presented clinically as a palpable pelvic mass. The dense central sinus echo pattern, uniform parenchymal echo and characteristic reniform shape should indicate the diagnosis. Oblique scans are usually necessary to define the long axis of the kidney. In the presence of calyceal deformity the sinus echo pattern may appear more bizarre, with the dilated and deformed calyces appearing as transonic areas (Rosenthal *et al.*, unpublished). Irregularity of the normally smooth renal outline may be present. Awareness of this possibility in the presence of an unusual pelvic mass, and subsequent demonstration of an empty renal fossa, serve to confirm the diagnosis.

THE ABNORMAL UTERUS

Uterine fibromyoma

The most commonly demonstrated abnormality of the uterus is that of a uterine fibromyoma. Fibromyomas are present in 10–20% of all females over 35 years of age and represent the commonest of female pelvic tumours. They are mostly found in the body of the uterus, less than 5% occurring in the cervical area. The number of fibromyomas present may vary considerably and, when they are multiple, it may be difficult to establish exactly how many are present (von Micsky, 1974). The uterus is usually increased in size, and shows some irregularity or lobulation of its outline, although the uterine borders still show good definition. The normal appearance of a fibromyoma is of a transonic area within the uterine outline (Fig. 14.4). Small fibromyomas may cause no contour abnormality of the uterus. A large fibromyoma which is causing marked irregularity of the uterine outline is distinguished from an adnexal lesion by demonstrating its continuity with the uterus. Where the tumour is anechoic the lack of posterior enhancement will confirm its solid nature. An echogenic line between the tumour and the remainder of the uterus may be seen and is due to a pseudo-capsule, although it is usually not complete. Areas of infarction or degeneration are represented by

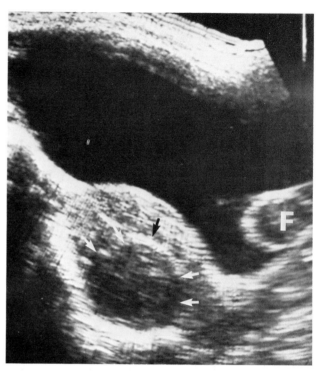

FIG. 14.4   Saggital scan showing the appearances of a small uterine fibroid (white arrows) with distortion of the endometrial cavity (black arrow). A Foley catheter (F) is present in the bladder.

discrete focal echoes of varying size within the tumour. Distortion of the endometrial cavity echo may occur (Fig. 14.4) and this may help in identifying the small submucous tumour. The endometrial cavity may appear prominent due to associated menorrhagia.

If calcification has occurred acoustic reverberation and shadowing will be demonstrated posterior to the areas of calcification (Fig. 14.5). Malignant degeneration within the tumour does not show any characteristic ultrasonographic features. A sudden increase in size of the tumour or loss of the normal regular uterine outline with evidence of an extrauterine pelvic mass will indicate the diagnosis. Similarly, enlargement of a fibroid in a postmenopausal uterus will suggest this possibility.

Fibromyomas within the retroverted uterus may be difficult to diagnose because the degree of attenuation present prevents visualization of the normal uterine echo pattern, which may then show a more transonic

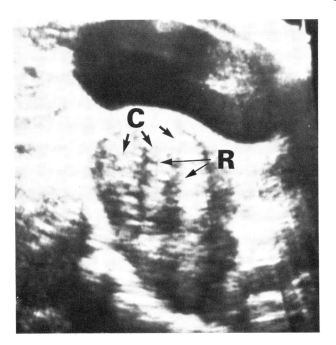

FIG. 14.5   Saggital scan showing a calcified uterine fibroid. The reverberation (R) is present posterior to the areas of calcification (C).

appearance. Other features such as enlargement or irregularity of outline should be demonstrated before a confident diagnosis is made.

Fibromyomas may increase in size during pregnancy. This may not be an apparent feature on serial scans due to the concomitant growth of the uterus, and there may in fact be an apparent reduction in the size of the fibromyoma. In these circumstances there will be persistent irregularity of the uterine outline. Follow-up examination at regular intervals is indicated in these patients due to the known complications which may occur with a fibromyomatous uterus and associated pregnancy. The possibility of pregnancy within a fibromyomatous uterus in any patient of childbearing age should always be borne in mind, as an early gestational sac may be difficult to identify in a uterus containing multiple fibroids (Fig. 14.6).

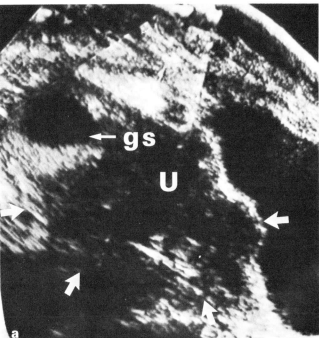

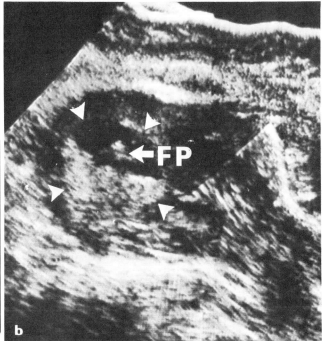

FIG. 14.6   (a) Saggital scan showing enlarged fibroid uterus (U) (arrows) containing a small gestational sac (gs) which is difficult to identify.

(b) a scan 1 cm adjacent to this shows the gestational sac (arrows) containing a fetal pole (FP).

There should be no difficulty with present-day equipment in distinguishing between a uterine fibroid and a hydatidiform mole. Even where extensive degeneration is present within a fibromyoma it does not show the same degree of echogenicity and cystic change seen with a hydatidiform mole. If difficulty in diagnosis does occur the presence of theca lutein cysts, seen in 50% of cases of molar degeneration, may aid in differentiation of the two entities. Clinical correlation and estimation of chorionic gonadotrophin levels will establish the diagnosis.

The uterus involutes in size after the menopause. Fibromyomas in this age group are more likely to show evidence of degenerative change and calcification. An increase in size is suggestive of malignant change although this is a relatively rare occurrence. Approximately 10% of fibroids may show some increase in size in this age group.

Adenomyosis of the uterus

Uterine endometriosis (adenomyosis) usually involves the body of the uterus. Internal and external endometriosis may occur together more frequently than has been previously indicated (Walsh et al., 1979). The uterus may be diffusely enlarged and small irregular cystic areas may be visualized in the myometrium due to the dilated glands containing menstrual products. The echo pattern of the endometrial cavity may be prominent. A combination of these ultrasonic findings in association with the clinical history should suggest the diagnosis.

Uterine malignancy

Early detection of malignancy involving the endometrium or the cervix is currently not possible by sonography. Carcinoma of the endometrium may cause an increased size of the uterus, and may be associated with a bizarre echo pattern replacing the normal uniform texture of the uterus. There will be loss of the normal uterine outline if extension of the growth has occurred outside the uterus, and the uterus will appear fixed within the pelvis. In addition, metastasis to the ovaries and to the pelvis and para-aortic lymph nodes can also be evaluated. Loculated ascites may be demonstrated, although this is more frequently seen with ovarian malignancies. Ultrasound is similarly useful in assessing Stage III and IV involvement in carcinoma of the cervix.

Hydatidiform mole

The classical bistable description of molar degeneration was that of an increased speckling with high gain (MacVicar & Donald, 1963) seen within the hydatidiform mole. Increasing experience with grey scale sonography indicates that there is a spectrum of appearances, the presence of a homogeneous vesicular texture being demonstrated in less than half of the cases of hydatidiform mole (Fleischer et al., 1978b; Baird et al., 1977). The clinical presentation may be similarly variable, the uterus being smaller than the expected gestational size in 25% of cases. A persistently elevated human chorionic gonadotrophin level may be due to other causes, such as multiple pregnancy, and may further confuse the diagnosis. While the most common appearance is that of a complex echo pattern of echogenic and transonic areas due to hydrophic villi (Fig. 14.7), the transonic areas may show considerable variability in size, and, where haemorrhage and clot formation coexist, large irregular transonic areas may also be present.

Fetal parts may occasionally be identified (Fig. 14.8) and in 1–2% of cases exhibit concomitant fetal growth. The presence of bilateral theca lutein cysts may assist in establishing the diagnosis, larger cysts showing a multi-locular appearance. Diagnostic difficulty was previously described in the differentiation of a mole from a fibromyoma, which showed a similar high gain appearance with bistable equipment. This problem is less frequently encountered using grey scale equipment. The major source of diagnostic error is in differentiation of an incomplete abortion, where the appearances of the disintegrated gestational sac may simulate haemorrhagic degeneration and associated trophoblastic disease. This may lead to diagnostic confusion of the two entities and subsequent inappropriate therapy.

Invasive trophoblastic disease and choriocarcinoma may show a more irregular echo pattern, with areas of high density echoes due to necrosis and haemorrhage. A rare complication encountered in the follow-up of patients with trophoblastic disease is resultant arteriovenous malformation (Fig. 14.9). This gives a somewhat confusing appearance as the uterus appears enlarged and contains transonic areas mimicking recurrent trophoblastic disease. Real time scanning in the illustrated case demonstrated pulsatility of the uterine outline.

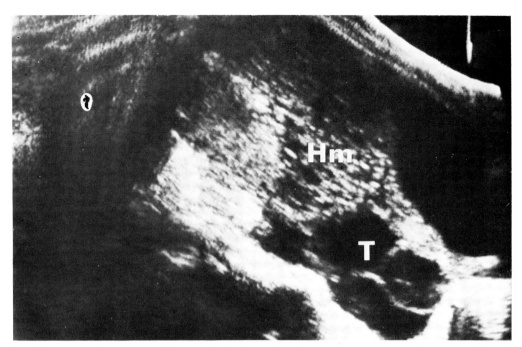

FIG. 14.7   Saggital scan showing a hydatidiform mole (Hm) showing characteristic vesicular echo pattern. Multiple theca lutein cysts are present (T).

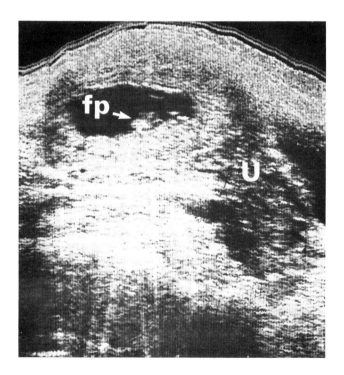

FIG. 14.8   Intact gestational sac in association with early trophoblastic disease (FP, fetal pole). A vesicular pattern is not identified but the trophoblastic margin is thickened and the uterine corpus (U) shows a mottled appearance. Diagnosis confirmed by amniography.

The role of ultrasound in the management of intrauterine devices

The intrauterine device has also an associated number of recognized complications. These include:

1. Irregular bleeding, menorrhagia and discomfort.
2. Pelvic inflammatory disease.
3. Loss of the thread or expulsion of the device.
4. Partial or complete perforation of the uterus.
5. Both intrauterine and ectopic pregnancy.

The more commonly used intrauterine devices may be recognized by their configuration on the ultrasound scan (Cochrane & Thomas, 1977).The Lippe's loop is still the more commonly used and shows a series of dense equally

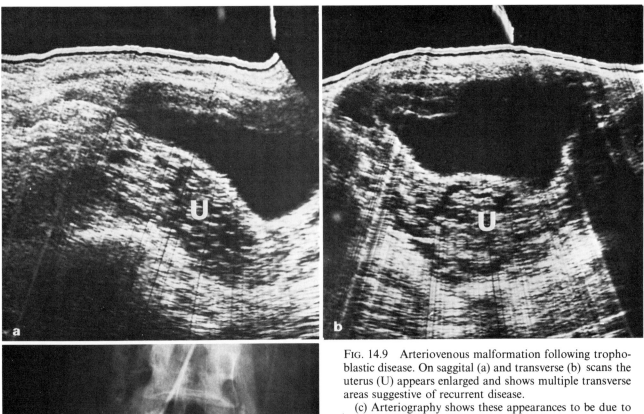

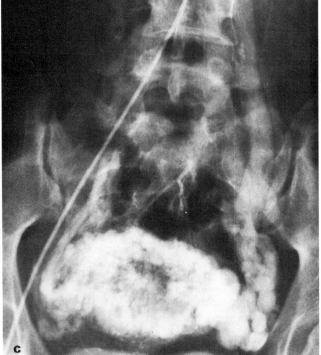

FIG. 14.9 Arteriovenous malformation following tropho-blastic disease. On saggital (a) and transverse (b) scans the uterus (U) appears enlarged and shows multiple transverse areas suggestive of recurrent disease.
(c) Arteriography shows these appearances to be due to arteriovenous malformation.

spaced echoes in the saggital axis of the uterus (Fig. 14.10), with a central echo within the uterine cavity on transverse section. The Saf-T-Coil is more difficult to delineate but adjacent sector scans should demonstrate the continuous echo of the central arm in the saggital axis, and interrupted echoes on the transverse scans. The Dalkon shield appears as a continuous dense linear echo on both saggital and transverse scans (Fig. 14.11). The Copper 7 and Copper T devices demonstrate a linear echo where the scan axis coincides with the axis of the arms of the device in both saggital and transverse sections with a single dense echo where the scan axis passes perpendicular to the device.

Ultrasound should now be the preliminary investiga-tion in the assessment of a lost intrauterine device. If the device is within the uterus, but the thread has been detached, it will be identified and further investigation

FIG. 14.10 Saggital scan showing the characteristic configuration of a Lippe's loop.

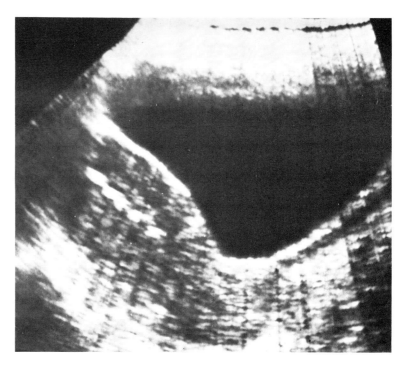

FIG. 14.11 A Dalkon shield (D) with an associated intrauterine gestation (arrowheads).

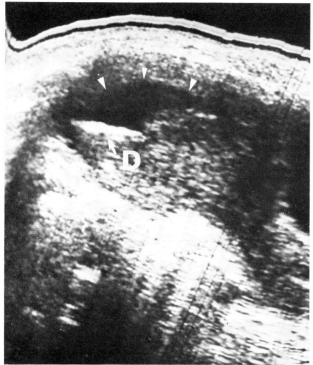

is unnecessary. A plain AP radiograph was previously the method of localization of a lost intrauterine device. However, the device may have been 'lost' due to expulsion, detachment of the nylon thread, uterine perforation, or uptake of the device association with pregnancy, in which case an AP film is an undesirable investigation.

Information as to the position of the device may also be obtained by ultrasonography. An experienced ultrasonographer will be able to detect perforation of the myometrium by the device because of its ectopic position. A low location of the device within the cervical os necessitates removal and re-insertion. If the device cannot be identified within the uterus and there is no evidence of an intrauterine gestation, it is unlikely that ultrasound will be able to demonstrate the device within the pelvis. It is in these circumstances that an AP radiograph will confirm that the device has penetrated the uterus and lies within the pelvis or abdomen, or if expulsion has occurred. When the device appears to be ectopic in position within the uterus, hysterosalpingography is indicated to assess the exact position and establish if partial perforation of the device has occurred (Dhall *et al.*, 1969).

The appearances of the postpartum uterus

Following parturition the uterus involutes in size over a period of 12 weeks. Abnormal sonographic appearances of the uterus have been correlated with retained products and fetal parts in both the postpartum and postabortion states (Robinson, 1972; Sanders, 1977), although the results are variable. The 'empty uterus' is a useful indicator that no retained products are present. However, a prominent series or echoes within the uterine cavity may or may not indicate the possibility of retained products, and the appearances must be taken in conjunction with clinical symptoms. Definite sonographic evidence of a retained portion of the placenta or fetal part may also be shown, curettage being indicated in these circumstances.

ASSESSMENT OF THE ADNEXA

The various pathological entities involving the adnexa may show extremely similar sonographic appearances, and it may only be possible to give a differential diagnosis with an indication as to which entity the sonographer feels is most likely to be present (Lawson & Albarelli, 1977; Fleischer *et al.*, 1978a; Brown *et al.*, 1978). Careful attention to the marginal characteristics and internal echogenicity of an abnormality, correlated with the clinical history and findings, may frequently lead to the correct diagnosis and greatly assist in the management of the patient.

Ectopic pregnancy

The early diagnosis of ectopic pregnancy has remained difficult despite the availability of a large number of diagnostic procedures. The routine pregnancy test may be negative in up to 50% of patients with ectopic gestation, and the diagnosis may not be suspected in up to two-thirds of patients at their initial presentation. In the United States the incidence of ectopic pregnancy is increasing, due to an increase in the incidence of pelvic infection and subsequent tubal adhesions. In addition, the use of the intrauterine contraceptive device does not protect the predisposed patient from ectopic gestation. Because the signs and symptoms are attributed to the presence of an IUD, the presence of an intrauterine device may delay and interfere with the diagnosis of an ectopic gestation.

Kobayashi *et al.* (1969), describing the bistable appear-ances of ectopic pregnancy, found a diagnostic error rate of 25%. A recent report has indicated the increased accuracy of grey scale imaging in this diagnosis (Maklad & Wright, 1978).

The superior resolution obtained with grey scale equipment has led to the diagnosis of ectopic pregnancy at an earlier stage and thus the frequency with which an unruptured ectopic gestation is diagnosed has increased. The delineation of an intact gestational sac containing a fetal pole is identified in a higher percentage of cases of unruptured ectopic pregnancy. The gestational sac is contained in a distended Fallopian tube which has sealed off during the evolution of the pregnancy. This shows an ovoid transonic appearance with posterior echo enhancement (Fig. 14.12). The gestational sac may appear somewhat fragmented and the fetal pole may be difficult to identify. Overlapping single sweep scans are mandatory. The uterus may be moderately enlarged in association with the ectopic gestation. It is usually displaced from the midline by the adnexal mass. Increased vascularity of the myometrium gives the uterus a more mottled appearance and the endometrial echo is prominent due to associated hyperplasia. Fetal heart motion is infrequently detected, but when present provides final confirmation of the diagnosis.

While acute rupture of an ectopic pregnancy is a surgical emergency, with ultrasound playing no part in its diagnosis, in chronic rupture a complex mass is demonstrated due to haematoma formation. The gestational sac is more difficult to identify, but a trophoblastic rim may still be delineated (Fig. 14.13). The uterus may be displaced by the mass, which is predominantly unilateral. The haematoma may extend to involve both adnexa and free fluid may be present in the cul-de-sac and adnexal areas. The uterus will again show evidence of increased myometrial vascularity and endometrial hypertrophy.

In both circumstances shedding of the decidua may have occurred which may lead to confusion clinically with a threatened abortion.

Pelvic inflammatory disease

Pelvic inflammatory disease may be due to gonococcal, pyogenic or, less frequently, tuberculous infection. Non-tuberculous forms, of which gonorrhoea is the commonest, are due to ascending infection, initially involving the endometrium and frequently affecting the Fallopian tubes. Adequate antibiotic therapy should result in

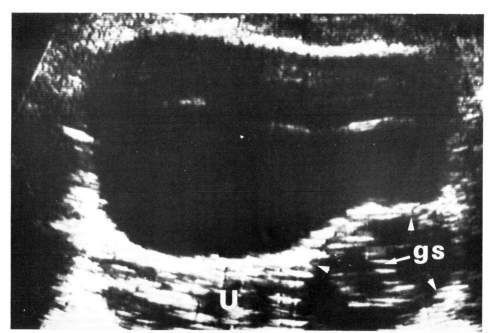

FIG. 14.12   Unruptured ectopic gestation. The gestational sac (gs) can be clearly identified within the distended Fallopian tube (arrowheads); U, uterus.

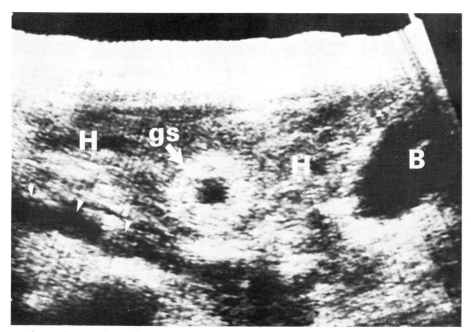

FIG. 14.13   Ruptured ectopic gestation. The intact gestational sac (gs) is identified within a large haematoma (H); B, bladder. Free fluid is present posteriorly in the pelvis (arrowheads).

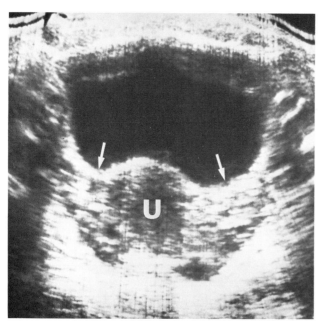

FIG. 14.14 Acute pelvic inflammatory disease. Bilateral symmetrical complex adnexal masses (arrowheads) are shown merging with the uterine outline (U). The uterus appears a little more transonic and there is increased transmission of the ultrasound beam through the adnexa.

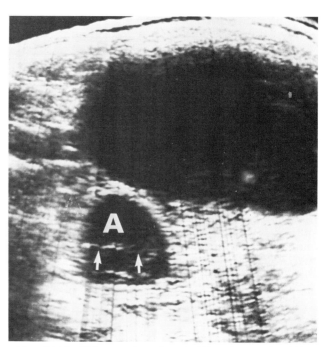

FIG. 14.15 Tubo-ovarian abscess. The abscess rim (A) shows a variable thickness with evidence of layering of debris (arrows) within the abscess cavity.

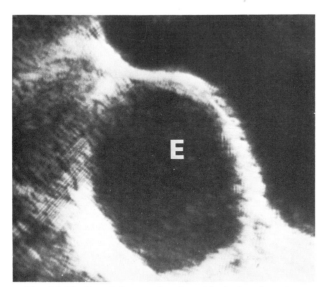

FIG. 14.16 Saggital scan of endometriosis showing a transonic cystic adnexal mass. Faint echoes are present within the endometrioma (E).

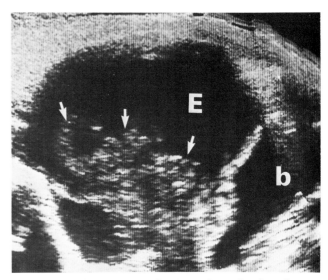

FIG. 14.17 Saggital scan of endometrioma showing a large endometriotic cyst (E) containing markedly irregular solid elements due to thrombus (arrows). The bladder (b) is compressed by the large mass.

complete resolution of the infection. If the organism is resistant to antibiotics, or if chemotherapy is inadequate, a chronic infection may ensue. Pyogenic inflammatory disease is commonest in the postpartum state, following curettage, or in association with insertion of an intrauterine device.

In the acute stage the uterus appears slightly enlarged and more transonic than normal. The endometrial echo pattern appears more prominent due to the associated endometritis, pus and debris within the uterine cavity. In both pyogenic and gonococcal forms of disease the adnexa appear prominent and have a complex echo pattern containing multiple small transonic areas of the adnexa and uterus (Fig. 14.14). This appearance is usually symmetrical, although a slight unilateral prominence may be present. The normal uterine outline cannot be clearly defined (Sample, 1977). Small or moderate amounts of free fluid may be present in the cul-de-sac and adjacent to the adnexa. Complete resolution of these appearances will occur with adequate therapy. If the infection proceeds to a more chronic state an adnexal abscess may occur. At this stage the disease may be predominantly unilateral in situation. The abscess shows a thick echogenic rim with a transonic centre (Ullrich & Sanders, 1976). The margin is often irregular and incomplete. Debris within the abscess cavity leads to a layering appearance which is gravity dependent (Fig. 14.15). Adequate antibiotic therapy at this stage may result in resolution of these appearances. Even with adequate therapy, hydrosalpinx may occur due to tubal adhesions. The hydrosalpinx demonstrates a completely transonic appearance and may be indistinguishable from an ovarian cyst. Adhesions within the hydrosalpinx may give the appearance of septation, again mimicking an ovarian cyst. Features which lead to the diagnosis of a hydrosalpinx are its elongated or tubular shape, the ability to distinguish the ovary adjacent to the pelvic wall separate from the cystic area, and the thickened wall of the hydrosalpinx.

Extrauterine endometriosis

Extrauterine endometriosis completes the triad of adnexal pathology which shows a wide and overlapping spectrum of ultrasonic appearances. A cystic, solid or mixed pattern may be identified. Where the cyst shows a predominantly transonic pattern careful adjustment of the gain setting may reveal an extremely subtle echo

pattern within the cavity (Fig. 14.16). When a mixed pattern is present, the solid elements often show a bizarre configuration which is distinguishable from the layering affect within an abscess, or the more regular margination of an ectopic pregnancy (Fig. 14.17). Examination of the uterus may be extremely useful in separating these entities. The cystic appearances which may be seen with endometriosis in up to 35% of cases (Walsh et al., 1979) are irregular, in contradistinction to the diffuse appearances seen with an ectopic pregnancy. The uterine changes have resolved at the stage of tubo-ovarian abscess formation in inflammatory disease, with the demonstration of a normal appearing uterus. Where endometrial disease is extensive, emptying of the full bladder may be useful in demonstrating fixity of the pelvic structures.

THE ABNORMAL OVARY
Assessment of ovarian function and development

Delineation of the normal ovaries is not only possible in the adult female but also in the pre-pubertal age group (Sample, 1977). Ultrasound examination of the paediatric pelvis is therefore useful in the assessment of precocious sexual development to exclude an ovarian tumour. In the adult female visualization of ovarian macrostructure allows demonstration of the ripening Graafian follicle and corpus luteum. The follicle is demonstrated as a cystic structure, 1–3 cm in size, protruding from the normal ellipsoid ovarian outline. Assessment of follicular development and its response to hormone therapy permits determination of the optimum time for induction of ovulation and conception (Hackeloer, 1977). A further application of ultrasound in relation to endocrinology is in the detection of the Stein-Leventhal syndrome, in which both ovaries typically appear enlarged and contain multiple small cysts.

Benign ovarian tumours

Following extrusion of the ovum, the corpus luteum may be identified as a small cystic structure, usually not more than 3 cm in size. The luteal cyst of a normal early pregnancy may be somewhat larger in size but does not normally exceed 6 cm.

When haemorrhage occurs into a luteal cyst, the clinical symptoms and signs may simulate an ectopic pregnancy. A little free fluid may be present when there is leakage

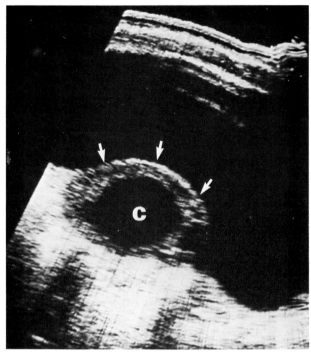

FIG. 14.18 Saggital scan of a haemorrhagic corpus lutein cyst (C). The cyst margins are clearly defined. The well-defined echogenic rim is felt to represent the attenuated ovary (arrows).

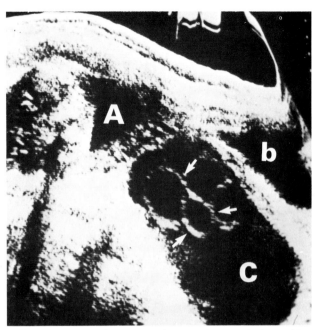

FIG. 14.19 Mucinous cystadenoma in association with intrauterine pregnancy. Multiple thin-walled septa (arrows) are present; C, cyst; A, amniotic sac; b, bladder.

of the cyst contents. The ultrasound appearances are those of a well-defined cyst with a thin wall. The ovary may be stretched around the cyst, giving apparent thickening of the cyst wall. There is no evidence of a trophoblastic margin or fetal pole, which helps to differentiate the haemorrhagic cyst from an ectopic gestation (Fig. 14.18).

Serous and mucinous cystadenomas are the most commonly encountered large cystic ovarian tumours. The serous cystadenomas show a thin well-defined wall with little or no evidence of septation. The mucinous cystadenoma shows a multilocular appearance (Fig. 14.19). Solid elements may be identified and are usually well circumscribed. A large hydrosalpinx may be indistinguishable from a serous cystadenoma. Rarely, a dermoid may present with an almost completely cystic appearance, and again presents difficulty in differentiation.

FIG. 14.20 Saggital scan of a cystic ovarian dermoid (D). Characteristic appearance of dense layering due to elements of sebum within the tumour are shown (arrows).

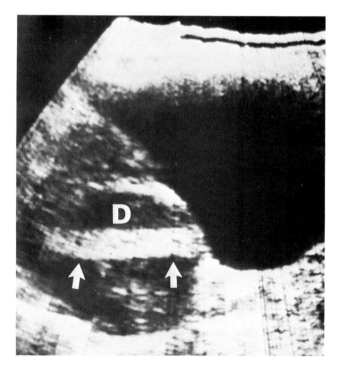

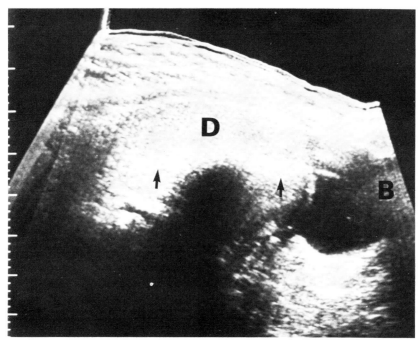

FIG. 14.21 Solid ovarian dermoid (D) showing the layering appearance (arrows) with posterior acoustic shadowing; B, bladder.

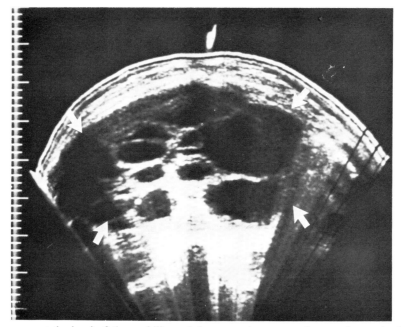

FIG. 14.22 Transverse scan at the level of the umbilicus. A large mucinous cystadenocarcinoma is shown arising out of the pelvis (arrows). Multiple solid elements are present within the tumour.

A fimbrial or para-ovarian cyst may similarly show a unilocular appearance.

Ovarian teratomas (dermoid) show a wide spectrum of appearances. There is no characteristic location for an ovarian dermoid. The smaller tumours are obviously encountered in the adnexal areas, but the larger tumour may extend to the pelvic brim and displace the normal pelvic anatomy. A characteristic ultrasonic sign which is seen in the majority of dermoid cysts is the presence of highly echogenic areas within the tumour whether it is partially cystic or solid. This pattern has been shown to be due to sebum present in the tumour (Guttman, 1977). Acoustic shadowing may be present posterior to the sebum which frequently shows a layered appearance (Figs. 14.20 and 14.21). Occasionally the more cystic element of the tumour may show an inverse relationship to the solid element.

There are a number of other solid ovarian tumours which are not distinguishable sonographically from each other. These include Brenner tumours, and granulosa cell tumours, both of which may occasionally be cystic. Fibromas of the ovary are a relatively frequent solid tumour and show similar echogenic characteristics to uterine fibromas. Separation of the uterine margin from the tumour should suggest the diagnosis.

Malignant ovarian tumours

Primary solid malignant tumours of the ovary show a less uniform echogenic pattern than their benign counterparts and generally show increased sonic transmission. Their outline is poorly defined, and there may be ascites.

Both serous and mucinous cystadenocarcinoma show loss of the tumour outline and contain irregular solid components with a more complex echo pattern (Fig. 14.22). Features which are suggestive of malignancy are a rapid increase in size of the tumour, extension across the midline or bilaterally, ascites, and fixity of the tumour in the pelvis (Morley & Barnett, 1977). Early detection of malignant change is still not feasible ultrasonographically, but the examination may be valuable in the assessment of pelvic and para-aortic nodal involvement.

REFERENCES

BAIRD A. M., BECKLEY D. E. & ROSS F. G. M. (1977) The ultrasound diagnosis of hydatidiform mole. *Clin. Radiol.*, **28**, 637–645.

BROWN T. W., FILLY R. A., LAING F. C. & BARTON J. (1978) Analysis of ultrasonic criteria in the evaluation of ectopic pregnancy. *Amer. J. Roentgenol.*, **131**, 967–971.

COCHRANE W. J. & THOMAS M. A. (1977) The value of ultrasound in the management of intrauterine devices. In *Ultrasonography in Obstetrics and Gynecology*, pp. 387–400, ed. R. C. Sanders & A. E. James. Appleton Century Crofts. New York.

DHALL K., DHALL G. I. & GUPTA B. B. (1969) Uterine perforation with the Lippe's loop. Detection by hysterography. *Obstet. Gynec.*, **34**, 266–270.

FLEISCHER A. C., JAMES A. E., KRAUSE A. D. & MILLIS J. B. (1978a). Sonographic patterns in trophoblastic disease. *Radiology*, **126**, 215–220.

FLEISCHER A. C., JAMES A. E., MILLIS J. B. & JULLIAN C. (1978b) Differential diagnosis of pelvic masses by grey scale sonography. *Amer. J. Roentgenol.*, **131**, 469–476.

FRIED A. M., OLIFF M., WILSON A. E. & WHISNANT J. (1978) Uterine anomalies associated with renal agenesis. Role of grey scale ultrasonography. *Amer. J. Roentgenol.* **131**, 973–975.

GUTTMAN P. H. (1977) In search of the elusive benign cystic ovarian teratoma. Application of the ultrasound 'tip of the iceberg' sign. *J. Clin. Ultrasound*, **5**, 403–406.

HACKELOER B. J. (1977) The ultrasonic demonstration of follicular development during the normal menstrual cycle and after hormone stimulation. In *Recent Advances in Ultrasonic Diagnosis*, pp. 122–128. Churchill Livingstone, Edinburgh.

HALL D. B., HANN L. E., FERRUCCI J. T., BLACK E. B., BRAITMAN B. S., CROWLEY W. F., NICURI N. & KELLEY J. A. (1979) Sonographic morphology of the normal menstrual cycle. *Radiology*, **113**, 185–188.

HALLER J., SCHNEIDER M., KASSNER G., STAIANO S. J. J., NOYES M. B., CAMPOS E. M. & MCPHERSON J. (1977) Ultrasonography in pediatric gynecology and obstetrics. *Amer. J. Roentgenol.*, **128**, 423–429.

KOBAYASHI M., HELLMAN L. M. & FILLISTI L. P. (1969) Ultrasound: an aid in the diagnosis of ectopic pregnancy. *Amer. J. Obstet. Gynec.*, **103**, 1131–1140.

LAWSON T. L. & ALBARELLI J. N. (1977) Diagnosis of pelvic masses by grey scale ultrasonography. Analysis of specificity and accuracy. *Amer. J. Roentgenol.*, **128**, 1003–1006.

MACVICAR J. & DONALD I. (1963) Sonar in the diagnosis of early pregnancy and its complications. *J. Obstet. Gynaec. Br. Cwth.*, **70**, 387–395.

MAKLAD N. F. & WRIGHT C. H. (1978) Grey scale ultrasonography in the diagnosis of ectopic pregnancy. *Radiology*, **126**, 221–225.

MORLEY P. & BARNETT E. (1977) The ovarian mass. In *Ultrasonography in Obstetrics and Gynecology*, pp. 333–335, ed. R. C. Saunders & A. E. James. Appleton Century Crofts, New York.

ROBINSON H. P. (1972) Sonar in the puerperium. *Scot. Med. J.*, **17**, 364.

ROSENTHAL S. J., LEVINE E., MAKLAD N. F. & WRIGHT C. H. Ultrasound appearance of the ectopic kidney. Unpublished.

SAMPLE W. F., LIPPE B. M., GYEPES M. T. (1977) Grey scale ultrasonography of the normal female pelvis. *Radiology*, **125**, 477–483.

SAMPLE W. F. (1977) Pelvic inflammatory disease. In *Ultrasonography in Obstetrics and Gynecology*, pp. 357–385, ed. R. C. Saunders & A. E. James. Appleton Century Crofts, New York.

SANDERS R. C. (1977) Post partum diagnostic ultrasound. In *Ultrasonography in Obstetrics and Gynecology*, pp. 285–295, ed. R. C. Saunders & A. E. James. Appleton Century Crofts, New York.

ULLRICH P. C. & SANDERS R. C. (1976) Ultrasonic characteristics of pelvic inflammatory disease. *J. Clin. Ultrasound*, **4**, 199–204.

VINSTEIN A. L. & FRANKEN E. A. (1972) Unilateral haematocolpos associated with agenesis of the kidney. *Radiology*, **102**, 652–672.

VON MICSKY L. I. (1974) Gynecologic sonography. In *Diagnostic Ultrasound*. pp. 207–241, ed. D. L. King. Mosby, St. Louis.

WALSH J. W., TAYLOR K. J. W. & ROSENFIELD A. T. (1979) Grey scale ultrasonography in the diagnosis of endometriosis and adenomyosis. *Amer. J. Roentgenol.*, **132**, 87–90.

ZEMLYN S. (1974) Comparison of pelvic ultrasonography and pneumography for ovarian size. *J. Clin. Ultrasound*, **2**, 331.

CHAPTER 15

Computed Tomography in Gynaecological Diagnosis

by C. H. Wright

The introduction of body computed tomography (CT) has added a further dimension to non-invasive imaging of the female pelvis. Since its introduction, a large number of publications have attested the value and relative merits of CT in the study of various organs, systems and pathologies. There is, as yet, relatively limited published experience in the assessment of abnormalities of the female pelvis, although the value of CT in the assessment of neoplastic abnormalities is becoming apparent (Table 15.1).

Computed tomography should be regarded as a complementary procedure to ultrasonography, rather than being a competitive technique. Although both modalities may provide similar information (Walsh *et al.*, 1978), ultrasonography remains the initial non-invasive diagnostic procedure of choice, while computed tomography may provide further information not readily available from the ultrasound scan (Carter *et al.*, 1976). Each technique has its advantages and limitations (Table 15.2).

With the introduction of faster scanners with angled

TABLE 15.1   Indications for pelvic CT in the female.

1. (A) Assessment and staging of neoplasms of the female genital organs.
   (B) Assessment of nodal involvement in lymphoma and neoplasia.
   (C) Localization of pelvic tumour for biopsy and radiotherapy planning.
2. Assessment of a pelvic abnormality where the bladder is absent or indistensible.
3. Identification and localization of a mass demonstrated but not definitely localized by ultrasound.
4. Staging of bladder neoplasms.
5. Determination of level and nature of ureteral obstruction.
6. Assessment of the extent of soft tissue and osseous abnormalities (tumour, abscess, lymphocoele and haematoma).

TABLE 15.2   Relative merits of computed tomography and ultrasound.

Ultrasound	CT
Non-ionizing No definite evidence of detrimental biological effects at diagnostic levels.	Moderate to high radiation dose depending on slice thickness and spacing.
Relatively cheap and rapid procedure.	Relatively expensive and time-consuming procedure.
Requires a full bladder to provide a sonic window for satisfactory examination.	Examination can be conducted without a full bladder, or if the bladder is absent.
Visualization of deep pelvic structures and pelvis side walls may be inadequate.	Excellent visualization of deep pelvic structures and bone detail.
Non-invasive (bladder may be catherized to ensure adequate filling).	Non-invasive (vaginal tampon, oral and rectal contrast, IV contrast and antiperistaltic agent may be indicated).
Bowel may prevent adequate examination or mimic a pelvic mass.	Bowel usually readily recognized.
Saggital, transverse and oblique scans may be obtained.	Scans limited to the transverse plane.

gantries, variable collimator sizes, and more refined saggital reconstruction techniques, a number of the disadvantages of CT scanning, such as the relative length and cost of the procedure and lack of a reasonable sagittal reconstruction at a moderate radiation dose, may be removed.

TECHNIQUE

To some extent this depends on the scanner available. In general, scans are obtained at fairly close intervals to include the pelvis from the superior ischial spine to the symphysis. In the assessment of a pelvic malignancy the scan is extended to include the para-aortic area and the liver. Using a 13 mm collimator, 15 mm cuts are recommended through the pelvis, with overlapping cuts if indicated. Twenty millimetre cuts are recommended to assess the para-aortic area and liver, unless there is suspicion of an hepatic abnormality when 15 mm cuts are indicated. The patient is scanned in the supine position. A full bladder is desirable, as this displaces bowel out of the pelvis and assists in delineation of the pelvic anatomy. An oral contrast agent is given to identify the small and large bowel. Ideally 500 cc of 2% Gastrografin is given at both three hours and half an hour before the examination. A vaginal tampon assists in localising the vagina (Cohen *et al.*, 1977). When oral Gastrografin has failed to delineate the distal colon adequately, rectal contrast may be useful in defining the rectum and sigmoid segment. Depending on the scan time, an intravenous anti-peristaltic agent (30 mg of Buscopan, 0.25 mg of Glucagon) is necessary to prevent streak artefacts from bowel movement. Intravenous contrast (Conray 420, 50 ml) will delineate the line of the ureters and their relationship to any abnormality present, although it does cause quite dense layering in the bladder, and therefore should not be used routinely. To obtain the maximum information and patient benefit from the investigation, the full clinical history and findings, and results of other radiological and imaging investigations, should be available to the radiologist in order to determine the most appropriate technique, slice spacing, and extent of the CT evaluation required.

ANATOMY

Computed tomography clearly delineates the pelvic musculature and bony contours. Evaluation of an abnormality is assisted by the bilateral nature of much of the anatomy (Ledley *et al.*, 1977). Sufficient fat is usually present to permit delineation of the tissue planes, and bowel peristalsis and respiratory movement rarely degrade the resultant image. The sacrum, sacro-iliac joints, ileum, pelvic wall and gluteal muscles are identified at the pelvic brim. Loops of small bowel lie anterior and superior to the bladder. The sigmoid colon lies along the left lateral wall of the pelvis, and the vascular bundles and lymphatics are seen on the surface of the ilio-psoas muscle. The arteries may be identified if calcification is present, but the veins and lymphatics may be indistinguishable. The iliacus and psoas muscles show a variable size and level of fusion depending on the patient's build. At the level of the sciatic notch the bladder lies anterior in the pelvis, with the uterine fundus posterior to the bladder. The broad ligaments may be visualized as lateral extensions of the uterine outline. The ovaries may be seen adjacent to the posterior aspect of the ileum but in practice the normal ovary is rarely visualized (Redman, 1977) (Fig. 15.1). At the level of the femoral heads the pelvic floor musculature is seen to encompass

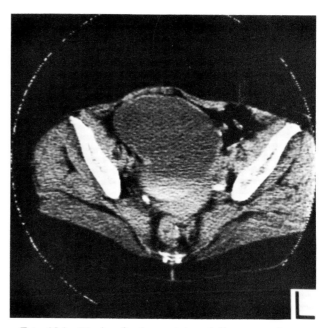

Fig. 15.1 Uterine fundus and broad ligaments shown posterior to the bladder containing a little contrast medium. Both ureters are clearly seen.

the rectum and uterine cervix. Caudad to this the vagina and bladder neck lie posterior to the symphysis pubis.

STAGING OF TUMOURS OF FEMALE GENITAL ORGANS

The previous chapter has demonstrated the ability of ultrasound to localize and differentiate the various pathologies affecting the uterus, adnexa and ovaries. The ability to obtain transverse and sagittal scans permits a ready appreciation of the three dimensional contours of an abnormality. CT, essentially confined to cross-sectional depiction, gives a more limited appreciation of variations of normal anatomy of some pelvic structures such as the uterus.

The wide range of position of the normal uterus frequently results in the scan being at an oblique angle to the vertical axis of the uterus (Fig. 15.2). Uterine enlargement and variation in contour may be identified but the change of texture of a uterine fibroid, usually readily demonstrable on an ultrasound scan, may not be

reflected by a significant density difference with CT. Calcification is easily identified (Fig. 15.3). Staging of endometrial and cervical carcinoma may be assisted by CT (Brizel *et al.*, 1979). Published works as to the value of CT in assessing local spread more accurately than ultrasound vary (Brizel *et al.*, 1979; Walsh *et al.*, 1978), but it would appear that CT is valuable not only in assessing the extent of spread of the pelvic malignancy (Fig. 15.4), but in determining the type and extent of treatment indicated.

Due to the accurate localization of abnormal pelvic masses, successful biopsy may be undertaken with CT guidance (Jacques *et al.*, 1978). Nodal involvement may be evaluated in addition to the local extent of tumour. Whilst nodal enlargement is frequently shown in patients with abdominal lymphoma with involvement of the pelvic nodes (Lee *et al.*, 1978a) (Fig. 15.5), nodal involvement may not infrequently be present from a pelvic malignancy without demonstrable nodal enlargement. Thus a patient whose scans show no evidence of nodal enlargement still requires lymphangiography for complete staging. Although a significant percentage of false negative examinations may occur with lymphangiography, a combination

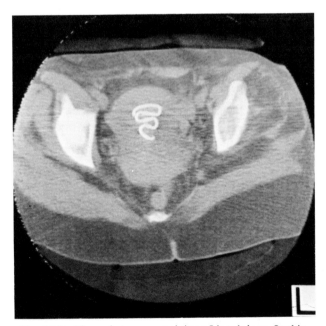

FIG. 15.2 Normal uterus containing a Lippe's loop. In this case the uterus is perpendicular to the scan plane.

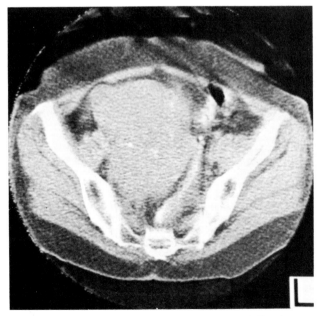

FIG. 15.3 Large fibroid uterus containing calcification.

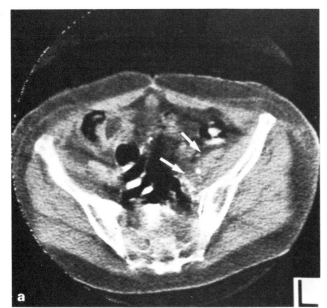

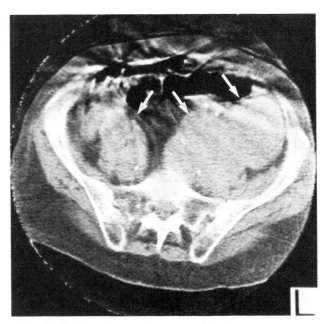

FIG. 15.5   Lymphoma with gross nodal enlargement more marked on the left (arrows).

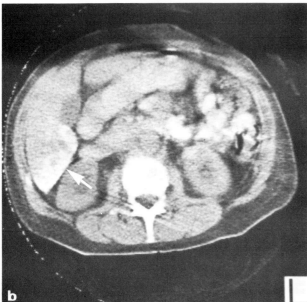

FIG. 15.4   (a) Carcinoma of the cervix. A soft tissue mass is shown on the left lateral pelvic wall (arrows). Some opacification is seen in lymph nodes following lymphangiography.

(b) Contrast medium is present in the right lobe of the liver (arrow) presumably due to a lymphaticovenous communication.

of both techniques will hopefully result in a lower false negative rate (Lee *et al.*, 1978b).

Difficulty may be encountered with ultrasound in the assessment of large cystic or mixed ovarian tumours, in determining both the presence or the absence of local invasion (Fig. 15.6) and the origin of the tumour, when it is displaced upward into the abdominal cavity (Fig. 15.7). Associated ascites may be identified within the abdominal and pelvic cavity. The presence of fat within the tumour, as determined by the attenuation value, may lead to a confident diagnosis of a dermoid. A tumour extending to involve the pelvic side walls may invade or compress the ureter. The intravenous urogram indicates obstruction if the kidney is functioning but does not show the size and extent of the associated soft tissue mass, and may not clearly demonstrate the level of obstruction. This can be readily accomplished by CT (Fig. 15.8). In the patient with a non-functioning kidney the size and level of the obstruction may still be determined, and scans taken to assess the para-aortic area will also demonstrate the kidney and the presence of hydronephrosis (Fig. 15.9a). In addition to the reservations expressed in the determination of lymph node involvement, a further

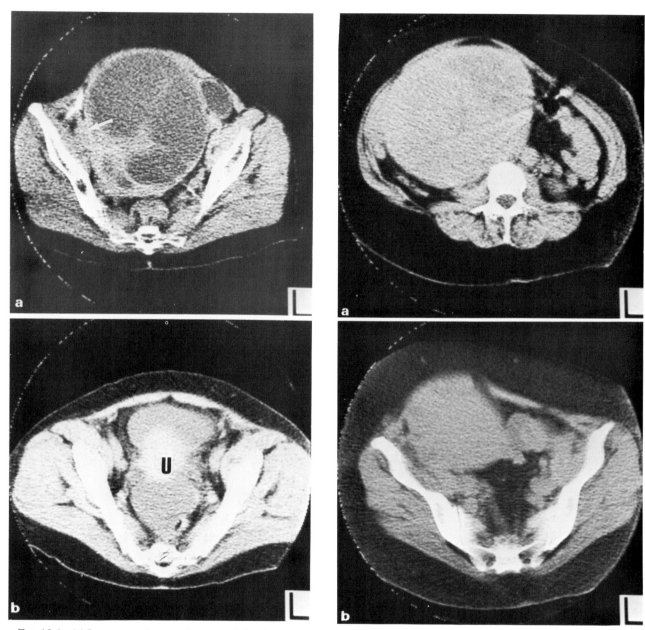

FIG. 15.6   (a) Large cystadenocarcinoma with local spread into the ilio-psoas (arrow).

   (b) Pelvic ascites. The uterus (U) is displaced forward. The uniform appearance and demonstration of ascites within the abdominal cavity should enable differentiation from a cystic ovarian tumour.

FIG. 15.7   (a) A large mixed ovarian tumour extending into the abdominal cavity.

   (b) More caudad scans demonstrate the ovarian origin of the tumour.

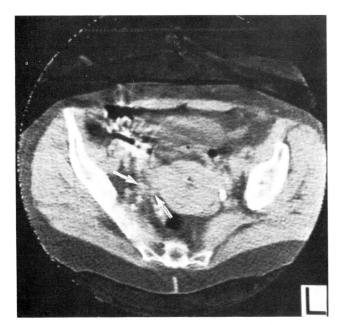

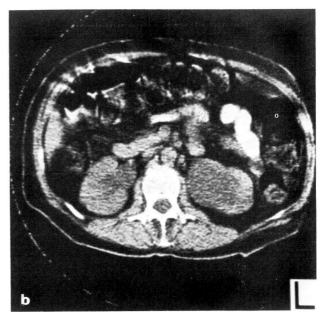

FIG. 15.8   Carcinoma of the cervix. The left ureter is shown. There is lateral extension of the tumour on the right (arrows) and the ureter is not visualized.

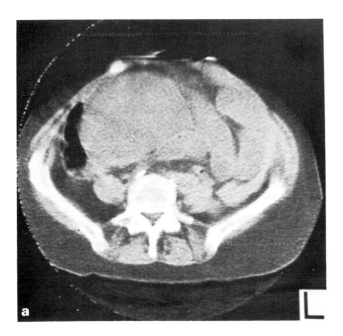

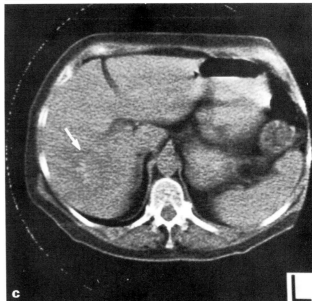

FIG. 15.9   (a) Recurrent colonic carcinoma with diffuse infiltration in the pelvis. Bilateral hydronephrosis, more marked on the left, is shown.

(b) Dilated loops of bowel are present in the pelvis.

(c) An ill-defined metastasis containing calcification is present in the liver (arrow).

consideration is the inability of CT to detect microscopic infiltration by malignant disease (Levitt *et al.*, 1978) (Fig. 15.9 b and c).

The ability of CT to give attenuation values enables differentiation between pelvic lipomatosis and an abnormal mass. In the patient whose bladder has been removed, or who has had a limited bladder capacity, CT provides a more useful examination in the assessment of the pelvis. The presence or absence of recurrence of malignancy may be determined by CT.

STAGING OF BLADDER NEOPLASMS

Computed tomography enables more accurate differentiation of the extent of bladder neoplasms (Siedelmann *et al.*, 1977). Tumour staging into clinically significant types B, C and D can be established although it is not possible to differentiate accurately between mucosal, submucosal and mural involvement (Fig. 15.10a). A full bladder is necessary for the examination. Intravenous contrast medium may cause dense layering within the bladder, and if ureteral involvement has occurred, scans taken following the introduction of intravenous contrast medium to assess the extent of and level of obstruction should be obtained following an initial non-contrast examination. Introduction of air or carbon dioxide, and positional change to assess fixity and invasion of the tumour into the peri-vesical fat, may prove useful where the initial scan is felt to be equivocal. The cardinal sign of extra-vesical spread is obliteration of the peri-vesical fat line by tumour. Local invasion of the pelvic side wall or organs can be obvious (Fig. 15.10b), but a gravity dependent scan may be indicated to differentiate between the effects of compression by the tumour bulk and actual invasion.

EVALUATION OF EXTRA-GENITO-URINARY PATHOLOGY

The unique ability of CT to visualize both the muscle and bony structures has greatly aided the diagnosis and extent of soft tissues and bony tumours (Levine *et al.*, 1979; Gilula *et al.*, 1979). CT not only gives a better indication of tumour location and extent than other conventional imaging procedures, but provides anatomical information of tumour relationship to nerves and vessels. With a primary bone lesion the absence of presence and

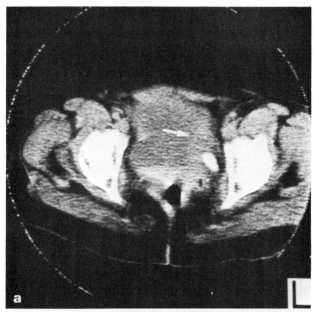

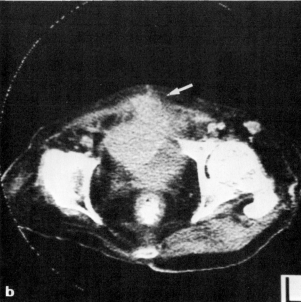

FIG. 15.10   (a) Bladder tumour on the left lateral bladder wall (arrow). Slight stasis in the contrast opacified ureter is shown.

(b) Bladder tumour invading the anterior abdominal wall (arrow).

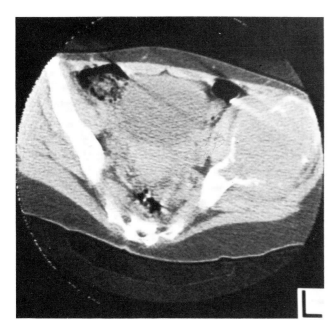

FIG. 15.11   Metastasis from a renal carcinoma. The extent
of bony destruction and soft tissue margins of the tumour
are clearly delineated.

extent of extra-osseous spread may be determined (Fig.
15.11). Both the intra- and extra-pelvic extent of tumour
may be demonstrated with a soft tissue lesion.

The attenuation value of a soft tissue abnormality may
enable differentiation between an abscess, haematoma or
lymphocoele and other cystic lesions. A spectrum of
appearances may be seen and the density characteristics
of these soft tissue abnormalities may overlap. Correlation with the clinical history and findings is of value.
Determination of the site and possible origin of the abnormality also assist in the final diagnosis.

The presence of gas within an abscess is pathognomic
of its identity (Callen, 1979). The appearances of a
haematoma and a tumour may be extremely similar, as
both may show evidence of a soft tissue mass containing
low density areas. Depending on the length of time the
haematoma has been present, a more uniform appearance
may be seen. A soft tissue tumour involving the pelvis
usually shows a more irregular and lobulated appearance,
but if the tumour is infiltrating along the muscle planes,
it can appear extremely similar to an abscess of
haematoma (Fig. 15.12).

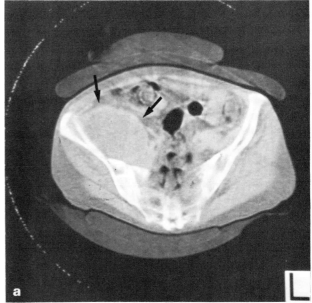

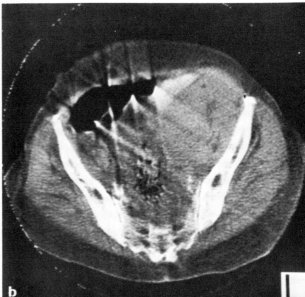

FIG. 15.12   (a) Recurrent colonic carcinoma containing
central low density areas (arrow).

(b) Leaking aortic aneurysm. A haematoma extends into
the left psoas muscle.

Computed tomography has also been shown to be of value in evaluating the sacrum and sacro-iliac joints (Gilula *et al.*, 1979) and may be preferable to conventional tomography when there are equivocal appearances on plain radiographs. The presence or absence of a soft tissue abnormality such as an anterior sacral meningocoele, or a lipoma, occurring in association with a congenital bony abnormality, may be readily diagnosed by computed tomography. The attenuation value of the abnormality will readily indicate the nature of this mass.

REFERENCES

BRIZEL E. H., LIVINGSTON P. A., GRAYSON E. U. (1979) Radiotherapeutic applications of pelvic CT. *J. Comp. Asst. Tomography*, **3**, 453–466.

CALLEN P. W. (1979) Computed tomographic evaluation of abdominal and pelvic abscesses. *Radiology*, **131**, 171–175.

CARTER B. L., KAHN P. C., WOLPERT S. M., HAMMERSCHLAG S. B., SCHWARTZ A. M. & SCOTT R. M. (1976) Unusual pelvic masses. A comparison of computed tomographic scanning and ultrasonography. *Radiology*, **121**, 383–386.

COHEN W. H., SEIDELMAN F. E. & BRYAN P. J. (1977) The use of a tampon to enhance vaginal localisation in computed tomography. *Amer. J. Roentgenol.*, **128**, 1064–1065.

GILULA L. A., MURPHY W. A., TAILOR C. C. & PATEL R. B. (1979) Computed tomography of the osseous pelvis. *Radiology*, **132**, 107–114.

JACQUES P. F., STAAB E., RICHEY W., PHOTOPULOS G. & Swanton M. (1978) CT assisted pelvic and abdominal biopsy in gynecological lesions. *Radiology*, **128**, 651–655.

LEDLEY R., HUANG H. K. & MAZZIOTTA J. C. (1977) *Cross Sectional Anatomy – An Atlas for Computerised Tomography*. Williams and Wilkins, Baltimore.

LEE J. K. T., STANLEY R. J., SAGEL S. S. & LEVITT R. G. (1978a) Accuracy of computed tomography in detecting intra-abdominal and pelvic lymphadenopathy in lymphoma. *Amer. J. Roentgenol.*, **131**, 311–315.

LEE J. K. T., STANLEY R. J., SAGEL S. S. & MCLENNAN B. (1978b) Accuracy of CT in detecting intra-abdominal and pelvic lymph node metastasis from pelvic cancer. *Amer. J. Roentgenol.*, **131**, 675–679.

LEVINE E., LEE K. R., NEFF J., MAKLAD N. F., ROBINSON R. G. & PRESTON D. F. (1979) Comparison of computed tomography and other imaging modalities in the evaluation of musculoskeletal tumours. *Radiology*, **131**, 431–437.

LEVITT R. G., SAGEL S. S., STANLEY R. J. & EVENS R. G. (1978) Computed tomography of the pelvis. *Seminars in Roentgenology*, **13**.

REDMAN H. C. (1977) Computed tomography of the pelvis. *Radiol. Clin. N. Amer.*, **15**, 441–448.

SEIDELMANN F. E., COHEN W. N. & BRYAN P. J. (1977) Computed tomographic staging of bladder neoplasms. *Radiol. Clin. N. Amer.*, **15**, 419–440.

WALSH W. J., ROSENFIELD A. T., JAFFE C. C., SCHWARTZ P.E., SIMEONE J., DEMBER A. G. & TAYLOR K. J. W. (1978) Prospective comparison of ultrasound and computed tomography in the evaluation of gynaecologic pelvic masses. *Amer. J. Roentgenol.*, **131**, 955–960.

Index